Esophageal Diseases

P. Marco Fisichella • Marco E. Allaix
Mario Morino • Marco G. Patti
Editors

Esophageal Diseases

Evaluation and Treatment

Springer

Editors
P. Marco Fisichella, MD, MBA, FACS
Department of Surgery
Boston Veteran Administration
Healthcare System
West Roxbury, MA
USA

Department of Surgery
Brigham and Women's Hospital
Harvard Medical School
Boston, MA
USA

Marco E. Allaix, MD
Department of Surgical Sciences
University of Torino
Torino
Italy

Division of Biological Sciences
University of Chicago
Chicago, IL
USA

Mario Morino, MD
Department of Surgical Sciences
University of Torino
Turin
Italy

Marco G. Patti, MD, FACS
Department of Surgery
Center for Esophageal Diseases
University of Chicago Pritzker
School of Medicine
Chicago, IL
USA

ISBN 978-3-319-35247-3 ISBN 978-3-319-04337-1 (eBook)
DOI 10.1007/978-3-319-04337-1
Springer Cham Heidelberg New York Dordrecht London

Printed on acid-free paper

Springer is part of Springer Science+Business Media (www.springer.com)

To Carlos Alberto Pellegrini, MD, mentor, role model, friend.

The Editors

Contents

1 **Esophageal Anatomy and Physiology** ... 1
Marco E. Allaix and Marco G. Patti

2 **Esophageal Diseases: Radiologic Images** ... 11
Bernardo A. Borraez, Aruna Gasparaitis, and Marco G. Patti

3 **Gastroesophageal Reflux Disease: Pathophysiology** ... 41
Antonio Carlos Valezi, Fernando A.M. Herbella, and Jorge Mali Junior

4 **Gastroesophageal Reflux Disease: Diagnostic Evaluation** ... 53
Marco E. Allaix, Bernardo A. Borraez, and Marco G. Patti

5 **Gastroesophageal Reflux Disease: Treatment** ... 69
Marco E. Allaix, Bernardo A. Borraez, and Marco G. Patti

6 **Treatment of Paraesophageal Hernias** ... 83
Anahita Jalilvand, Justin B. Dimick, and P. Marco Fisichella

7 **Extraesophageal Manifestation of Gastroesophageal Reflux Disease** ... 95
Fernando A.M. Herbella and Attila Dubecz

8 **Epiphrenic Diverticulum** ... 109
Anahita Jalilvand and P. Marco Fisichella

9 **Evaluation and Treatment of Zenker's Diverticulum** ... 119
Cheryl C. Nocon and Louis D. Portugal

10 **Achalasia: Pathophysiology and Diagnostic Evaluation** ... 133
Benedetto Mungo and Daniela Molena

11 **Achalasia: Treatment** ... 143
Marco E. Allaix, Fabrizio Rebecchi, Claudio Giaccone, and Mario Morino

12 Benign Esophageal Tumors: Evaluation and Treatment 153
Anahita Jalilvand and P. Marco Fisichella

13 Gastroesophageal Reflux Disease: From Heartburn to Cancer..... 165
Marco E. Allaix, Bernardo A. Borraez, and Marco G. Patti

14 Barrett's Esophagus: Treatment Options 177
Ajaypal Singh and Irving Waxman

15 Esophageal Cancer: Evaluation 189
Henner M. Schmidt and Donald E. Low

16 Esophageal Cancer: Surgical Treatment...................... 207
Henner M. Schmidt and Donald E. Low

17 Esophageal Cancer: Neoadjuvant and Adjuvant Therapy 227
Shuang Qin Zhang and Victoria M. Villaflor

Index 241

Contributors

Marco E. Allaix, MD Department of Surgical Sciences, University of Torino, Torino, Italy

Division of Biological Sciences, University of Chicago, Chicago, IL, USA

Bernardo A. Borraez, MD Department of Surgery, Center for Esophageal Diseases, University of Chicago Pritzker School of Medicine, Chicago, IL, USA

Justin B. Dimick, MD, MPH, FACS Department of Surgery, University of Michigan Health System, Ann Arbor, MI, USA

Attila Dubecz, MD Department of General and Thoracic Surgery, Klinikum Nürnberg Nord, Nürnberg, Germany

P. Marco Fisichella, MD, MBA, FACS Department of Surgery, Boston Veteran Administration Healthcare System, West Roxbury, MA, USA

Department of Surgery, Brigham and Women's Hospital, Harvard Medical School, Boston, MA, USA

Aruna Gasparaitis, MD Department of Radiology, Center for Esophageal Diseases, University of Chicago Pritzker School of Medicine, Chicago, IL, USA

Claudio Giaccone, MD Department of Surgical Sciences, University of Torino, Torino, Italy

Fernando A.M. Herbella, MD Department of Surgery, Federal University of São Paulo, São Paulo, Brazil

Anahita Jalilvand, MD Department of Surgery, Loyola University Medical Center and Loyola Stritch School of Medicine, Maywood, IL, USA

Jorge Mali Junior, MD Department of Surgery, State University of Londrina, Londrina, Brazil

Donald E. Low, MD, FACS, FRCS(c) Department of General, Thoracic and Vascular Surgery, Virginia Mason Medical Center, Seattle, WA, USA

Esophageal Center of Excellence, Digestive Disease Institute, Seattle, WA, USA

Daniela Molena, MD Division of Thoracic Surgery, Department of Surgery, Johns Hopkins Medical School, Baltimore, MD, USA

Mario Morino, MD Department of Surgical Sciences, University of Torino, Torino, Italy

Benedetto Mungo, MD Division of Thoracic Surgery, Department of Surgery, Johns Hopkins Medical School, Baltimore, MD, USA

Cheryl C. Nocon, MD Section of Otolaryngology-Head and Neck Surgery, The University of Chicago Medical Center, Chicago, IL, USA

Department of Surgery, University of Chicago Medicine, Chicago, IL, USA

Marco G. Patti, MD, FACS Department of Surgery, Center for Esophageal Diseases, University of Chicago Pritzker School of Medicine, Chicago, IL, USA

Louis D. Portugal, MD Section of Otolaryngology-Head and Neck Surgery, University of Chicago Medical Center, Chicago, IL, USA

Fabrizio Rebecchi, MD Department of Surgical Sciences, University of Torino, Torino, Italy

Henner M. Schmidt, MD Department for General, Thoracic and Vascular Surgery, Virginia Mason Medical Center, Seattle, WA, USA

Ajaypal Singh, MD Department of Medicine, Center for Esophageal Diseases, University of Chicago Pritzker School of Medicine, Chicago, IL, USA

Antonio Carlos Valezi, MD Department of Surgery, State University of Londrina, Londrina, Brazil

Victoria M. Villaflor, MD Division of Medical Oncology, Department of Medicine, Center for Esophageal Diseases, University of Chicago Pritzker School of Medicine, Chicago, IL, USA

Department of Internal Medicine, Section of Hematology/Oncology, University of Chicago Medicine, Chicago, IL, USA

Irving Waxman, MD, FASGE Department of Medicine, Center for Esophageal Diseases, University of Chicago Pritzker School of Medicine, Chicago, IL, USA

Shuang Qin Zhang, MD Division of Medical Oncology, Department of Medicine, Center for Esophageal Diseases, University of Chicago Pritzker School of Medicine, Chicago, IL, USA

Introduction

The United States has been the largest recipient country in the world of Italian immigrants. They have outnumbered immigrants from any other European nation, driven by the search for better opportunities.

Irrespective of their backgrounds and professions, Italians have always proven themselves diligent and hard workers, capable of establishing harmonious relations wherever they go.

Today, a new wave of Italians is pursuing opportunities in the United States to improve their education, skills, and chances for a brighter career. They represent a new breed of inspired and well-educated Italians, who chose to become citizens of the world, motivated by the desire to succeed in their profession, not only for the benefit of their own careers but also for their country of birth and their new country of residence.

Italians abroad are the ambassadors of our excellence, and thanks to their collaboration from the new host country with many Italian academic institutions, they help transfer their experience and expertise to their colleagues in Italy.

This book by Drs. Fisichella, Allaix, Morino, and Patti represents an excellent example of such collaboration. Two of the authors (Fisichella and Patti) left Italy after completing medical school, trained in surgery in the United States, where they eventually started a career at prestigious academic institutions. Today, Dr. Fisichella is Associate Professor of Surgery at Harvard Medical School, Associate Chief of Surgery at the Boston Veterans Administration Medical Center, and Associate Surgeon at Brigham and Women's Hospital in Boston. Dr. Patti is Professor of Surgery and Director of the Center for Esophageal Diseases at the University of Chicago Pritzker School of Medicine. Dr Patti has served as President of the International Society of Digestive Surgery and is the President Elect of the International Society of Surgery. Dr Allaix trained at the University of Torino and was sent by Professor Morino to Chicago to spend 18 months working with Dr Patti in order to improve his skills in the diagnosis and treatment of esophageal disorders. Today, Dr Allaix is back in Torino, where he has brought back to the excellent Department led by Professor Morino the experience gained in the States.

To all of them, our thanks and best wishes for a brighter future and a continuous collaboration.

February 14, 2014
Chicago, USA

Adriano Monti
Consul General of Italy, Chicago

Chapter 1
Esophageal Anatomy and Physiology

Marco E. Allaix and Marco G. Patti

Abstract The esophagus can be divided into three anatomic segments: the cervical, thoracic, and abdominal esophagus. Three layers form the esophageal wall: the mucosa, the submucosa, and the muscle layer, with an inner circular and an outer longitudinal layer. The lymphatic drainage is not segmental: lymph can flow for a long distance in the plexus before crossing the muscular layer and reaching the paraesophageal lymph nodes.

Keywords Cervical esophagus • Thoracic esophagus • Abdominal esophagus • Vagus nerves • Upper esophageal sphincter • Lower esophageal sphincter • Esophageal peristalsis

Anatomy of the Esophagus

The esophagus originates at the level of the sixth cervical vertebra, posterior to the cricoid cartilage, and extends to the eleventh thoracic vertebra. It is divided into three anatomic segments. The *cervical esophagus* lies just left of the midline,

Conflict of Interest
The authors have no conflicts of interest to declare.

M.E. Allaix, MD
Department of Surgical Sciences, University of Torino,
Corso A.M. Dogliotti 14, Torino 10126, Italy

M.G. Patti, MD, FACS (✉)
Department of Surgery, Center for Esophageal Diseases,
University of Chicago Pritzker School of Medicine, 5841 S. Maryland Ave,
MC 5095, Room G-207, Chicago, IL 60637, USA
e-mail: mpatti@surgery.bsd.uchicago.edu

P.M. Fisichella et al. (eds.), *Esophageal Diseases*,
DOI 10.1007/978-3-319-04337-1_1,

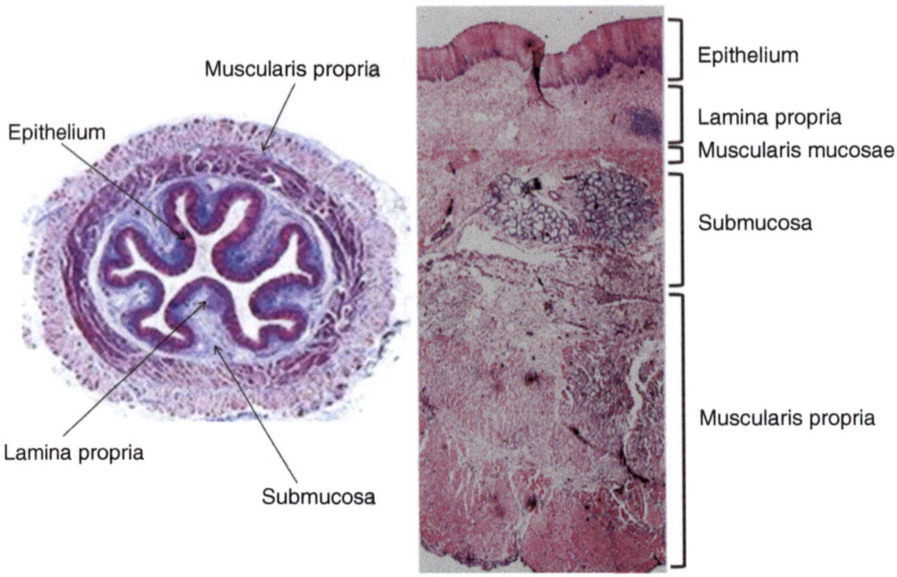

Fig. 1.1 Layers in the esophageal wall

posterior to the larynx and trachea, and anterior to the prevertebral layer of the cervical fascia.

The upper portion of the *thoracic esophagus* curves slightly to the right and passes behind the tracheal bifurcation and the left mainstem bronchus. The lower portion of the thoracic esophagus lies behind the pericardium and the left atrium, where it bends to the left and enters the abdomen through the esophageal hiatus.

The *abdominal esophagus* is 2–4 cm long and ends at its junction with the stomach.

There are three points of anatomical narrowing of the esophageal lumen: (1) at the level of the cricoid cartilage, (2) at the left main bronchus and the aortic arch, and (3) at the esophageal hiatus of the diaphragm.

Architecture of the Esophageal Wall

The epithelium of the esophagus is composed of stratified squamous cells that overlay the lamina propria and muscularis mucosa that is mainly formed by longitudinal muscular fibers (Fig. 1.1). The squamous epithelium joins the junctional columnar epithelium of the gastric cardia at the Z-line.

The *submucosal layer* contains elastic and fibrous tissue and is the strongest layer of the esophageal wall.

The *muscular layer* consists of an inner circular and an outer longitudinal layer. The upper esophageal sphincter is formed by the cricopharyngeal muscle and fibers from the esophageal wall and the inferior constrictors of the pharynx.

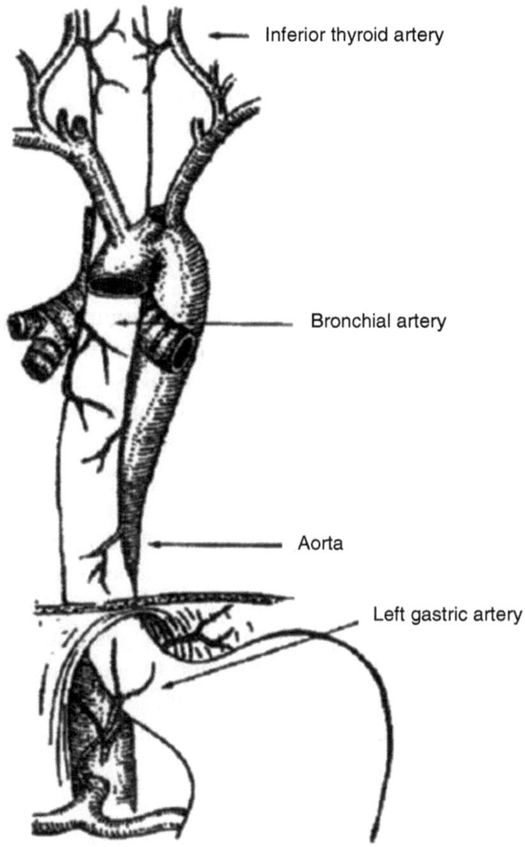

Fig. 1.2 Arterial blood supply to the esophagus

The *lower esophageal sphincter* is not a well-defined anatomic structure, even though a thickening of the circular esophageal musculature at the level of the manometric high-pressure zone has been reported.

Contrary to the rest of the gastrointestinal tract, the esophagus is not covered by a serosal layer.

Blood Supply

The cervical segment of the esophagus receives blood supply by branches of the inferior thyroid arteries.

The upper thoracic segment is supplied by the bronchial arteries, while the mid-thoracic segment receives blood by esophageal branches that originate from the aorta. The intercostal arteries may also contribute.

The arterial supply of the lower thoracic, diaphragmatic, and abdominal segments includes the left inferior phrenic artery and the esophageal branches of the left gastric artery (Fig. 1.2).

The submucosal venous drainage is more complex and variable. The veins that drain the cervical esophagus are tributary of the inferior thyroid veins; the veins from the thoracic esophagus drain into the hemiazygos and azygos veins. The most important veins are those that drain the lower esophagus. Blood from this region passes into the esophageal branches of the coronary vein, which is a tributary of the portal vein.

Lymphatic Drainage

Abundant lymphatic vessels form a dense submucosal plexus. Lymph usually flows longitudinally, running proximal in the upper two thirds and distal in the lower third of the esophagus. Lymph from the cervical esophagus drains mostly into the cervical and paratracheal lymph nodes, while lymph from the lower thoracic and abdominal esophagus reaches preferentially the retro-cardiac and celiac nodes. However, the drainage is not segmental; therefore, lymph can flow for a long distance in the plexus before crossing the muscular layer and reaching the paraesophageal lymph nodes.

The thoracic duct originates from the cysterna chili that is located in the abdominal cavity, at the level of the second lumbar vertebra. The duct enters the chest through the aortic hiatus and runs in the posterior mediastinum to the right of the midline between the esophagus and the azygos vein. At the level of the fifth thoracic vertebra, it crosses the midline behind the esophagus and reaches the base of the neck. Then, it curves to the right to drain into the internal jugular vein. A single thoracic duct is described in about 70 % of people, while two or more are present in the remainder individuals (Fig. 1.3).

Innervation

The striated muscle of the pharynx and upper esophagus receives nerves fibers that originate in the brain stem at the level of the nucleus ambiguous. The distal esophagus and LES are innervated by nerves that originate in the dorsal motor nucleus of the vagus and end in ganglia in the myenteric plexus. The myenteric plexus is located between the longitudinal and the circular muscle layers and receives efferent impulses from the brain stem and afferent impulses from the esophagus. Two main types of effector neurons are found in this plexus: (1) excitatory neurons and (2) inhibitory neurons that mediate contraction of the musculature via cholinergic receptors and via vasoactive intestinal polypeptide and nitric oxide.

The vagus nerves run along each side of the neck until they reach the thoracic esophagus, where they form an extensive plexus. Above the diaphragm, they form two trunks. The left trunk runs anterior, while the right trunk is more posterior once they cross the esophageal hiatus. The anterior vagus then divides and gives rise to the hepatic branch and the anterior nerve of Latarjet, while the posterior vagus gives rise to the celiac branch and the posterior nerve of Latarjet. The posterior nerve of Latarjet runs parallel but deeper to the anterior counterpart in the gastrohepatic ligament about 1 cm from the lesser curvature of the stomach.

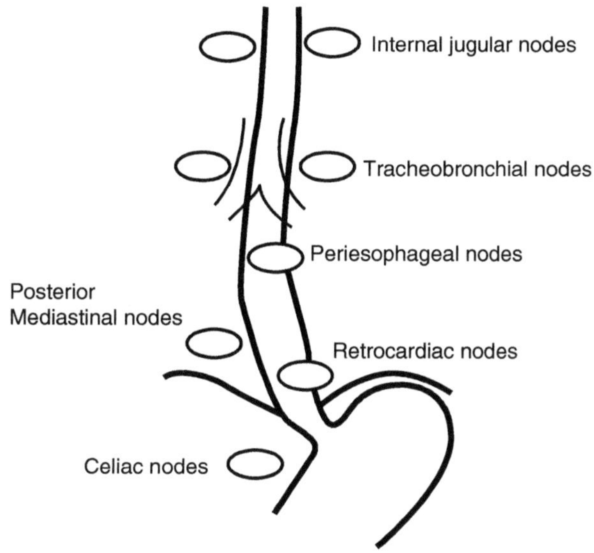

Fig. 1.3 Lymphatic drainage of the esophagus

Branches of the superior and inferior cervical ganglia in the neck, the splanchnic nerves, and the celiac plexus in the chest and in the abdomen provide the sympathetic innervations. These nerves do not have a motor function and mainly modulate the activity of other neurons.

Right Thoracoscopic View

The thoracoscopic approach to the right chest provides an excellent view of the esophagus from the thoracic inlet to the gastroesophageal junction (Fig. 1.4). In order to obtain adequate exposure, the right lung is deflated and retracted anteriorly, while the inferior pulmonary ligament is divided. After incision of the mediastinal pleura, most thoracic esophagus is exposed. The upper thoracic part of the esophagus is crossed anteriorly by the right brachiocephalic vessels. At the level of the right mainstem bronchus, the azygos vein passes from a paravertebral position anteriorly to enter the superior vena cava, crossing over the esophagus. Distal to the inferior pulmonary vein, the esophagus lies between the heart and the descending aorta. The sympathetic chain and ganglia run vertically, parallel and lateral to the azygous vein, crossing over the intercostals vessels.

Left Thoracoscopic View

Left thoracoscopy provides a good view of the esophagus from the aortic arch to the gastroesophageal junction (Fig. 1.5). After deflation and anterior retraction of the lung, the inferior pulmonary ligament is divided and the mediastinal pleura opened. The esophagus can be identified in the space between the pericardium and the

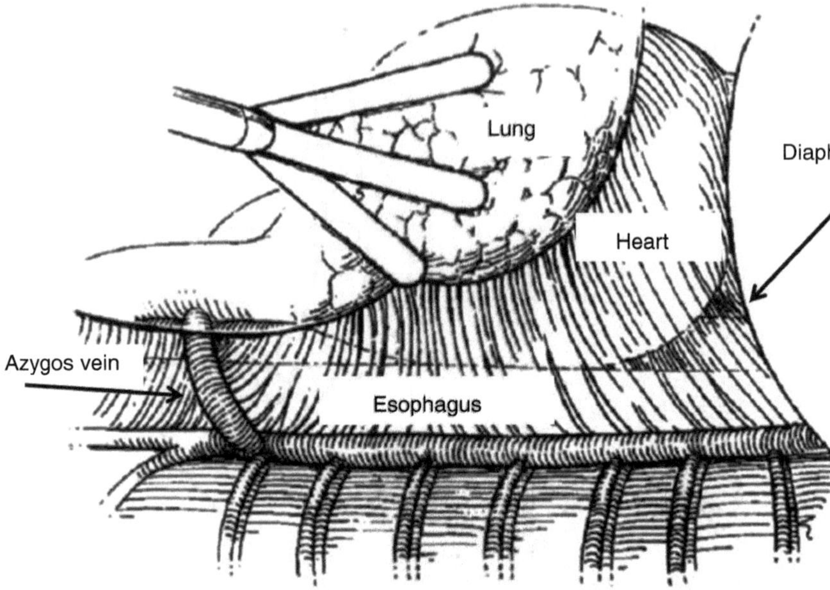

Fig. 1.4 Right thoracoscopic view

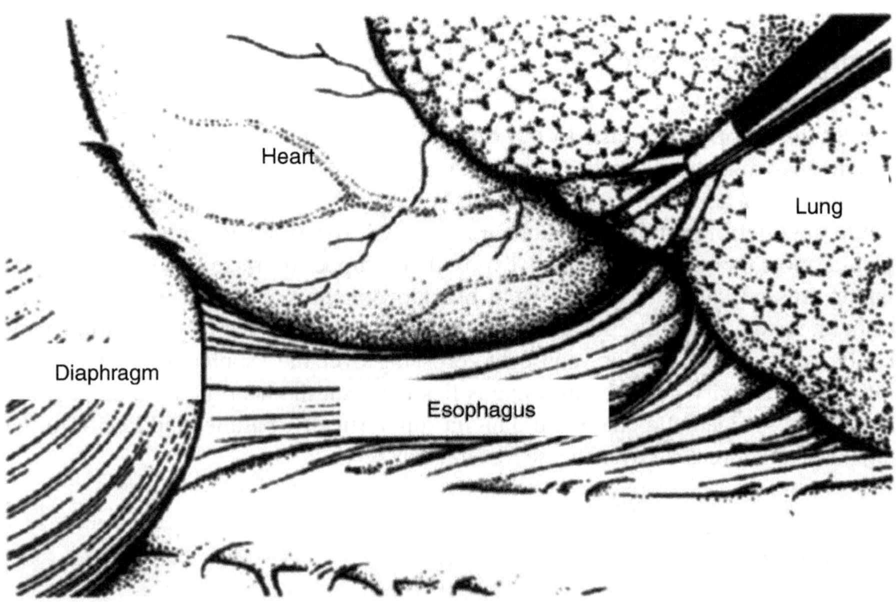

Fig. 1.5 Left thoracoscopic view

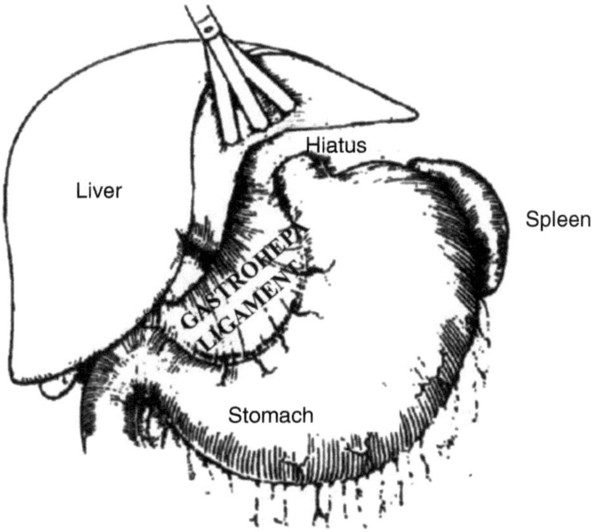

Fig. 1.6 Laparoscopic view

descending aorta. Behind and lateral to the aorta, the hemiazygos vein runs along the anterolateral aspect of the vertebral bodies, draining the left intercostal veins. It crosses behind the esophagus to join the azygos vein on the right at the level of the eighth thoracic vertebra.

Sympathetic chain's anatomy on the left is similar to that on the right.

Laparoscopic View

The left lobe of the liver must be retracted anteriorly and to the right in order to have the esophageal hiatus and abdominal esophagus exposed (Fig. 1.6). The phreno-esophageal membrane covers the hiatus and the intra-abdominal esophagus. If the gastrohepatic ligament is stretched flat by pulling the stomach caudad and to the left, the caudate lobe of the liver and a portion of the inferior vena cava can be seen through the transparent upper part. The hepatic branch of the anterior vagus is visible in the gastrohepatic ligament, sometimes close to an accessory left hepatic artery arising from the left gastric artery.

After dividing the gastrohepatic ligament and the phreno-esophageal membrane, the right border of the crus and the intra-abdominal esophagus are clearly visible (Fig. 1.7). The anterior vagus nerve can be identified on the anterior aspect of the esophagus. Its bifurcation is usually covered by the gastroesophageal fat pad. The posterior vagus nerve becomes evident after blunt dissection of the space between the esophagus and right pillar of the crus and anterior lift of the esophagus, since it passes through the hiatus posterior to the esophagus. Variations of the typical anatomy are present in about 10 % of patients, consisting of extension of the esophageal plexus into the abdomen or early bifurcation of the two trunks above the diaphragm.

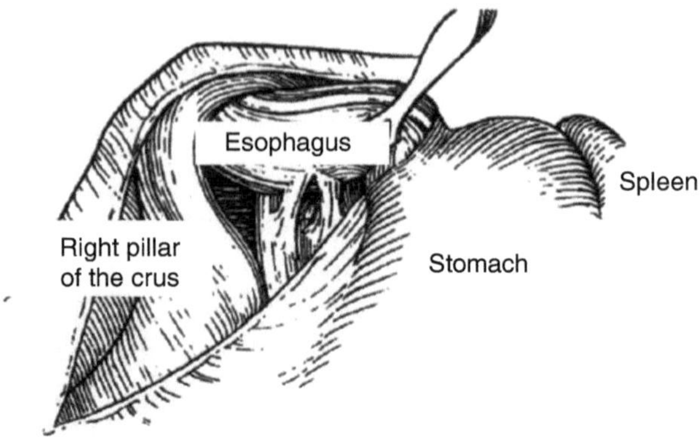

Fig. 1.7 Dissection of the right and left pillars of the crus

Physiology

The coordinated activity of the upper esophageal sphincter (UES), the esophageal body, and the lower esophageal sphincter (LES) is responsible for the motor function of the esophagus and the progression of the bolus from the pharynx to the stomach.

Upper Esophageal Sphincter

The UES receives motor innervation directly from the nucleus ambiguus. The sphincter is in a state of continuous tonic contraction. The UES prevents passage of air from the pharynx into the esophagus and reflux of contents from the esophagus into the pharynx. During a swallow, the tongue moves a bolus into the pharynx, which contracts while the UES relaxes. After the bolus has reached the esophagus, the UES regains its resting tone.

Esophageal Body

When a bolus passes through the UES, a contraction originates at the level of the upper esophagus and progresses distally toward the stomach. This wave, which is initiated by swallowing and is called *primary peristalsis*, travels at a speed of 3–4 cm/s with amplitudes of 60–140 mmHg in the distal esophagus. Local stimulation of sensory receptors in the esophageal body by distention elicits a peristaltic wave at the point of stimulation that moves distally. It is called *secondary peristalsis* and aims to improve esophageal emptying when the lumen is not completely cleared of ingested food by the primary waves or when gastric contents reflux into the esophagus. *Tertiary waves* are non-propulsive contractions. They are considered abnormal and are frequently diagnosed in asymptomatic elderly people or in patients with esophageal motility disorders.

Lower Esophageal Sphincter

The main function of the lower esophageal sphincter (LES) is to prevent reflux of gastric contents into the esophagus. The LES is 3–4 cm long, its pressure profile is slightly asymmetric, and the resting pressure ranges between 15 and 35 mmHg. When a swallow occurs, the LES relaxes for 5–10 s to allow the bolus to enter the stomach, and then it returns to its resting tone.

LES relaxation is mediated by non-adrenergic, non-cholinergic neurotransmitters, such as vasoactive intestinal peptide and nitric oxide. The resting tone mainly depends on the intrinsic myogenic activity. During fasting, the LES presents cyclic phasic contractile activity synchronous with phases II and III of the interdigestive motor complex.

The LES has periodic relaxations independently from swallowing. They are called *transient lower esophageal sphincter relaxations* to distinguish them from relaxations secondary to swallows. The cause of these transient relaxations is not known, but gastric distention is thought to play a role. Transient LES relaxations are responsible for the physiologic gastroesophageal reflux present in any individual. When they are more frequent and prolonged, they are the most common cause of abnormal reflux in patients with gastroesophageal reflux disease (GERD) and normotensive LES. Decreased LES length and/or pressure is responsible for pathologic reflux in the remaining patients with GERD.

The crus of the diaphragm at the level of the esophageal hiatus contributes to the LES resting pressure. This pinchcock action of the diaphragm protects against reflux caused by sudden increased intra-abdominal pressure. This synergistic action of the diaphragm is lost in presence of a sliding hiatal hernia, as the gastroesophageal junction is located above the diaphragm.

Summary

- The esophagus is divided into three anatomic segments: cervical, thoracic, and abdominal esophagus.
- There are three areas of anatomical narrowing of the esophageal lumen: (1) at the level of the cricoid cartilage, (2) at the left main bronchus and the aortic arch, and (3) at the esophageal hiatus of the diaphragm.
- The mucosal lining of the esophagus consists of stratified squamous epithelium that overlies the lamina propria and muscolaris mucosa.
- The muscular layer consists of an inner circular and an outer longitudinal layer.
- The esophagus is not covered by a serosal layer.
- The lymphatic drainage is not segmental.
- The UES prevents passage of air from the pharynx into the esophagus and reflux of contents from the esophagus into the pharynx.
- The peristaltic wave that is initiated by swallowing is called *primary peristalsis*.

- Local stimulation of sensory receptors in the esophageal body by distention elicits a peristaltic wave at the point of stimulation that is called *secondary peristalsis*
- Non-propulsive contractions are called *tertiary waves* and are frequently diagnosed in asymptomatic elderly people or in patients with esophageal motility disorders.

Selected Reading

1. Aggestrup S, Uddman R, Sundler F, Fahrenkrug J, Håkanson R, Sørensen HR, Hambraeus G. Lack of vasoactive intestinal polypeptide nerves in esophageal achalasia. Gastroenterology. 1983;84:924–7.
2. Akiyama H, Tsurumaru M, Kawamura T, Ono Y. Principles of surgical treatment for carcinoma of the esophagus: analysis of lymph node involvement. Ann Surg. 1981;194(4):438–46.
3. Bonavina L, Evander A, DeMeester TR, Walther B, Cheng SC, Palazzo L, Concannon JL. Length of the distal esophageal sphincter and competency of the cardia. Am J Surg. 1986;151(1):25–34.
4. Collard JM, Lengele B, Otte JB, Kestens PJ. En bloc and standard esophagectomies by thoracoscopy. Ann Thorac Surg. 1993;56(3):675–9.
5. Cuschieri A. Endoscopic vagotomy for duodenal ulcer disease: procedures and appraisal. Adv Surg. 1996;29:291–302.
6. Dent J, Dodds WJ, Sekiguchi T, Hogan WJ, Arndorfer RC. Interdigestive phasic contractions of the human lower esophageal sphincter. Gastroenterology. 1983;84(3):453–60.
7. Holloway RH, Kocyan P, Dent J. Provocation of transient lower esophageal sphincter relaxations by meals in patients with symptomatic gastroesophageal reflux. Dig Dis Sci. 1991;36(8):1034–9.
8. Liebermann-Meffert D, Allgöwer M, Schmid P, Blum AL. Muscular equivalent of the lower esophageal sphincter. Gastroenterology. 1979;76(1):31–8.
9. Orringer MB, Bluett M, Deeb GM. Aggressive treatment of chylothorax complicating transhiatal esophagectomy without thoracotomy. Surgery. 1988;104(4):720–6.
10. Patti MG. Minimally invasive esophageal procedures. In: Souba WW, Fink MP, Jurkovich GJ, Kaiser LR, Pearce WH, Pemberton JH, Soper N, editors. ACS surgery. Principles & practice. 6th ed. New York: WebMD Professional Pub; 2007.
11. Patti MG, Goldberg HI, Arcerito M, Bortolasi L, Tong J, Way LW. Hiatal hernia size affects lower esophageal sphincter function, esophageal acid exposure, and the degree of mucosal injury. Am J Surg. 1996;171:182–6.
12. Pellegrini C, Wetter LA, Patti M, Leichter R, Mussan G, Mori T, Bernstein G, Way L. Thoracoscopic esophagomyotomy. Initial experience with a new approach for the treatment of achalasia. Ann Surg. 1992;216(3):291–6.
13. Skandalakis LJ, Donahue PE, Skandalakis JE. The vagus nerve and its vagaries. Surg Clin North Am. 1993;73(4):769–84.
14. Stein HJ, DeMeester TR, Naspetti R, Jamieson J, Perry RE. Three-dimensional imaging of the lower esophageal sphincter in gastroesophageal reflux disease. Ann Surg. 1991;214(4):374–83.
15. Zaninotto G, DeMeester TR, Schwizer W, Johansson KE, Cheng SC. The lower esophageal sphincter in health and disease. Am J Surg. 1988;155:104–11.

Chapter 2
Esophageal Diseases: Radiologic Images

Bernardo A. Borraez, Aruna Gasparaitis, and Marco G. Patti

Abstract Esophageal diseases are functional disorders (gastroesophageal reflux disease (GERD), achalasia, esophageal diverticula), congenital abnormalities (esophageal duplication cyst), or tumors (leiomyoma, gastrointestinal stromal tumors (GIST), cancer). In the evaluation of these disorders, no single test provides all the needed information, but the final diagnosis and treatment plan are based on information provided by multiple tests. For instance, in patients with GERD, a barium swallow describes the anatomy of the esophagus and stomach (hiatal hernia, Schatzki's ring, stricture); an upper endoscopy determines if mucosal injury is present and excludes gastric and duodenal pathology; esophageal manometry defines pressure, length, and position of the lower esophageal sphincter; quality of esophageal peristalsis; and pressure of the upper esophageal sphincter and its coordination with the pharyngeal contraction; ambulatory pH monitoring determines if abnormal gastroesophageal reflux is present, if reflux extends to the proximal esophagus and pharynx, and if there is a temporal correlation between episodes of reflux and symptoms experienced by the patient.

Keywords Barium swallow • Computerized tomography (CT scan) • Positive emission tomography (PET) • Gastroesophageal reflux • Hiatal hernia • Achalasia • Diffuse esophageal spam • Zenker's diverticulum • Epiphrenic diverticulum • Esophageal leiomyoma • Esophageal cancer

---

Conflict of Interest
The authors have no conflicts of interest to declare.

B.A. Borraez, MD • M.G. Patti, MD, FACS (✉)
Department of Surgery, Center for Esophageal Diseases,
University of Chicago Pritzker School of Medicine,
5841 S. Maryland Ave, MC 5095, Room G-207, Chicago, IL 60637, USA
e-mail: mpatti@surgery.bsd.uchicago.edu

A. Gasparaitis, MD
Department of Radiology, Center for Esophageal Diseases,
University of Chicago Pritzker School of Medicine,
5841 S. Maryland Ave, MC 5095, Room G-207, Chicago, IL 60637, USA

P.M. Fisichella et al. (eds.), *Esophageal Diseases*,
DOI 10.1007/978-3-319-04337-1_2, © Springer International Publishing Switzerland 2014

Introduction

Esophageal diseases are functional disorders (gastroesophageal reflux disease (GERD), achalasia, esophageal diverticula), congenital abnormalities (esophageal duplication cyst), or tumors (leiomyoma, gastrointestinal stromal tumors (GIST), cancer). In the evaluation of these disorders, no single test provides all the needed information, but the final diagnosis and treatment plan are based on information provided by multiple tests. For instance, in patients with GERD, a barium swallow describes the anatomy of the esophagus and stomach (hiatal hernia, Schatzki's ring, stricture); an upper endoscopy determines if mucosal injury is present and excludes gastric and duodenal pathology; esophageal manometry defines pressure, length, and position of the lower esophageal sphincter; quality of esophageal peristalsis; and pressure of the upper esophageal sphincter and its coordination with the pharyngeal contraction; ambulatory pH monitoring determines if abnormal gastroesophageal reflux is present, if reflux extends to the proximal esophagus and pharynx, and if there is a temporal correlation between episodes of reflux and symptoms experienced by the patient. In patients with esophageal cancer, an endoscopy with biopsies establishes the diagnosis; a barium swallow determines the location and length of the cancer; an endoscopic ultrasound, a CT scan, and a PET scan determine the stage of the disease at the time of presentation.

The following chapter illustrates each disease through radiologic images, correlating those with the findings of other tests.

Gastroesophageal Reflux Disease (GERD)

A barium swallow is a key test for physicians treating patients with GERD. It is the best test to assess the anatomy of the esophagus, the gastroesophageal junction, and the stomach. Some authors feel that this test is also useful for establishing the diagnosis of GERD. Specifically they feel that GERD is present if reflux is demonstrated during the test. However, in a recent study from the University of Chicago, Bello and colleagues tested this hypothesis and reached the opposite conclusion. Specifically they showed that even when reflux is demonstrated during a barium swallow, it does not mean that abnormal reflux will be found on an ambulatory pH monitoring, the gold standard for the diagnosis of GERD. In their study, a cohort of 134 patients underwent barium swallow and pH monitoring. Based on the results of the pH monitoring, they were divided in two groups: GERD+and GERD-. On barium esophagography, gastroesophageal reflux was identified in 47 % of patients in the GERD+group and in 30 % of the GERD-, while no reflux was noted in 53 % of GERD+patients and in 70 % of GERD- patients ($p=0.050$), accounting for a sensitivity of 47 %, a specificity of 70 %, a positive predictive value of 68.5 %, and a negative predictive value of 49 %. The overall accuracy was 57 %. In addition, there was no difference in the presence of hiatal hernia between GERD+and GERD- patients (40 % vs. 32 % ($p=0.368$)). Similarly, Chen and colleagues demonstrated

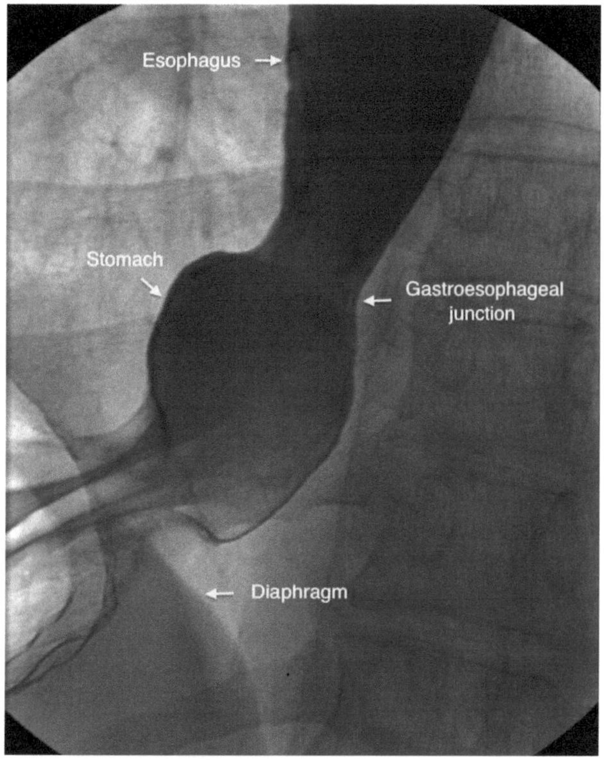

Fig. 2.1 Barium swallow. Sliding hiatal hernia

radiologic abnormalities in only 30 % of patients with an abnormal pH study. Based on these data, a barium swallow should not be considered a diagnostic test for GERD, but rather a complement to other tests, particularly before antireflux surgery. Its great value is providing anatomic information, such as the presence and type of a hiatal hernia, a Schatzki's ring, or a stricture.

Hiatal Hernia

The hernias of the esophageal hiatus are divided in four types (I, II, III, IV):

- Type I hiatal hernia occurs when the gastroesophageal junction (GEJ) and the upper stomach are herniated into the chest. The GEJ maintains its position above the herniated stomach (Figs. 2.1 and 2.2). It is also called "sliding" hiatal hernia as it can slide in and out of the thoracic cavity so that the presence and size of the hernia can vary over time. This is the most common type of hernia, accounting for more than 85 % of all hiatal hernias.
- Type II paraesophageal hiatal hernia. This type of hernia (also known as "rolling hernia) occurs when the stomach rolls in the posterior mediastinum next to the GEJ (usually left lateral) which maintains its normal position (Fig. 2.3).

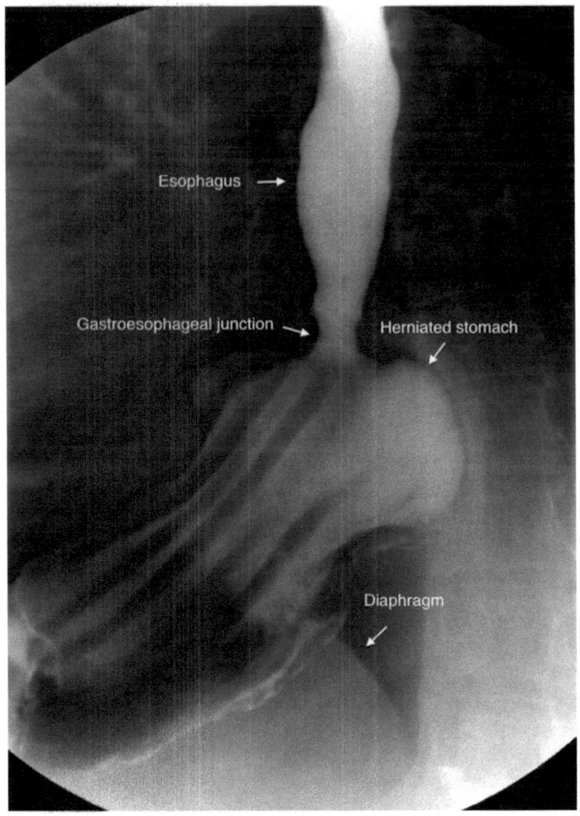

Fig. 2.2 Barium swallow. Sliding hiatal hernia

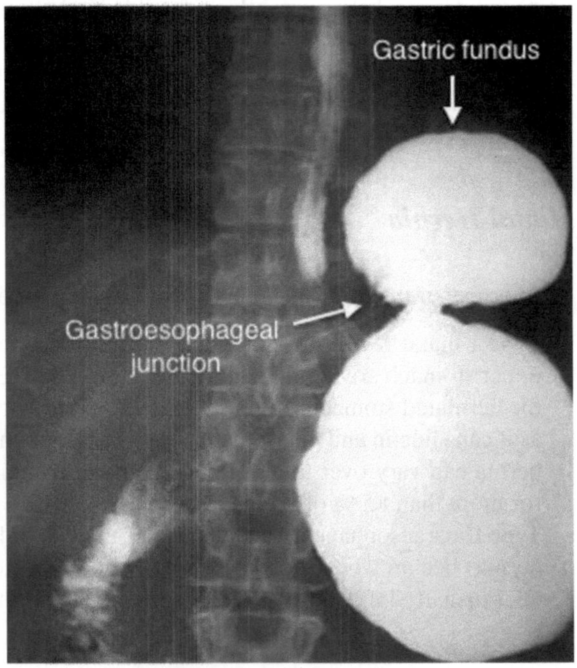

Fig. 2.3 Barium swallow. Paraesophageal hernia

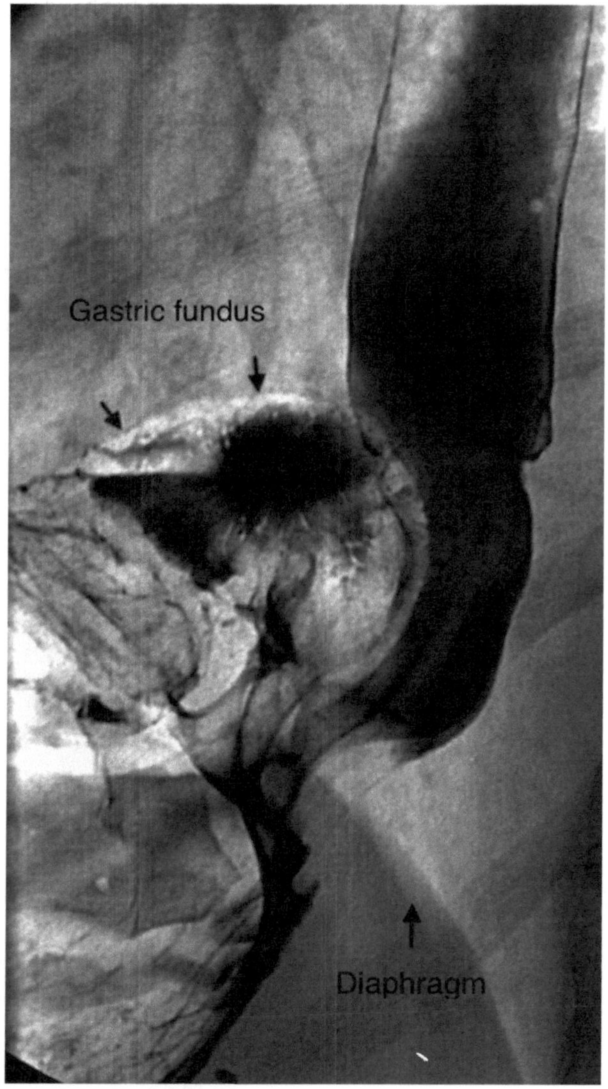

Fig. 2.4 Barium swallow. Paraesophageal hernia

- Type III paraesophageal hernia. This is also known as "mixed" hiatal hernia, a combination of sliding and rolling as both the GEJ and the stomach are herniated in the chest, with the stomach located next to the esophagus (Fig. 2.4). These hernias can be very large, and sometimes they can be identified in plain upright chest radiograph (Fig. 2.5). These hernias can be associated with a gastric volvulus (Figs. 2.6 and 2.7).
- Type IV. These hernias occur when not only the stomach but other upper abdominal organs (colon, spleen, omentum, small bowel) are herniated into the chest (Fig. 2.8).

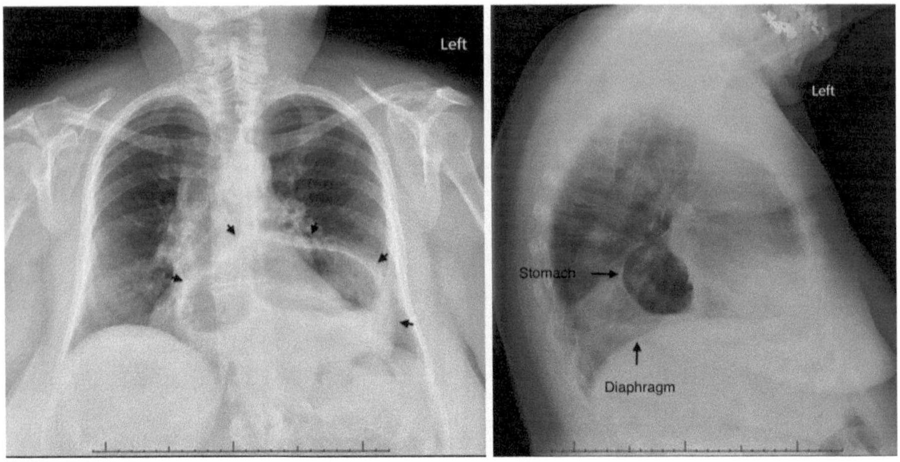

Fig. 2.5 Chest x-ray. Paraesophageal hernia with stomach above the diaphragm (*short arrows*)

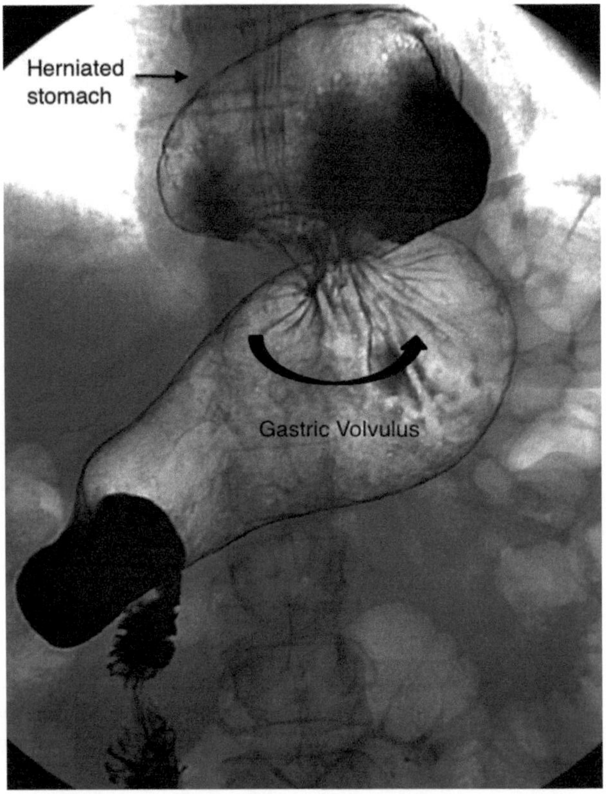

Fig. 2.6 Barium swallow. Paraesophageal hernia with gastric volvulus

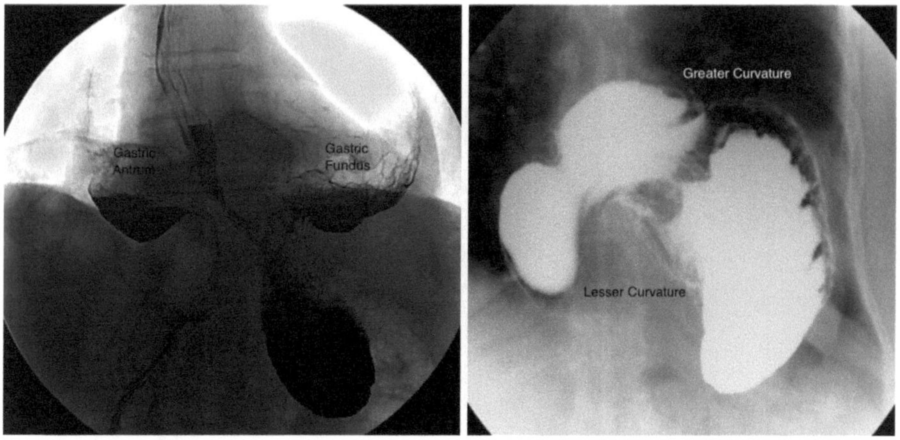

Fig. 2.7 Barium swallow. Paraesophageal hernia with gastric volvulus

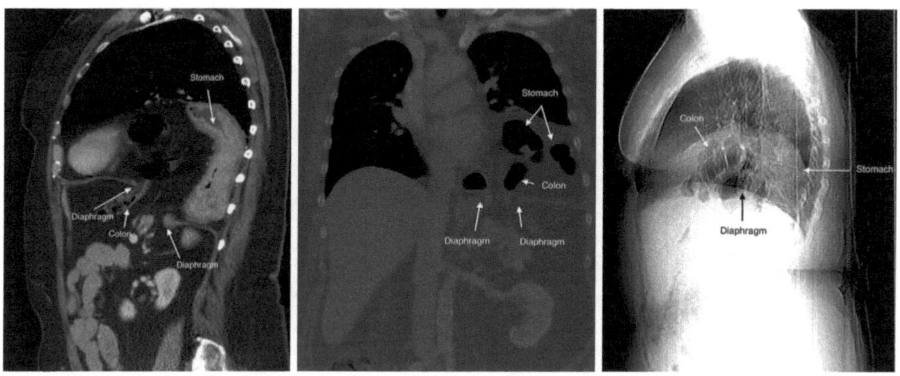

Fig. 2.8 Chest and abdominal CT scan. Type IV hiatal hernia with stomach and colon herniated into the chest

Schatzki's Ring

Schatzki's rings are found at the level of the GEJ or just above it. They consist of annular membranes of mucosa and submucosa, and they are usually associated with pathologic gastroesophageal reflux (Figs. 2.9 and 2.10).

Achalasia

Achalasia is a primary esophageal motility disorder characterized by failure of the lower esophageal sphincter to relax appropriately in response to swallowing and absent esophageal peristalsis. The classic radiologic findings include a) distal

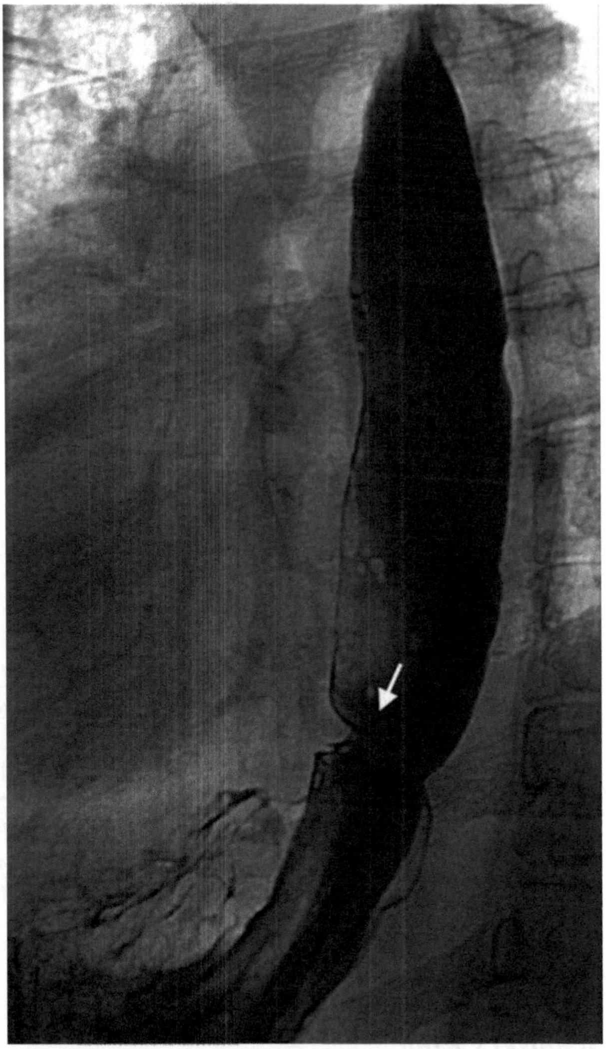

Fig. 2.9 Barium swallow. Schatzki's ring (*arrow*)

esophageal narrowing ("bird beak"); an air-fluid level, residual food in the esophagus; and slow emptying of the barium from the esophagus into the stomach (Fig. 2.11). In long-standing cases, the esophagus may become dilated and assume a sigmoid shape (Figs. 2.12 and 2.13). These findings are very important as treatment (pneumatic dilatation or surgery) is usually less effective when the esophagus is massively dilated and sigmoid, and an esophageal resection, may be indicated.

Diffuse esophageal spasm (DES) is another esophageal motility disorder, less frequent than achalasia. In DES the pressure of the lower esophageal sphincter may be normal or elevated, and normal peristalsis is mixed with simultaneous contractions. This disorder is often intermittent so that the esophagus can sometimes look normal while other times shows the characteristic "corkscrew" appearance (Figs. 2.14 and 2.15).

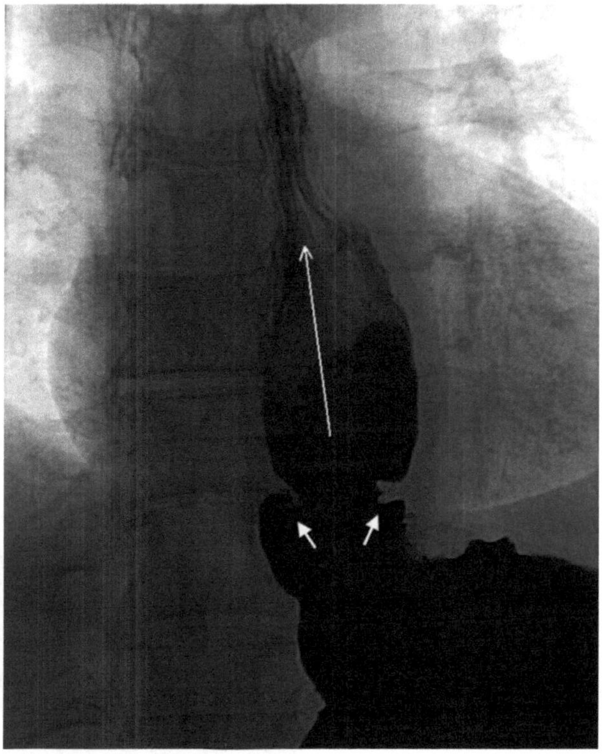

Fig. 2.10 Barium swallow. Schatzki's ring (*short arrows*), spontaneous reflux of gastric barium (*long arrow*)

Esophageal Diverticula

Zenker's Diverticulum

This diverticulum forms in the Killian's triangle, limited superiorly by the inferior constrictors of the pharynx and inferiorly by the cricopharyngeus muscle (Figs. 2.16 and 2.17). A functional obstruction, such as a hypertensive upper esophageal sphincter (UES) or a lack of coordination between the pharyngeal contraction and the UES, probably causes the formation of this diverticulum.

Epiphrenic Diverticulum

This diverticulum is located in the distal esophagus above the diaphragm, more commonly on the right side (Figs. 2.18, 2.19, and 2.20). This diverticulum is usually associated with a primary esophageal motility disorder such as achalasia or diffuse esophageal spasm.

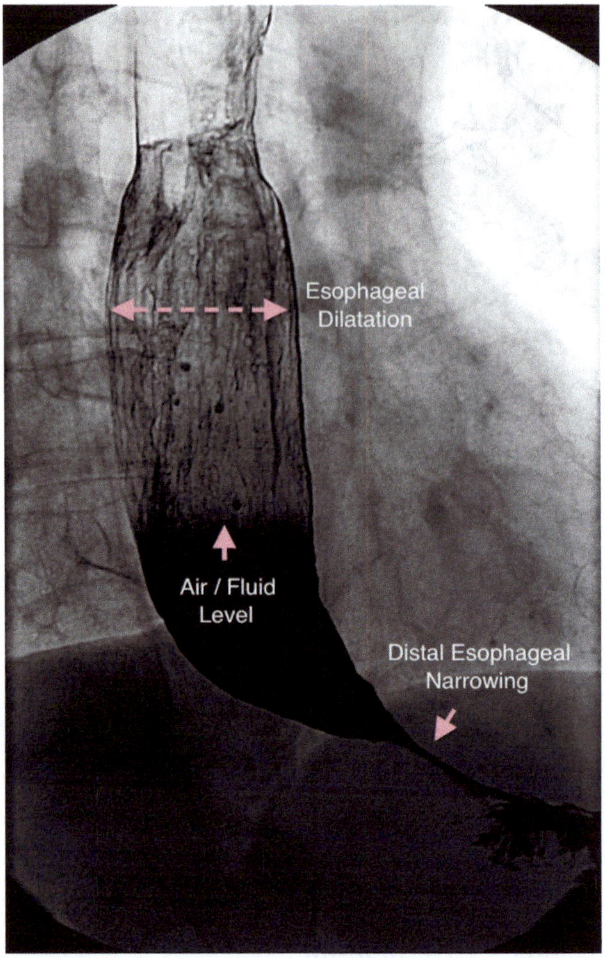

Fig. 2.11 Barium swallow. Esophageal achalasia

Benign Esophageal Tumors

Polyps

Fibrovascular polyps are benign mesenchymal tumors. They usually present as a pedunculated intraluminal mass (Fig. 2.21). They are well diagnosed by endoscopy and endoscopic ultrasound (Fig. 2.22).

Leiomyomas

They are the most common benign submucosal tumors in the esophagus (Fig. 2.23). They present as an intraluminal defect, and they are well defined by endoscopy and endoscopic ultrasound (Fig. 2.24).

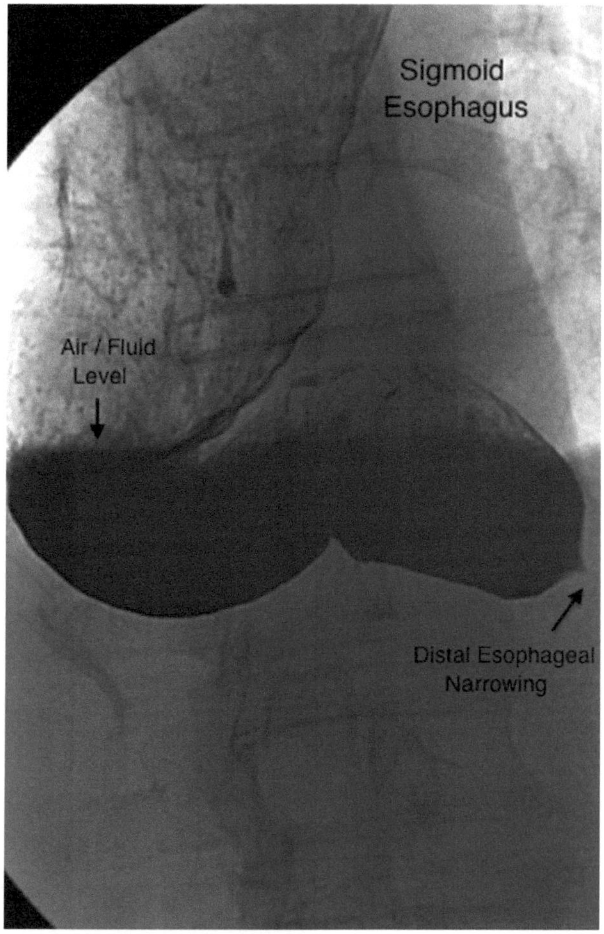

Fig. 2.12 Barium swallow. Esophageal achalasia with dilated and sigmoid-shaped esophagus

Malignant Esophageal Tumors

Esophageal Cancer

The squamous cell cancer is usually localized in the mid-thoracic esophagus (Figs. 2.25 and 2.26), while the adenocarcinoma is more frequently located in the distal esophagus arising from a background of Barrett's esophagus (Figs. 2.27 and 2.28). The diagnosis is established by endoscopy with biopsies. The staging of the cancer relies on endoscopic ultrasound to define the depth of the tumor (T) and the presence of pathologic periesophageal lymph nodes (N) (Fig. 2.29) and on a CT scan (Figs. 2.30, 2.31, and 2.32) and a PET scan to identify distant metastases (Figs. 2.33, and 2.34).

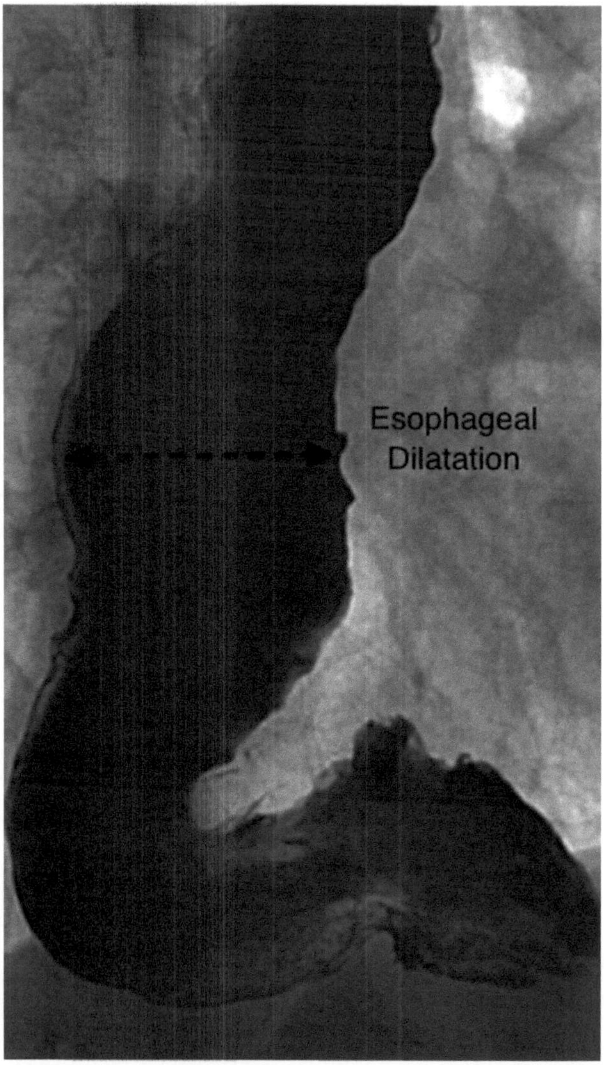

Fig. 2.13 Barium swallow. Esophageal achalasia with dilated and sigmoid-shaped esophagus

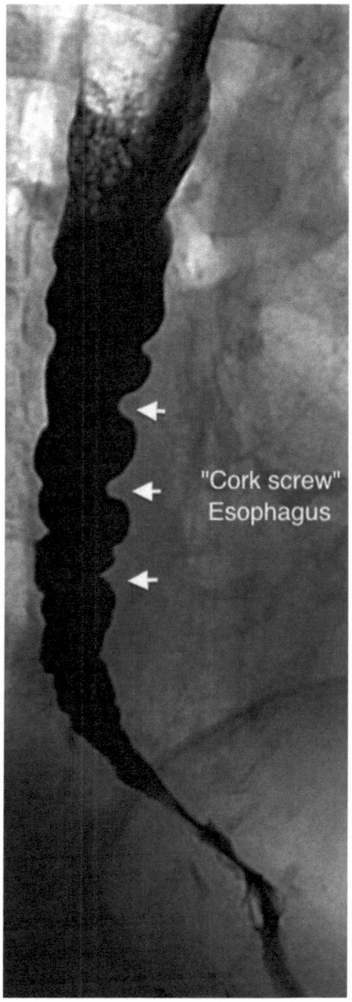

Fig. 2.14 Barium swallow. Diffuse esophageal spasm, "Corkscrew" esophagus (*arrows*)

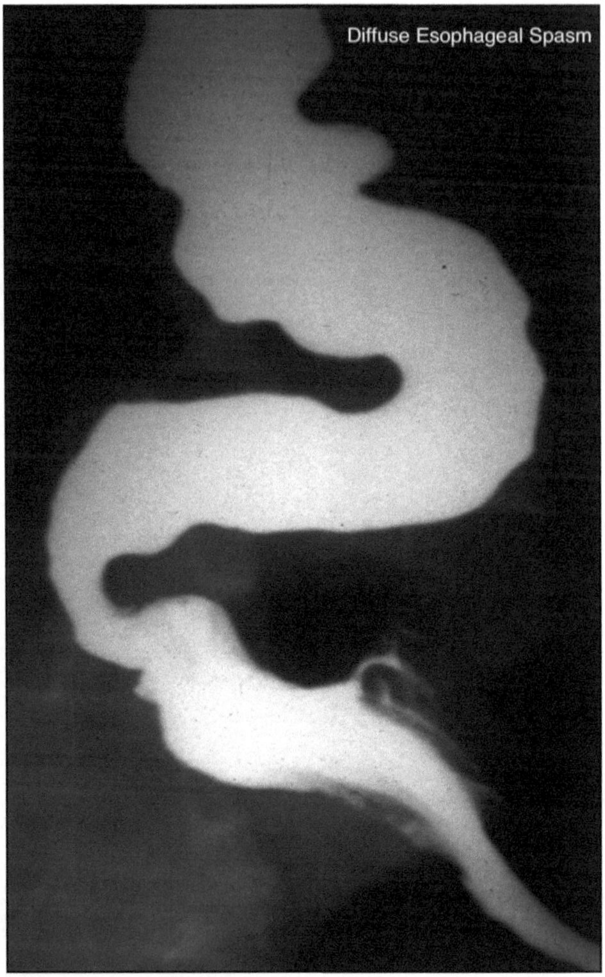

Fig. 2.15 Barium swallow. Diffuse esophageal spasm

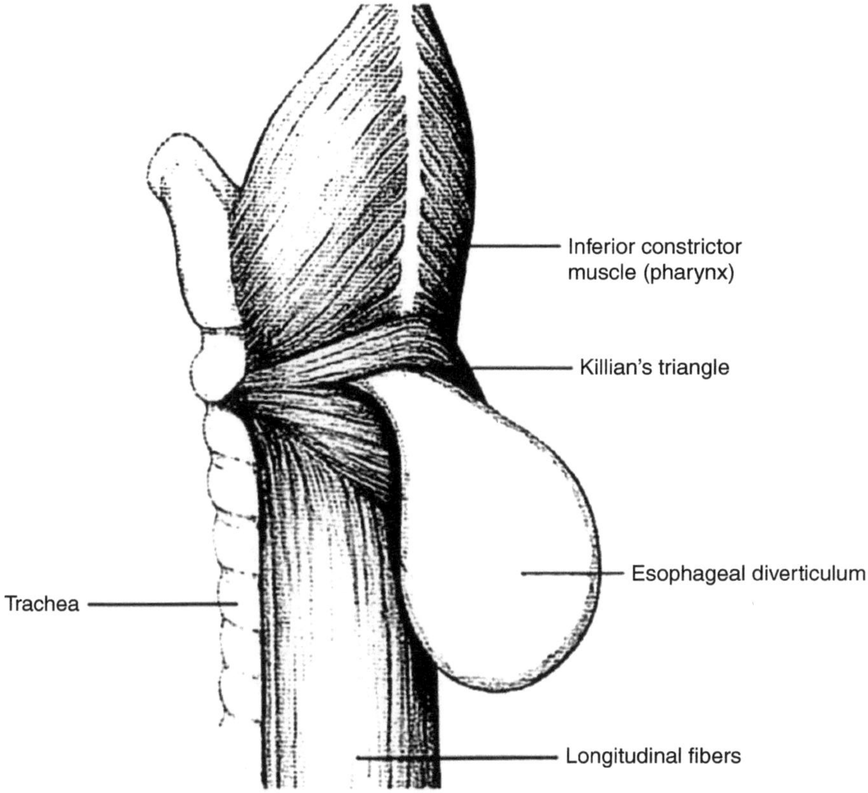

Fig. 2.16 Zenker's diverticulum

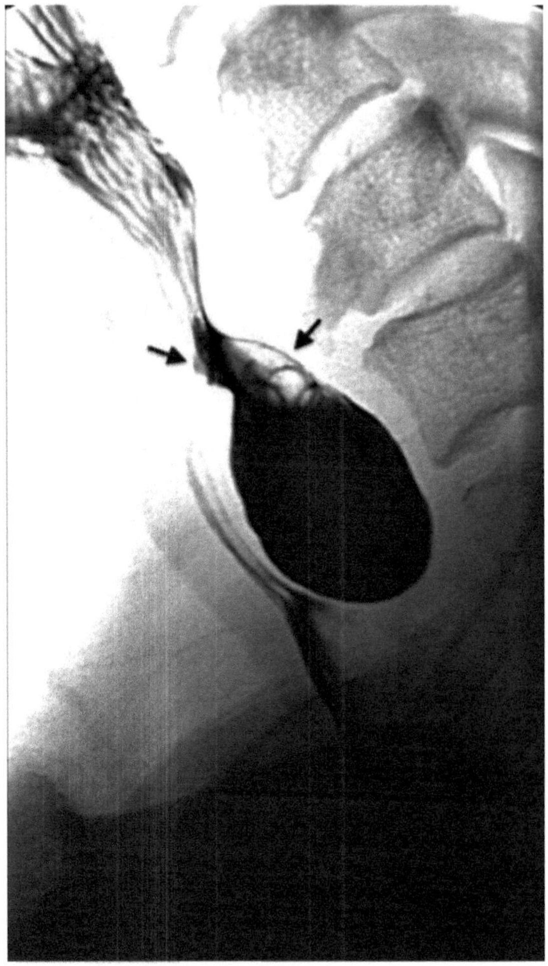

Fig. 2.17 Barium swallow. Zenker's diverticulum, barium filled sac (*arrows*)

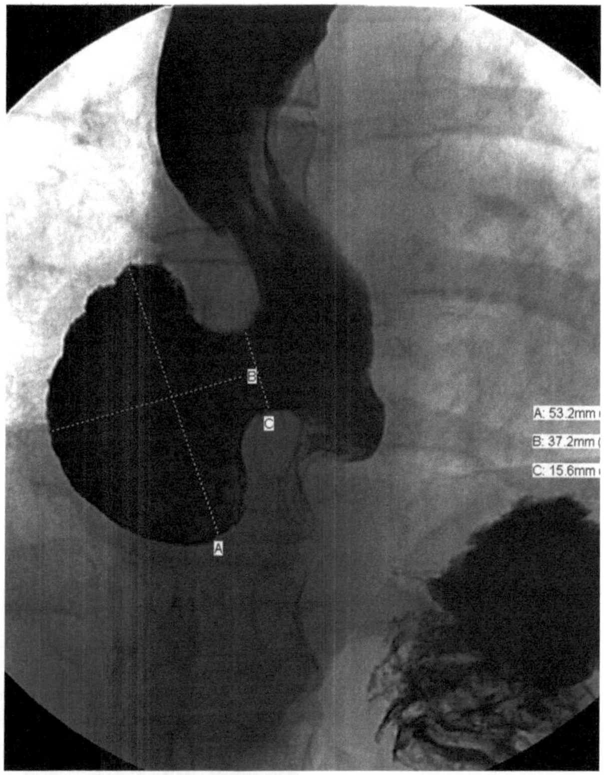

Fig. 2.18 Barium swallow. Epiphrenic diverticulum

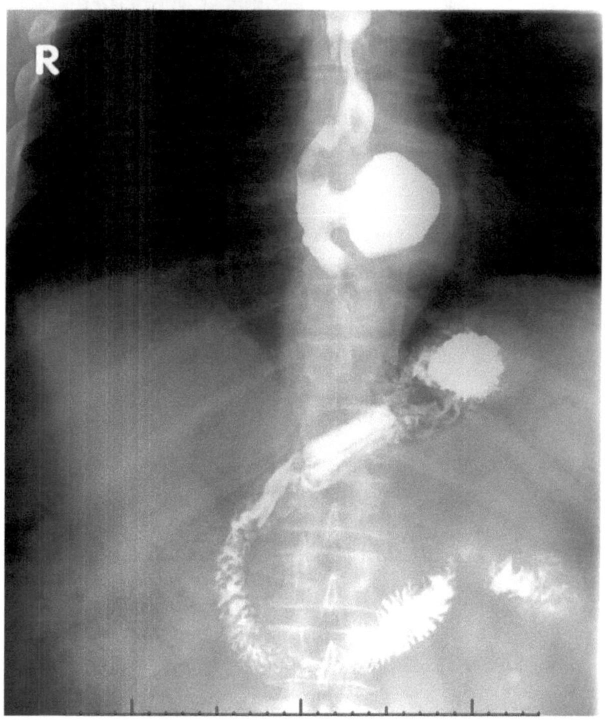

Fig. 2.19 Barium swallow. Epiphrenic diverticulum

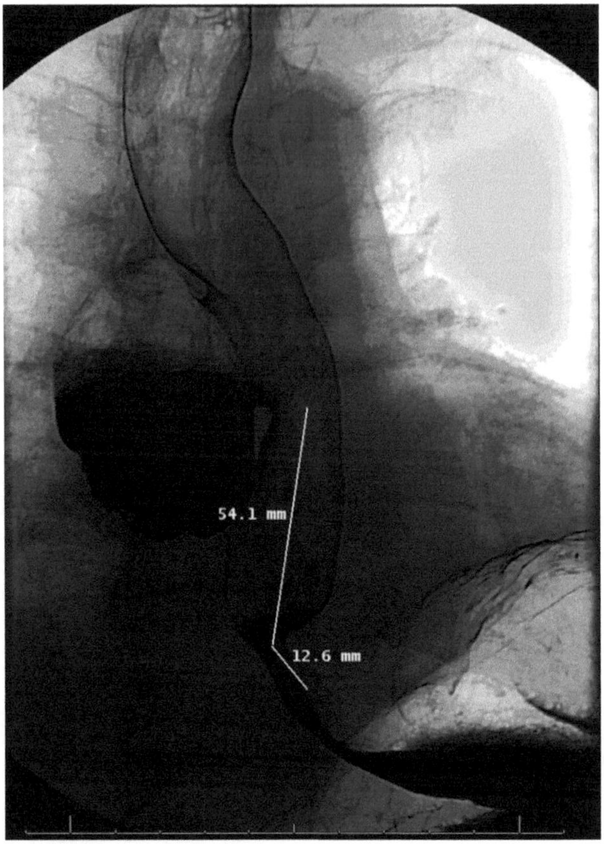

Fig. 2.20 Barium swallow. Epiphrenic diverticulum

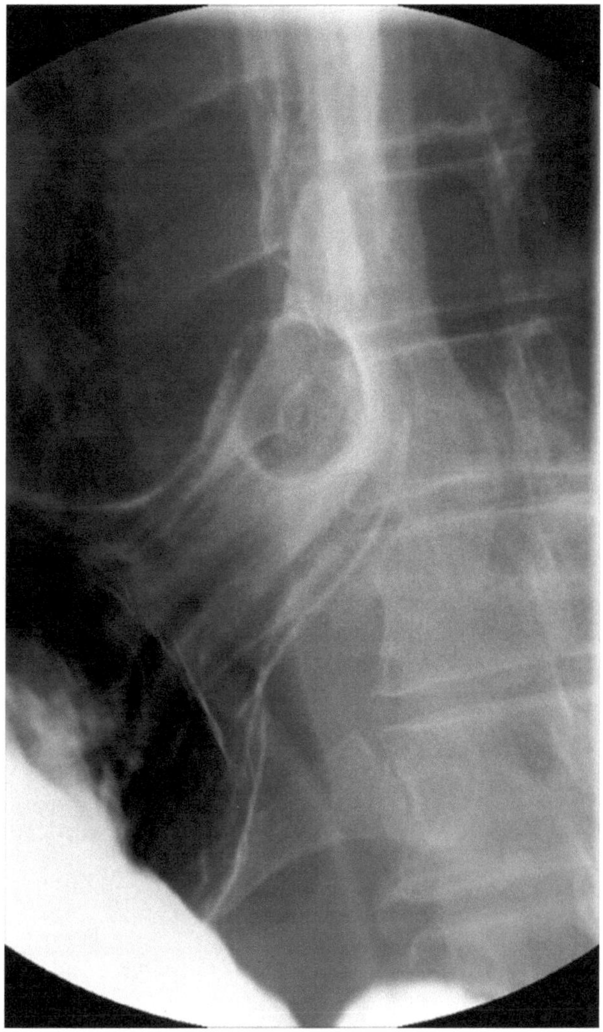

Fig. 2.21 Barium swallow. Esophageal polyp

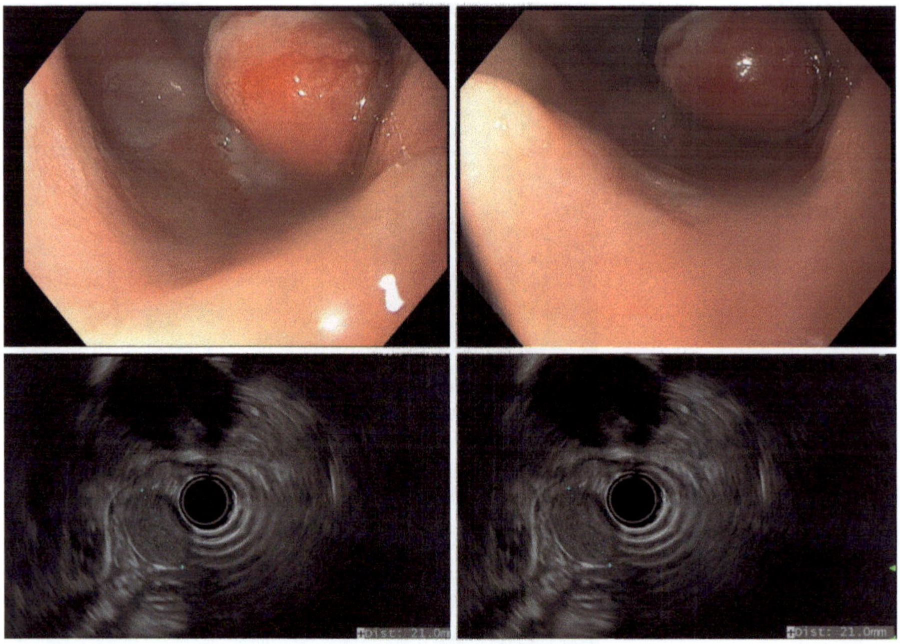

Fig. 2.22 Endoscopy with endoscopic ultrasound. Esophageal polyp

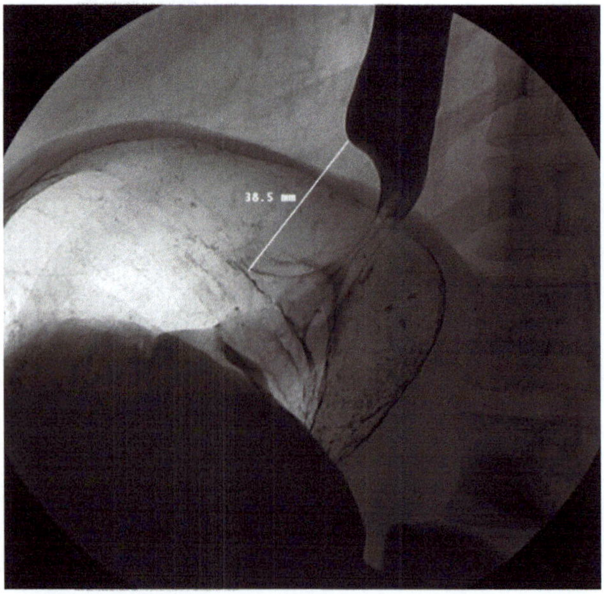

Fig. 2.23 Barium swallow. Esophageal leiomyoma

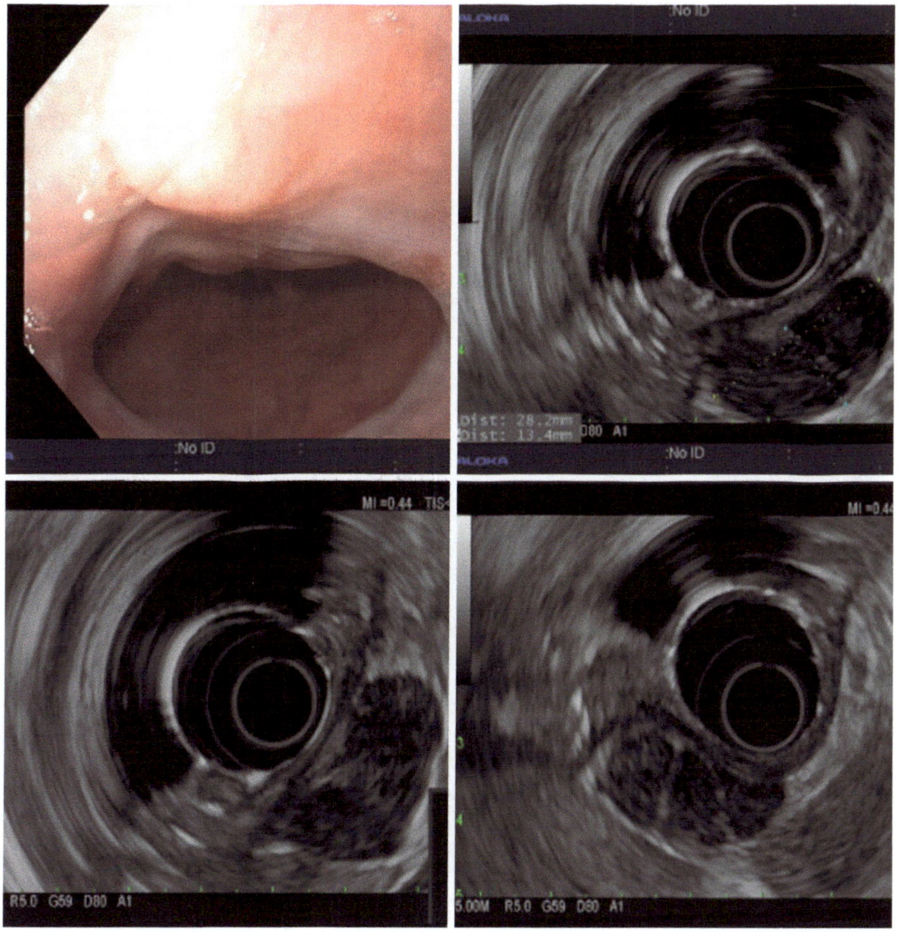

Fig. 2.24 Endoscopy with endoscopic ultrasound. Esophageal leiomyoma

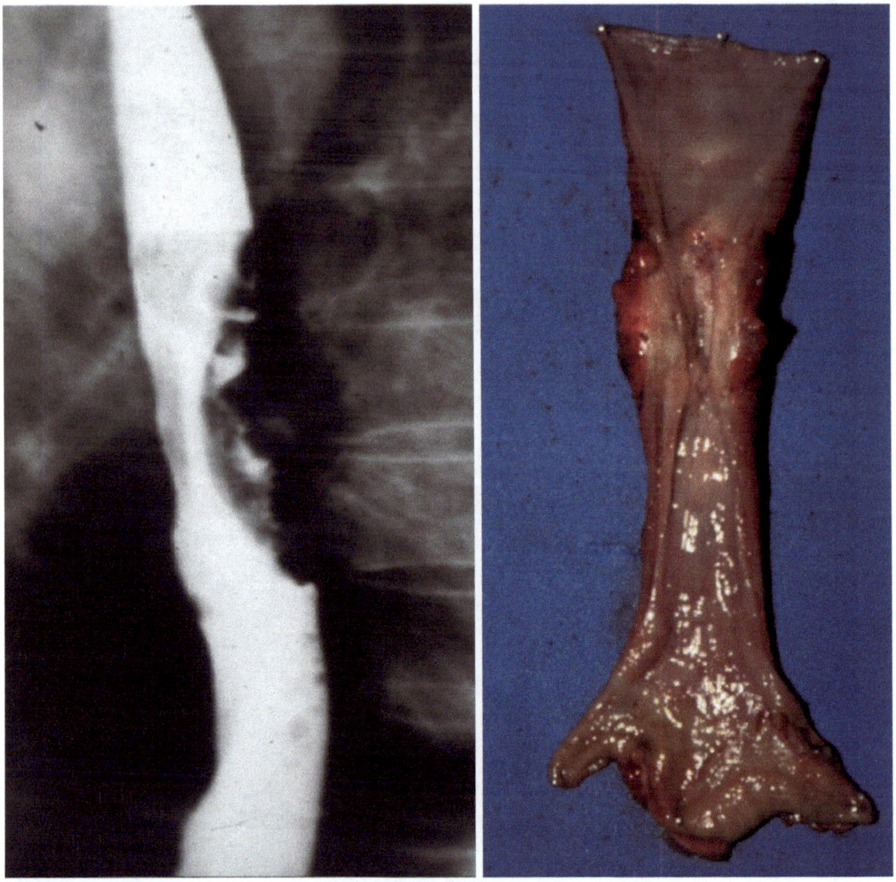

Fig. 2.25 Barium swallow and pathology. Mid-thoracic esophageal squamous cell cancer

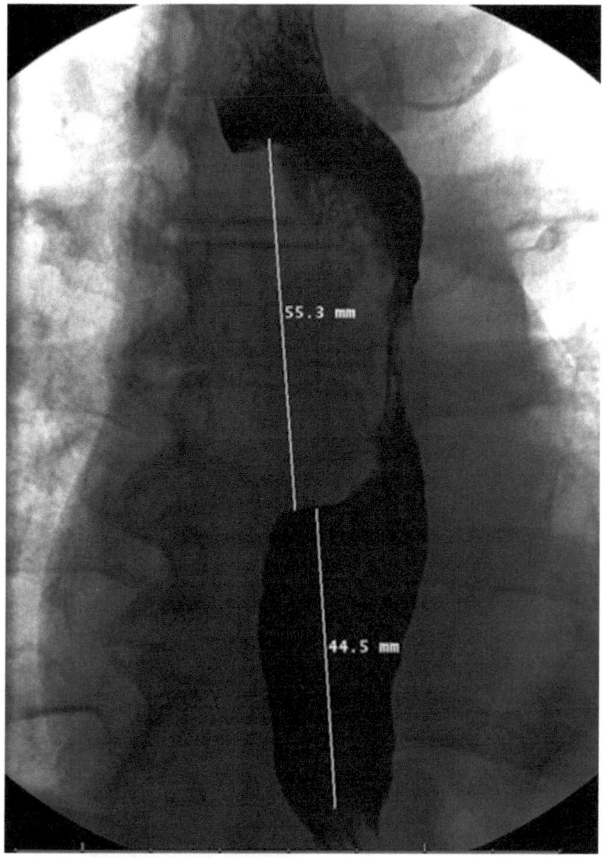

Fig. 2.26 Barium swallow. Mid-thoracic esophageal squamous cell cancer

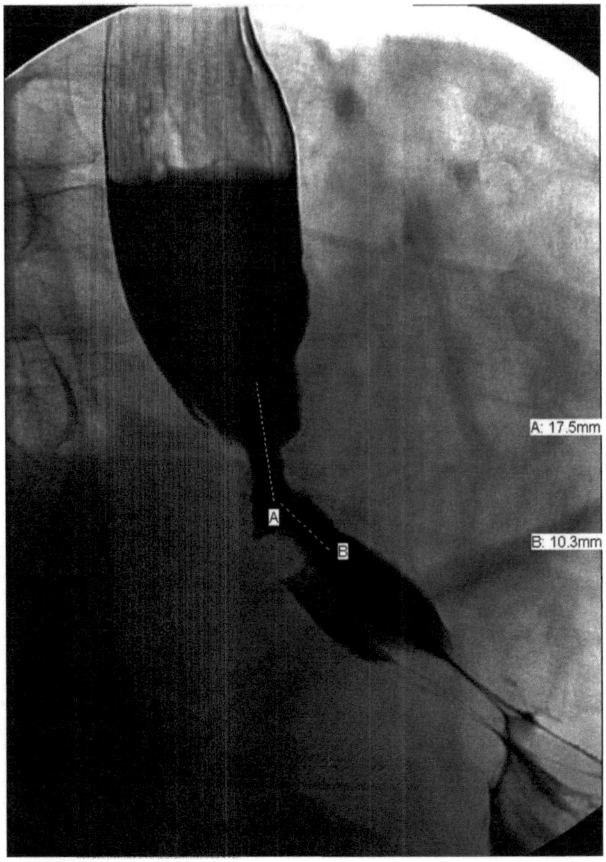

Fig. 2.27 Barium swallow. Distal esophageal adenocarcinoma

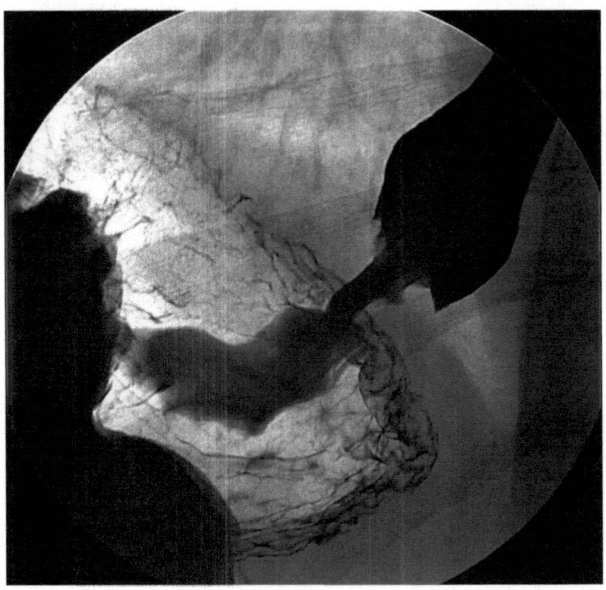

Fig. 2.28 Barium swallow. Distal esophageal adenocarcinoma

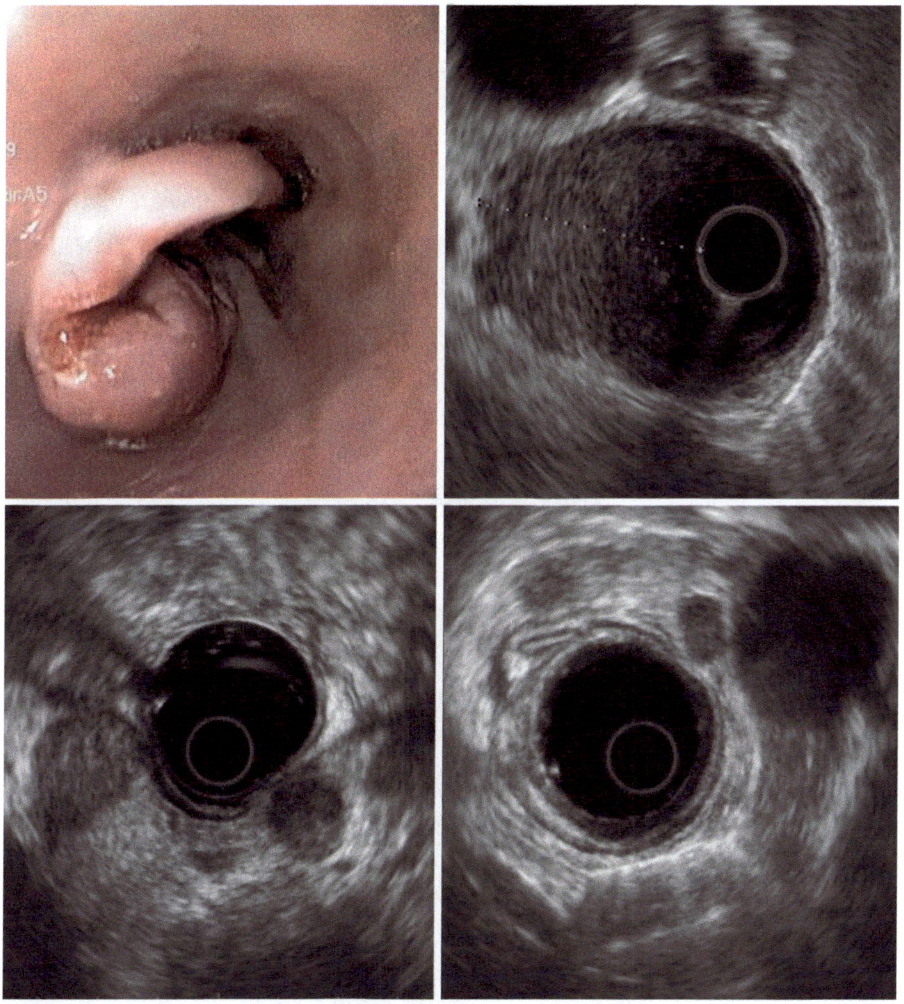

Fig. 2.29 Endoscopy and endoscopic ultrasound. Distal esophageal adenocarcinoma

Fig. 2.30 Chest/abdominal CT scan. Distal esophageal adenocarcinoma

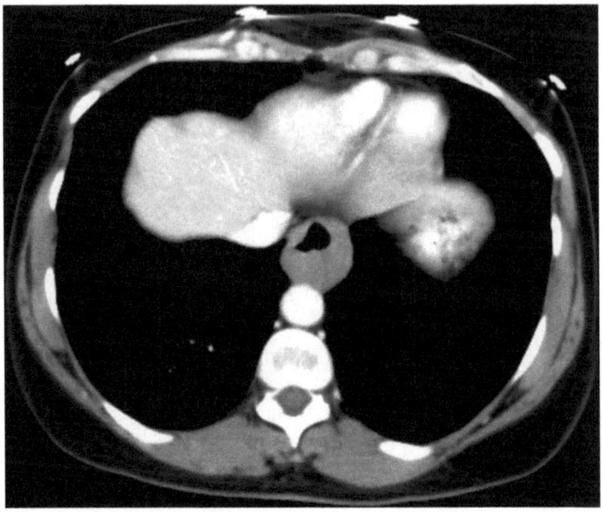

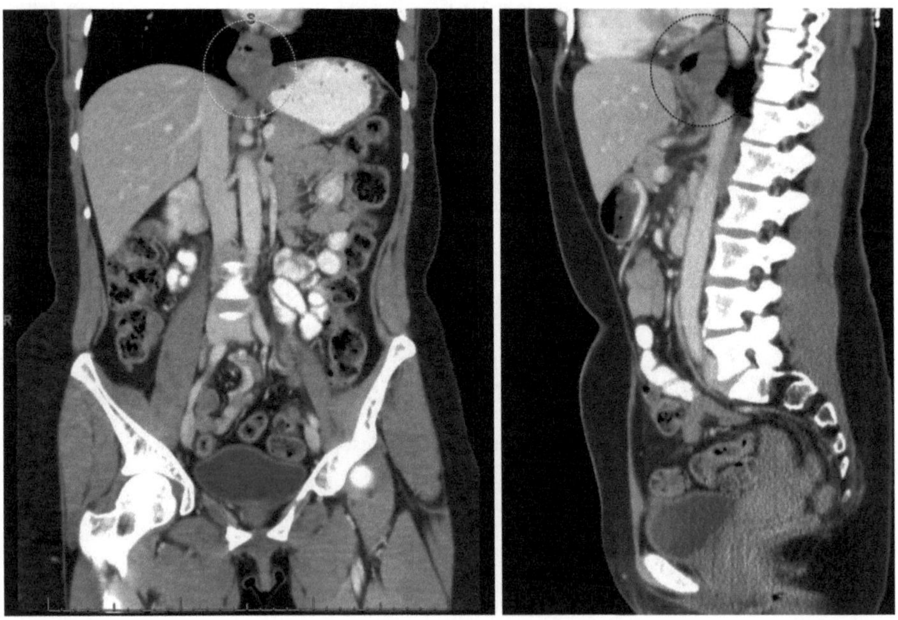

Fig. 2.31 Chest/abdominal CT scan. Distal esophageal adenocarcinoma, coronal view (*white circle*) and lateral view (*black circle*)

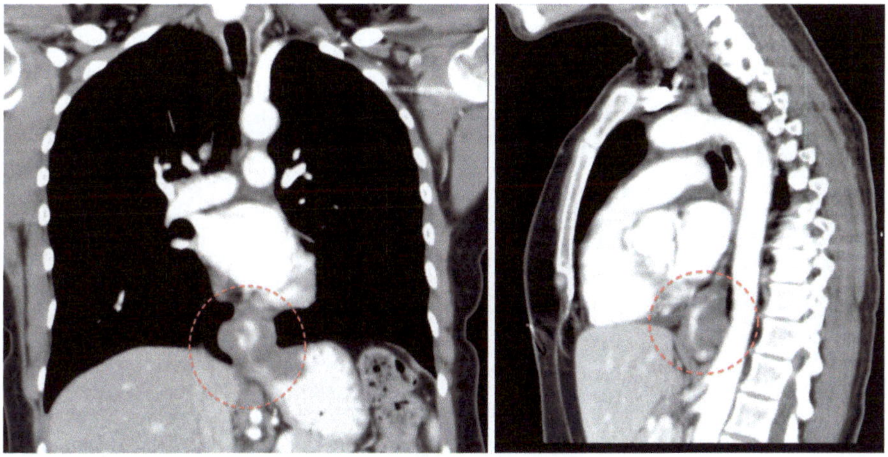

Fig. 2.32 Chest/abdominal CT scan. Distal esophageal adenocarcinoma, coronal and lateral view (*red circles*)

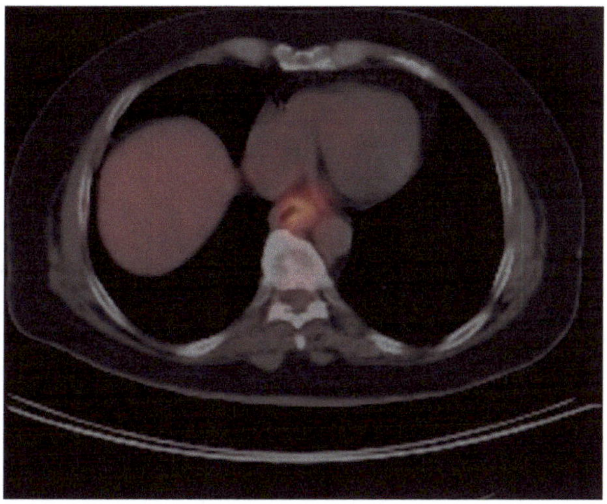

Fig. 2.33 PET scan. Distal esophageal adenocarcinoma

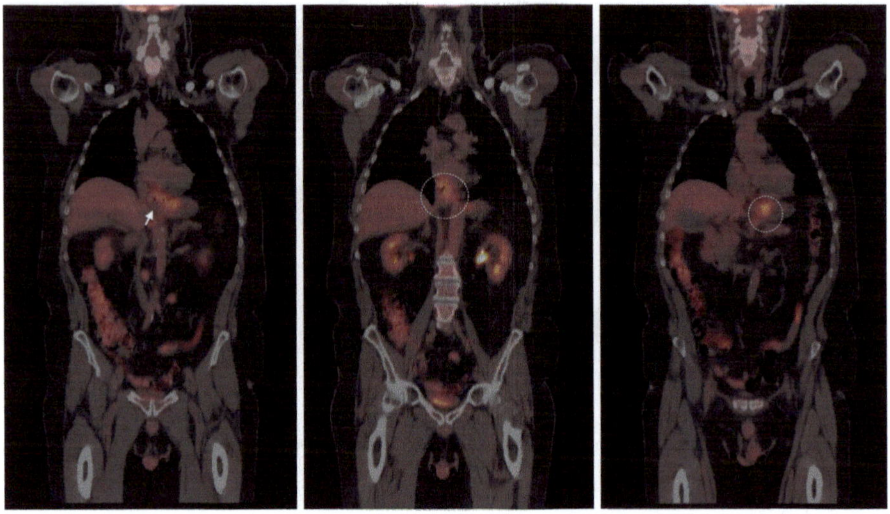

Fig. 2.34 PET scan. Distal esophageal adenocarcinoma (*white arrow* and *white circles*)

Selected Reading

1. Allaix ME, Patti MG. Laparoscopic paraesophageal hernia repair. Surg Laparosc Endosc Percutan Tech. 2013;23:425–8.
2. Allaix ME, Herbella FA, Patti MG. The evolution of the treatment of esophageal achalasia: a look at the last two decades. Updates Surg. 2012;64:161–5.
3. Baker ME, Einstein DM, Herts BR, Remer EM, Motta-Ramirez GA, Ehrenwald E, Rice TW, Richter JE. Gastroesophageal reflux disease: integrating the barium esophagram before and after antireflux surgery. Radiology. 2007;243:329–39.
4. Bello B, Zoccali M, Gullo R, et al. Gastroesophageal reflux disease and antireflux surgery. What is the proper preoperative work-up? J Gastrointest Surg. 2013;17:14–20.
5. Bruzzi JF, Munden RF, Truong MT, et al. PET/CT of esophageal cancer: its role in clinical management. Radiographics. 2007;27:1635–52.
6. Chen MYM, Ott DJ, Sinclair PA, et al. Gastroesophageal reflux disease: correlation of esophageal pH testing and radiographic findings. Radiology. 1992;185:483–6.
7. Cole TJ, Turner MA. Manifestations of gastrointestinal disease on chest radiographs. Radiographics. 1993;13:1013–34.
8. Dean C, Etienne D, Carpentier B, et al. Hiatal hernias. Surg Radiol Anat. 2012;34:291–9.
9. Gullo R, Herbella FA, Patti MG. Laparoscopic excision of esophageal leiomyoma. Updates Surg. 2012;64:315–8.
10. Hansford BG, Mitchell MT, Gasparaitis A. Water flush technique: a noninvasive method of optimizing visualization of the distal esophagus in patients with primary achalasia. Am J Roentgenol. 2013;200:818–21.
11. Herbella FA, Patti MG, Del Grande JC. Hiatal mesh repair—current status. Surg Laparosc Endosc Percutan Tech. 2011;21:61–6.
12. Jobe BA, Richter JE, Hoppo T, et al. Preoperative diagnostic work up before antireflux surgery: an evidence and experience-based consensus of the esophageal diagnostic advisory panel. J Am Coll Surg. 2013;217:586–97.

13. Lee SS, Ha HK, Byun JH, et al. Superficial esophageal cancer: esophagographic findings correlated with histopathologic findings. Radiology. 2005;236:535–44.
14. Levine MS. Benign tumors of the esophagus. In: Gore RM, Levine MS, editors. Textbook of gastrointestinal radiology. Second edition: WB Saunders; 2000.
15. Levine MS, Rubesin SE. Diseases of the esophagus: diagnosis with esophagography. Radiology. 2005;237:414–27.
16. Levine MS, Chu P, Furth EE, et al. Carcinoma of the esophagus and esophagogastric junction: sensitivity of radiographic diagnosis. Am J Roentgenol. 1997;168:1423–6.
17. Levine MS, Rubesin SE, Laufer I. Barium esophagography: a study for all seasons. Clin Gastroenterol Hepatol. 2008;6:11–25.
18. Muller M, Gockel I, Hedwig P, et al. Is the Schatzki ring a unique esophageal entity? World J Gastroenterol. 2011;17:2838–43.
19. Patel B, Han E, Swan K. Richard Schatzki: a familiar ring. Am J Roentgenol. 2013;201:678–82.
20. Patti MG, Herbella FA. Achalasia and other esophageal motility disorders. J Gastrointest Surg. 2011;15:703–7.
21. Patti MG, Waxman I. Gastroesophageal reflux disease: from heartburn to cancer. World J Gastroenterol. 2010;16:3743–4.
22. Patti MG, Gorodner MV, Galvani C, et al. Spectrum of esophageal motility disorders: implications for diagnosis and treatment. Arch Surg. 2005;140:442–8.
23. SAGES Guidelines Committee. Guidelines for the management of hiatal hernia. Surg Endosc. 2013;27(12):4409–28.
24. Soares R, Herbella FA, Prachand VN, Ferguson MK, Patti MG. Epiphrenic diverticulum of the esophagus: from pathophysiology to treatment. J Gastrointest Surg. 2010;14:2009–15.

Chapter 3
Gastroesophageal Reflux Disease: Pathophysiology

Antonio Carlos Valezi, Fernando A.M. Herbella, and Jorge Mali Junior

Abstract Gastroesophageal reflux disease (GERD) is a common disease with a variable prevalence ranging from 5 % in the Eastern population to 25 % in the West. Moreover, GERD incidence seems to be escalating.

Gastroesophageal reflux occurs daily in normal individuals (physiological reflux); however, it may become "a disease which develops when the reflux of stomach contents causes troublesome symptoms and/or complications" – or GERD – as defined by an International Consensus.

Keywords Gastroesophageal reflux disease • Pathophysiology • Acid reflux • Non-acid reflux • Esophageal manometry • Ambulatory pH

Introduction

Gastroesophageal reflux disease (GERD) is a common disease with a variable prevalence ranging from 5 % in the Eastern population to 25 % in the West. Moreover, GERD incidence seems to be escalating.

Gastroesophageal reflux occurs daily in normal individuals (physiological reflux); however, it may become "a disease which develops when the reflux of stomach contents causes troublesome symptoms and/or complications" – or GERD – as defined by an International Consensus.

A.C. Valezi, MD • J.M. Junior, MD
Department of Surgery, State University of Londrina,
Av. Robert Koch, 60, Londrina 86038-440, Brazil
e-mail: valezi@sercomtel.com.br; jmalijr@yahoo.com.br

F.A.M. Herbella, MD (✉)
Department of Surgery, Federal University of São Paulo,
Rus Diogo de Faria 1087 cj 301, São Paulo, Brazil
e-mail: herbella.dcir@epm.br

P.M. Fisichella et al. (eds.), *Esophageal Diseases*,
DOI 10.1007/978-3-319-04337-1_3,

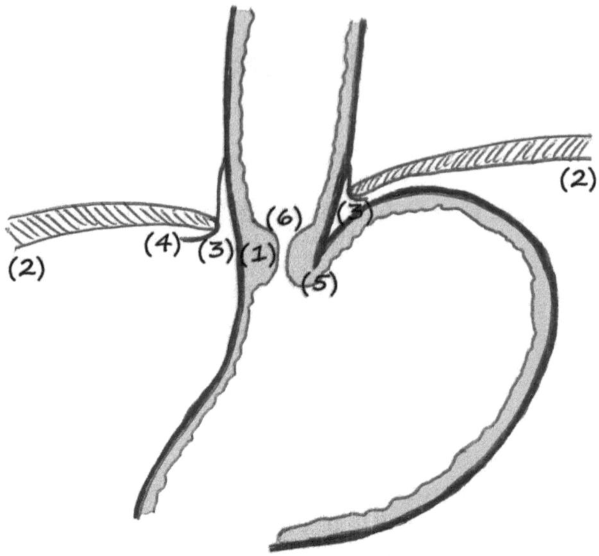

Fig. 3.1 Gastroesophageal barrier – natural antireflux mechanisms. The gastroesophageal barrier is a complex mechanism formed by different components: (*1*) the lower esophageal sphincter, which creates a high-pressure zone between the esophagus and the stomach; (*2*) the diaphragm, which acts as an external sphincter during rises in intra-abdominal pressure; (*3*) the abdominal portion of the esophagus, submitted to abdominal pressure; (*4*) the phrenoesophageal membrane, which acts transmitting the abdominal pressure high up in the mediastinum; (*5*) the angle of His, which separates between gastric fundus and cardia; and (*6*) the Gubaroff valve which represents the cushion effect of the esophageal mucosa at the gastroesophageal junction

Gastric hydrochloric acid has long been recognized as harmful to the esophagus; however, the gastroesophageal refluxate contains a variety of other noxious agents, including bile, pancreatic enzymes, and pepsin.

GERD pathophysiology is multifactorial and linked to a disbalance between the aggressiveness of the refluxate into the esophagus or adjacent organs and the failure of the esophagogastric barrier and protective mechanisms. This chronic pathologic backflow of gastroduodenal contents leads to a spectrum of symptoms, with or without tissue damage. The degree of the disease gravity depends on the frequency, duration, and quality of the exposure of the refluxate into the esophagus or adjacent organs.

This chapter reviews GERD pathophysiology.

Antireflux Mechanisms

The esophagogastric junction (EGJ) area has a specialized valve mechanism formed by the lower esophageal sphincter (LES) and abdominal esophagus, the diaphragm, the angle of His, the Gubaroff valve, and the phrenoesophageal membrane (Fig. 3.1).

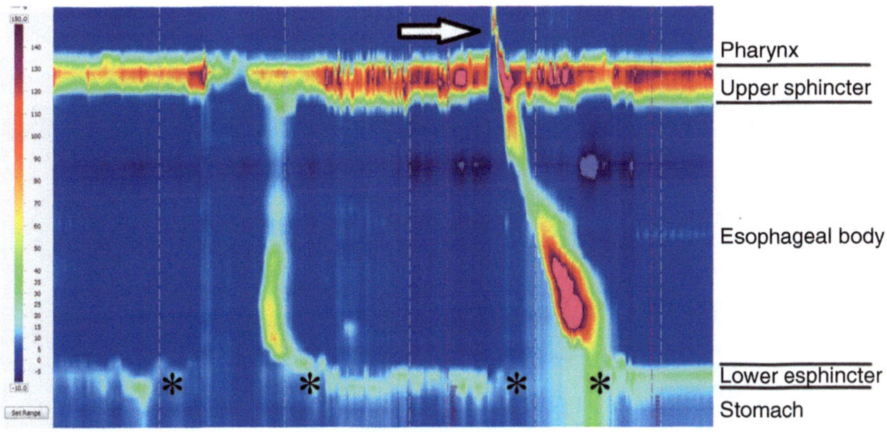

Fig. 3.2 High-resolution manometry images of the lower esophageal relaxation (between*) during transient relaxation (*left*) and swallow (*right*). The *arrow* points to swallow

Lower Esophageal Sphincter and Abdominal Esophagus

The LES creates a high-pressure zone at the level of the EGJ without a clear anatomic representation. This smooth muscle sphincter maintains a sustained tone that is disrupted only in two moments: (1) *swallowing*, to allow food transit to the stomach, and (2) *gastric fundus distention*, to allow gas ventilation and eructation.

An effective LES must have an adequate resting pressure and total and intra-abdominal length. It is intuitive that the resting pressure of the LES must be higher than the thoracoabdominal pressure gradient. Also, reflux control is linked to the extension of the LES, since gastric distension may alter the shape of the proximal stomach leading to a shorter LES. Moreover, the intra-abdominal portion of the LES is submitted to a positive abdominal pressure that forces the sphincter to collapse and close. The same mechanism applies to the presence of an abdominal portion of the esophagus, not found in a hiatal hernia (HH).

Even though most patients with GERD have a defective LES, a normal LES pressure does not exclude GERD, since the pathophysiology may be linked to abnormal relaxations.

Periodic relaxation of the LES or transient lower esophageal sphincter relaxation (TLESR) – to distinguish it from relaxation triggered by swallowing – explains physiological reflux found in normal subjects.

This relaxation is longer, and it is associated to diaphragm inhibition and contraction of the longitudinal muscular layer of the esophagus, when compared to swallow-induced relaxations (Fig. 3.2). It may contribute to reflux disease, when more frequent and prolonged. It explains the reflux seen in the 40 % of patients with GERD whose resting LES pressure is normal.

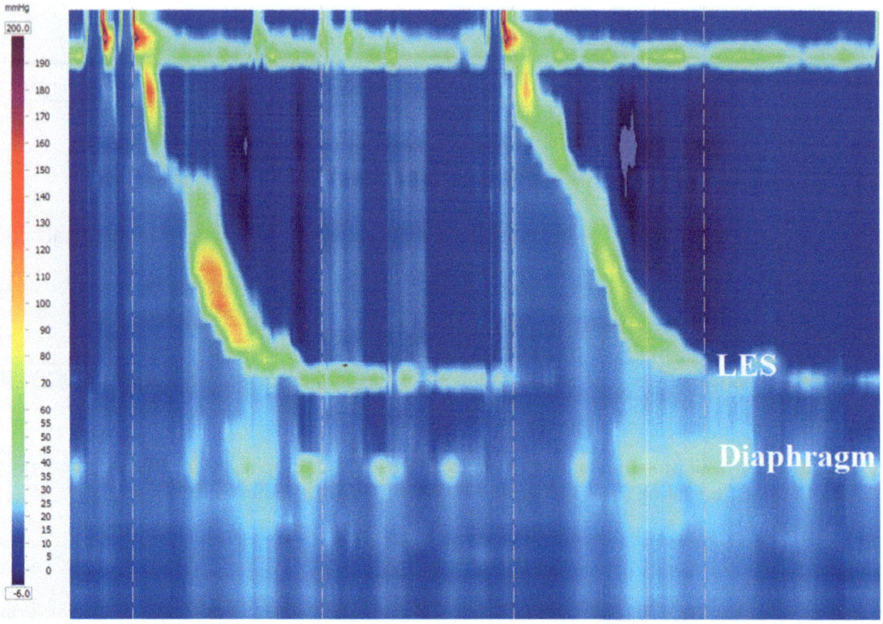

Fig. 3.3 High-resolution manometry images of two high-pressure zones at the level of the esophagogastric junction in a patient with hiatal hernia corresponding to the lower esophageal sphincter and the diaphragm. *LES* lower esophageal sphincter

Diaphragm

The esophagus crosses from the thorax to the abdomen through the esophageal hiatus formed by the right crus of the diaphragm. Thus, the esophagus is compressed during diaphragm contraction. The crus of the diaphragm provides an extrinsic component to the gastroesophageal barrier. This pinchcock action of the diaphragm is particularly important as a protection against reflux induced by sudden increases in intra-abdominal pressure.

Very interestingly, high-resolution manometry is able to show the distinct action of the diaphragm in patients with hiatal hernia (Fig. 3.3), and a high pressure zone is observed at this level even in patients after distal esophagectomy when the LES was resected.

Angle of His and Gubaroff Valves

The acute angle formed between the esophagus and the gastric fundus (His angle) creates a longer distance between the gastric fundus where the food is stored during feeding. Also, gastric distention projects the fundus in the direction of the esophagus accentuating the His angle and closing the EGJ (Fig. 3.4).

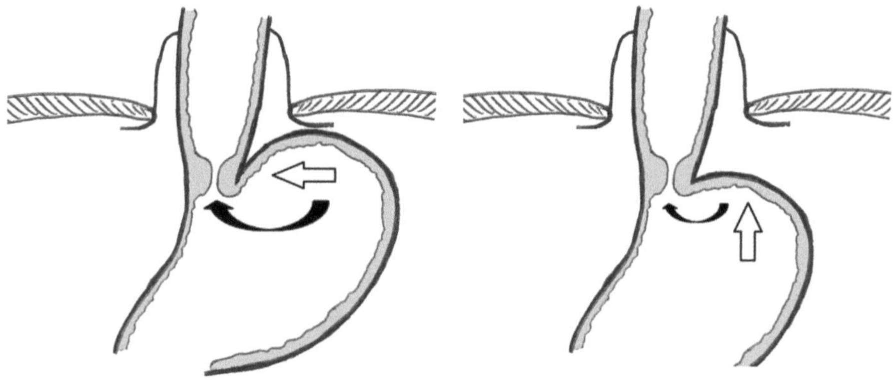

Fig. 3.4 Antireflux mechanism of the angle of His. The *white arrow* shows the vector of the intragastric pressure and the *black arrow* the path the food needs to follow to reflux with an acute His angle (physiological – *left*) or with an obtuse His angle (pathologic – *right*)

Gubaroff valves consisted in a cushion action of the distal esophageal mucosa at the level of the EGJ.

Phrenoesophageal Membrane

The phrenoesophageal membrane is a fibroelastic ligament consisting in the continuation of the transversalis fascia that leaves the diaphragm and surrounds the esophagus in a variable distance from the abdominal inlet. The membrane protects against reflux transmitting the positive abdominal pressure above the abdominal inlet into the esophageal walls. This effect creates a segment of the esophagus that is anatomically in the thorax but physiologically behaves like an abdominal segment (Fig. 3.5).

Protective Mechanisms

Some mechanisms protect the esophagus from injury when a reflux occurs.

Esophageal Clearance

The refluxate is likely to produce more mucosal injury if the contact time with the mucosa is prolonged. A rapid esophageal clearance minimizes the effect of the refluxate. Esophageal clearance is promoted by gravity, esophageal motility, and saliva production.

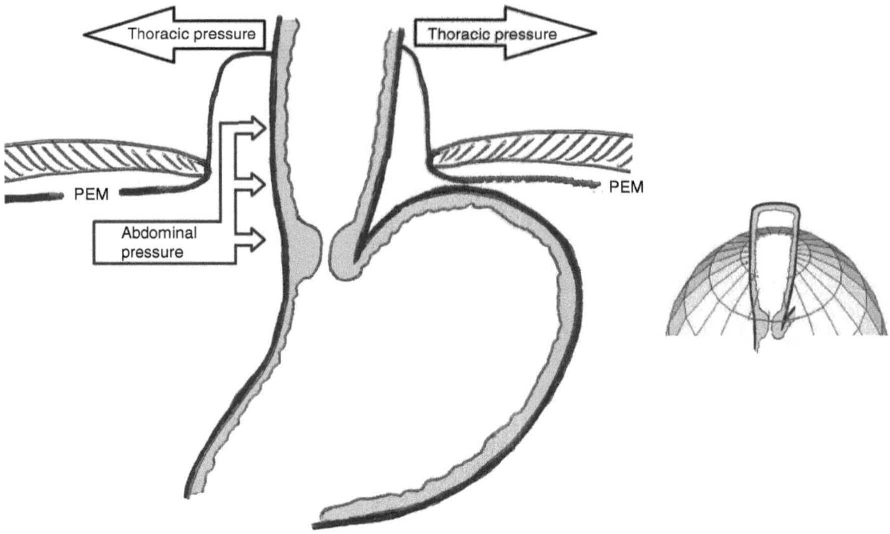

Fig. 3.5 Antireflux mechanism of the phrenoesophageal membrane. The abdominal pressure is transmitted to the insertion point of the membrane. *PEM* phrenoesophageal membrane

Esophageal Motility

Esophageal peristalsis is probably the most important component of the esophageal clearance of the refluxate. Thus, defective peristalsis is associated with more severe GERD with a higher intensity of symptoms and mucosal damage.

Saliva Production

The daily output of saliva is over 1 l. It has a dual protection effect on the esophagus: (1) mechanical, as it washes out the refluxate, and (2) chemical, as it buffers acid reflux due to the presence of bicarbonate.

Epithelial Protection

Esophageal epithelial cells have protective mechanisms against the noxious effects of reflux. These mechanisms may be divided in pre-epithelial, epithelial, or post-epithelial.

Esophageal mucus, produced by mucus cells localized at the epithelium surface and from the submucosal glands, acts as a pre-epithelial barrier against the refluxate. Under the mucus, a layer of bicarbonate-rich fluid also buffers acid that penetrates the mucus.

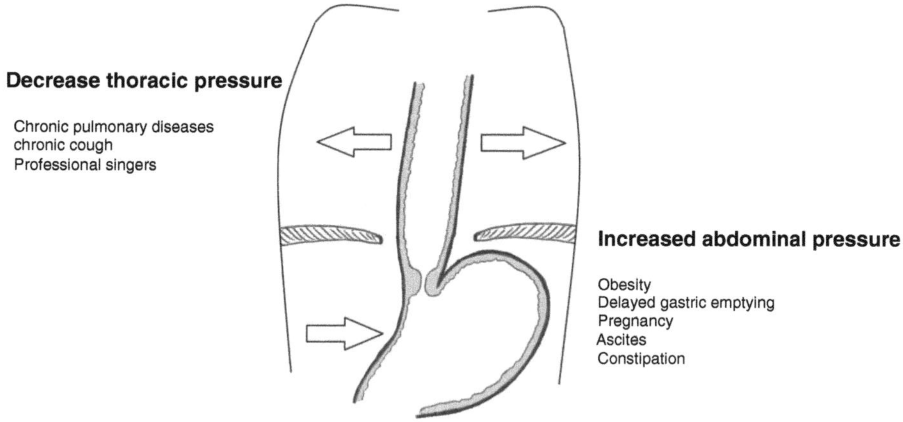

Fig. 3.6 Conditions that may affect the balance of the thoracoabdominal pressure gradient

Esophageal epithelial cells have specialized cellular membranes and intercellular junctions to prevent H+ ions to flow into the cells.

The post-epithelial protective mechanism is performed by the clearance of H+ ions to the blood.

Thoracoabdominal Gradient

The esophagus is placed in almost its totality in the thorax under a negative pressure. This promotes the upward extension of gastric contents. On the other side, the stomach lies within the positive pressure of the abdomen, compressing its walls and also forcing contents upwards. This thoracoabdominal gradient must be counterbalanced by the valve mechanism previously described, interposed between the esophagus and the stomach. An increase in abdominal (intragastric) pressure or a decrease in thoracic pressure (becoming more "negative") may alter this and lead to GERD (Fig. 3.6).

Obesity is probably the main cause for GERD due to increased abdominal pressure. It has been shown that there is a dose-response relationship between increasing body mass index (BMI) and prevalence of GERD and its complications. Abnormal gastric emptying might also contribute to GERD by increasing intragastric pressure.

The association of various pulmonary diseases and GERD has been demonstrated. It has been shown that patients with end-stage lung disease may have a prevalence of GERD in up to 70 %.

Others

Age

Although GERD symptoms are distributed equally in different ages, the prevalence and severity of GERD increase with aging. This fact may be attributed to decrease in the esophageal motility, decrease in the production of saliva, and a higher incidence of hiatal hernias.

Helicobacter pylori

Helicobacter pylori might influence GERD by leading to an atrophic gastritis and consequent achlorhydria, altering the nature of the refluxate. Some studies showed an inverse association between *H. pylori* infection and reflux esophagitis and increase in GERD symptoms after eradication of the bacteria. However, studies on the topic are not unanimous and the real interaction between GERD and *H. pylori* is still elusive.

Drugs, Diet, and Hormones

Many substances may alter the lower esophageal sphincter function and promote GERD (Table 3.1).

Table 3.1 Substances may alter the lower esophageal sphincter function and promote GERD

Drugs	Food	Hormones
Nitrates	Caffeine	Secretin
Ca++ channel blockers	Alcohol	Cholecystokinin
Morphine	Tobacco	Glucagon
Sildenafil	Chocolate	Progesterone
Meperidine	Mint	E2 prostaglandin
Beta-adrenergic agonist	Fat	
Aminophylline		
Benzodiazepines		
Barbiturates		
Tricyclic antidepressant		

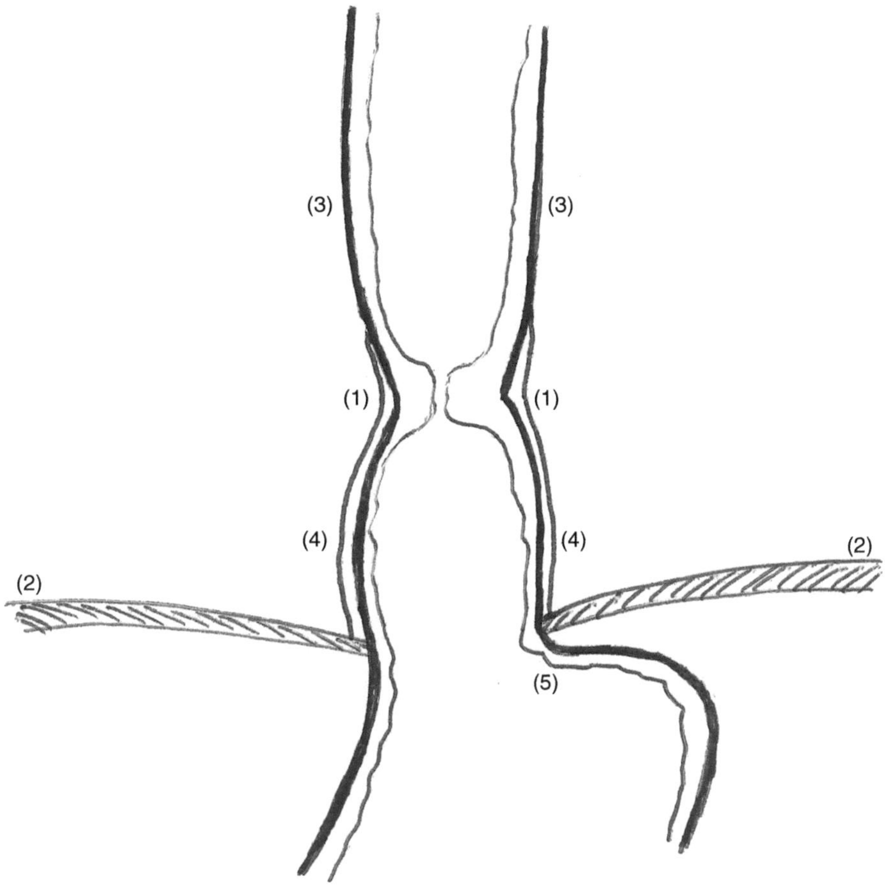

Fig. 3.7 Hiatal hernia and antireflux mechanisms. All natural antireflux mechanisms are absent or compromised when a hiatal hernia is present: (*1*) the lower esophageal sphincter is under negative thoracic pressure, (*2*) the diaphragm is below the esophagogastric junction, (*3*) the abdominal portion of the esophagus is not present, (*4*) the phrenoesophageal membrane is stretched and nonfunctional, and (*5*) the angle of His is obtuse

Hiatal Hernia

Hiatal hernia and GERD were considered synonyms in the past. Currently, it is well known that both conditions can exist independently; however, the presence and size of a hiatal hernia increase the chance of GERD by disrupting most of the natural antireflux mechanisms (Fig. 3.7). The presence and size of a hiatal hernia are also associated with more severe mucosal damage and increased acid exposure.

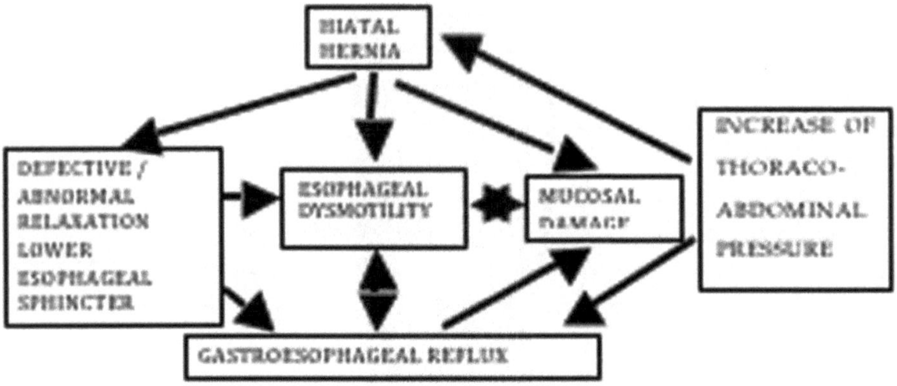

Fig. 3.8 Gastroesophageal reflux disease interaction among causative factors

Conclusions

GERD is a multifactorial disease, and there is a great interaction among causative factors (Fig. 3.8). Patients with suspected GERD must be carefully studied, and therapy should be based on the pathophysiology of the disease.

Summary

- GERD is defined as a condition which develops when the reflux of stomach contents causes troublesome symptoms and/or complications.
- Gastroesophageal reflux occurs daily in normal individuals.
- GERD pathophysiology is multifactorial and linked to a disbalance between the aggressiveness of the refluxate into the esophagus or adjacent organs and the failure of the esophagogastric barrier and protective mechanisms.
- Antireflux mechanisms include the lower esophageal sphincter and abdominal esophagus, the diaphragm, the His angle, the Gubaroff valve, and the phreno-esophageal membrane.
- Protective mechanisms include esophageal motility, saliva production, and epithelial protection.
- Age, drugs, hormones, *Helicobacter pylori* infection, increased abdominal pressure (especially obesity and delayed gastric emptying), a more negative thoracic pressure, and the presence of hiatal hernia all affect GERD.

Selected Reading

1. Armstrong D. Gastroesophageal reflux disease. Curr Opin Pharmacol. 2005;5:589–95. This paper highlights the symptoms and their relationship to the anatomical and physiological changes of the mechanisms that prevent GERD.
2. Armstrong D, Sifrim D. New pharmacologic approaches in gastroesophageal reflux disease. Gastroenterol Clin North Am. 2010;39:393–418. This paper discusses the mechanisms of GERD with emphasis on the LES and substances (pharmaceutical and food) that can change its pressure.
3. Bredenoord AJ, Pandolfino JE, Smout AJPM. Gastro-oesophageal reflux disease. Lancet. 2013;381:1933–42. This review focuses on the aspects of the esophagogastric junction dysfunction through manometry and pH monitoring.
4. Cram M. Hiatus hernia and gastro-oesophageal reflux disease. Medicine. 2010;39(3):132–6. Review on the relationship between hiatal hernia and GERD.
5. Fass R. Epidemiology and pathophysiology of symptomatic gastroesophageal reflux disease. Am J Gastroenterol. 2003;98(3):S2–7. This manuscript covers all etiopathogenic aspects of GERD. It states that there are subgroups of patients with distinct mechanisms in the pathophysiology of the disease.
6. Herbella FA, Sweet MP, Tedesco P, Nipomnick I, Patti MG. Gastroesophageal reflux disease and obesity. Pathophysiology and implications for treatment. J Gastrointest Surg. 2007;11(3):286–90. This study elucidates on the relationship between obesity and GERD, focusing on the etiopathogenic aspects.
7. Hom C, Vaezi MF. Extraesophageal manifestations of gastroesophageal reflux disease. Gastroenterol Clin North Am. 2013;42:71–91. Review on extra-esophageal manifestations of GERD and on the aggressive and defensive factors in the pathogenesis of GERD.
8. Kahrilas PJ, Lee TJ. Pathophysiology of gastroesophageal reflux disease. Thorac Surg Clin. 2005;15:323–33. Review paper that shows the relationship between antireflux mechanisms and severity of GERD.
9. Lee YY, McColl KEL. Pathophysiology of gastroesophageal reflux disease. Best Pract Res Clin Gastroenterol. 2013;27:339–51. Review paper on the normal physiology of the antireflux barrier.
10. Orlando RC. Pathogenesis of gastroesophageal reflux disease. Gastroenterol Clin North Am. 2002;31:33–44. Review paper with comments on the transient relaxation of the lower esophageal sphincter and on esophageal clearance. It focuses on the evolution from GER to GERD.
11. Pandolfino JE, Kwiatek MA, Kahrilas PJ. The pathophysiologic basis for epidemiologic trends in gastroesophageal reflux disease. Gastroenterol Clin Notrth Am. 2008;37:827–43. This paper focuses on relationship between GERD pathophysiology and epidemiology, focusing on the potential risk factors for GERD.
12. Patti MG, Perreta S. Gastro-oesophageal reflux disease: a decade of changes. Asian J Surg. 2003;26(1):4–6. The authors report that in the last decade there have been changes in the understanding, diagnosis and treatment of GERD.
13. Salvatore S, Vandenplas Y. Gastro-esophageal reflux disease and motility disorders. Best Pract Res Clin Gastroenterol. 2003;17(2):163–79. Relevant paper on esophageal motility. Discusses the epidemiology, natural history, pathophysiology and esophageal motility, focusing on the differences between different age groups.
14. Shafik A, Shafik I, El-Sibai O, Shafik AA. On the pathogenesis of gastroesophageal reflux: the concept of gastroesophageal dyssynergia. J Thorac Cardiovasc Surg. 2005;130:401–7. Importance of the diaphragm.
15. Weijenborg PW, Bredenoord AJ. How reflux causes symptoms; reflux perception in gastroesophageal reflux disease. Best Pract Res Clin Gastroenterol. 2013;27:353–64. Volume and composition of refluxate as being important for the perception of symptoms.

Chapter 4
Gastroesophageal Reflux Disease: Diagnostic Evaluation

Marco E. Allaix, Bernardo A. Borraez, and Marco G. Patti

Abstract The diagnosis of gastroesophageal reflux disease (GERD) is frequently based on symptoms and upper endoscopy only, with a wrong diagnosis of GERD that occurs in up to 30 % of patients. Since a correct diagnosis of GERD is necessary to avoid inappropriate medical therapy and to properly select patients who might benefit from laparoscopic antireflux surgery, the proper evaluation of patients with symptoms suggestive of GERD should always include esophageal manometry and ambulatory 24-h pH monitoring.

Keywords Gastroesophageal reflux disease • Heartburn • Upper endoscopy • Barium esophagogram • Esophageal manometry • Ambulatory 24-h pH monitoring • Multichannel intraluminal impedance • Radiolabeled gastric emptying study

---

Conflict of Interest
The authors have no conflicts of interest to declare.

M.E. Allaix, MD
Department of Surgical Sciences, University of Torino,
Corso A.M. Dogliotti 14, Torino 10126, Italy

B.A. Borraez, MD • M.G. Patti, MD, FACS (✉)
Department of Surgery, Center for Esophageal Diseases,
University of Chicago Pritzker School of Medicine, 5841 S. Maryland Ave,
MC 5095, Room G-207, Chicago, IL 60637, USA
e-mail: mpatti@surgery.bsd.uchicago.edu

P.M. Fisichella et al. (eds.), *Esophageal Diseases*,
DOI 10.1007/978-3-319-04337-1_4, © Springer International Publishing Switzerland 2014

Introduction

Gastroesophageal reflux disease (GERD) is the most prevalent disorder of the upper gastrointestinal tract in the Western countries. Heartburn is the most common symptom and it is usually assumed to be secondary to gastroesophageal reflux. As a consequence, medical therapy is often started without performing a more extensive diagnostic workup.

A careful evaluation of patients with symptoms suggestive of GERD is key for a correct diagnosis and treatment of the disease. The treatment options for GERD include medical therapy, such as proton pump inhibitor (PPIs), H2 blockers, and laparoscopic fundoplication. However, while antisecretory medications improve or eliminate heartburn by changing the pH of the gastric refluxate without stopping reflux, laparoscopic fundoplication stops any type of reflux by restoring the competence of the lower esophageal sphincter (LES), with excellent long-lasting results.

The preoperative evaluation aims to:

(a) Establish the presence of abnormal esophageal acid exposure.
(b) Correlate reflux events with symptoms.
(c) Identify anatomical and functional abnormalities secondary to reflux.

The complete workup includes:

- Symptomatic evaluation
- Upper endoscopy
- Barium esophagram
- High-resolution manometry (HRM)
- Ambulatory 24-h pH monitoring
- Multichannel intraluminal impedance (MII) (in selected cases)
- Radiolabeled gastric emptying study (in selected cases)

Table 4.1 summarizes the preoperative workup before antireflux surgery.

Table 4.1 Preoperative workup

Symptom evaluation
Upper endoscopy
Barium esophagram
Esophageal high-resolution manometry
Ambulatory 24-h pH monitoring
Multichannel intraluminal impedance pH monitoring[a]
Radiolabeled gastric emptying study[a]

[a]In selected patients

Symptomatic Evaluation

The preoperative evaluation starts with a meticulous medical history that assesses both the presence and severity of typical (heartburn, regurgitation, and dysphagia) and atypical (cough, hoarseness, chest pain, dental erosions) symptoms of GERD and use of antisecretory medications and their effect in terms of symptom relief. The presence of gas bloating, nausea, and diarrhea should be always investigated as they often suggest the presence of other diseases rather than GERD.

Many physicians feel that GERD can be diagnosed on the basis of symptoms evaluation only. Heartburn is usually considered secondary to GERD, and antisecretory medications are often prescribed without diagnostic studies. However, the sensitivity and specificity of typical symptoms is low, and a wrong diagnosis of GERD occurs in about one third of patients. For instance, Patti et al. found abnormal gastroesophageal reflux detected by 24-h ambulatory pH monitoring in only 70 % of patients referred for esophageal function tests after a clinical diagnosis of GERD based on symptoms and upper endoscopy. Heartburn and regurgitation were equally experienced in both patients with and without GERD, underlying that symptoms alone do not help distinguish between patients with and without pathologic reflux. Many patients with a normal pH monitoring study had been treated with expensive medications on the assumption that their symptoms were secondary to reflux, therefore misdiagnosing other diseases such as irritable bowel syndrome, gallstone disease, and coronary artery disease. In addition, some patients who had been referred for antireflux surgery were diagnosed with primary esophageal motility disorders, such as diffuse esophageal spasm and achalasia. Heartburn is experienced by about 40 % of achalasia patients because of stasis and fermentation of food in the distal esophagus. Since these patients are often thought to have GERD refractory to antisecretory medications, antireflux surgery may be performed in some of them if esophageal function tests are not obtained.

The clinical response to PPIs is a good predictor of abnormal reflux and has been demonstrated to be an independent outcome predictor after antireflux surgery, along with typical symptoms, and an abnormal DeMeester score at ambulatory 24-h pH monitoring.

Barium Esophagram

Barium esophagram provides information about:

- The length and diameter of the esophagus
- The presence, type, and size of a hiatal hernia
- The presence of a Schatzki ring or a stricture

Reflux of gastric content into the esophagus is seldom demonstrated during a barium esophagram even in symptomatic patients. On the other hand, even if reflux is radiologically observed, 24-h pH monitoring will not necessarily detect abnormal gastroesophageal reflux. In fact, while the barium esophagram evaluates the presence of reflux during a very short period of time (usually about 10 min), the ambulatory pH monitoring assesses the occurrence of reflux episodes during 24 h, both in the postprandial and fasting state and in the upright and supine position. For instance, Chen et al. found radiological abnormalities in only 30 % of patients with an abnormal pH study. Recently, Bello et al. reported similar findings, demonstrating the absence of any radiological sign of reflux in more than half of patients with GERD confirmed by ambulatory 24-h pH monitoring. In addition, the incidence of hiatal hernia did not differ significantly between patients with and without GERD.

In conclusion, the main goal of a barium esophagram is to define the anatomy of the esophagus, the gastroesophageal junction, and the stomach and not to establish the diagnosis of GERD.

Upper Endoscopy

Upper endoscopy is often the first test obtained to confirm a diagnosis of GERD based on symptoms. However, this approach has several limitations: for instance, endoscopic findings consistent with esophagitis are present in only about 50 % of patients with pathologic reflux. Patti et al. showed the absence of esophagitis on endoscopy in about 60 % of patients with a clinical diagnosis of GERD. In this study, patients with Barrett's esophagus were excluded. It is well known that major interobserver variation exists regarding the endoscopic evaluation of esophagitis, particularly for low-grade esophagitis. In addition, the extensive use of PPIs has dramatically reduced both the presence and severity of mucosal injury.

Therefore, the major goals of upper endoscopy is the detection of Barrett's esophagus which is usually present in up to 14 % of GERD patients, erosive esophagitis, and exclusion of gastric and duodenal diseases.

Esophageal Manometry

The most reliable tool to assess the function of upper esophageal sphincter (UES), esophageal body, and LES is the esophageal manometry.

The study is performed after an overnight fast. The probe is inserted trans-nasally and positioned in order to record from the pharynx to the stomach. Esophageal motility is assessed in the right lateral decubitus position, starting with a basal period without swallowing, followed by ten wet swallows of 5 ml of water. Data are then analyzed using a commercially available computer software.

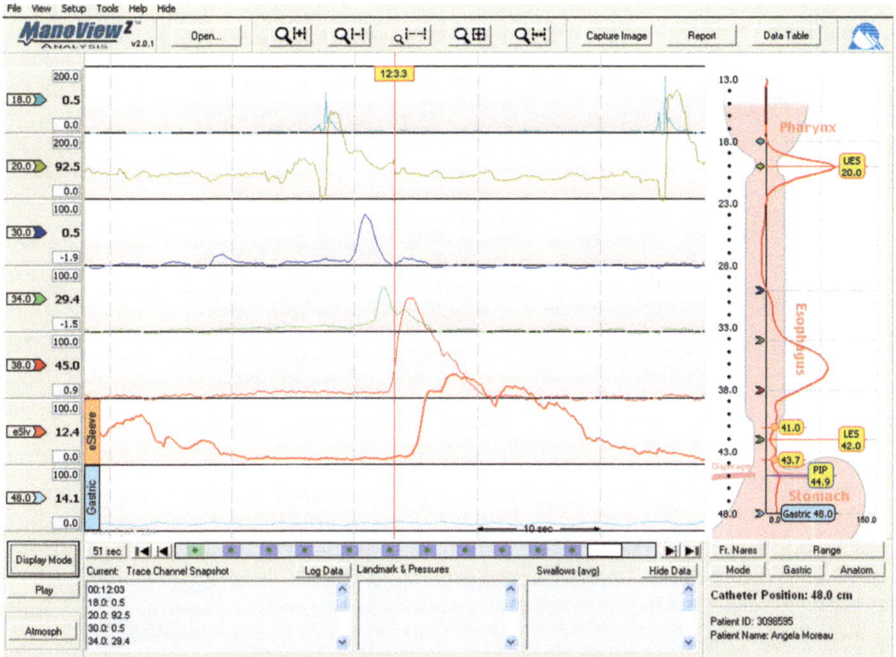

Fig. 4.1 Normal esophageal peristalsis by conventional manometry

The primary goals of esophageal manometry before antireflux surgery are:

1. To rule out a primary esophageal motility disorder such as achalasia, which may be misdiagnosed as GERD
2. To measure LES resting pressure, length, and relaxation
3. To assess amplitude and propagation of esophageal peristalsis
4. To measure the precise location of the LES for proper placement of the pH probe or MII catheter (5 cm above the upper border of the LES)
5. To evaluate the pressure and coordination of the hypopharynx and cricopharyngeal muscle

Recently, HRM using a solid-state catheter with 36 circumferential sensors spaced at 1-cm intervals has replaced the conventional manometry performed using an 8-channel water-perfused catheter. HRM provides detailed pressure topography of the esophagus (Figs. 4.1 and 4.2). It allows a better identification of segments of compartmentalized esophageal pressurization and better discrimination of conditions such as distal esophageal spasm, ineffective esophageal motility, and achalasia than conventional manometry (Figs. 4.3, 4.4, 4.5, and 4.6).

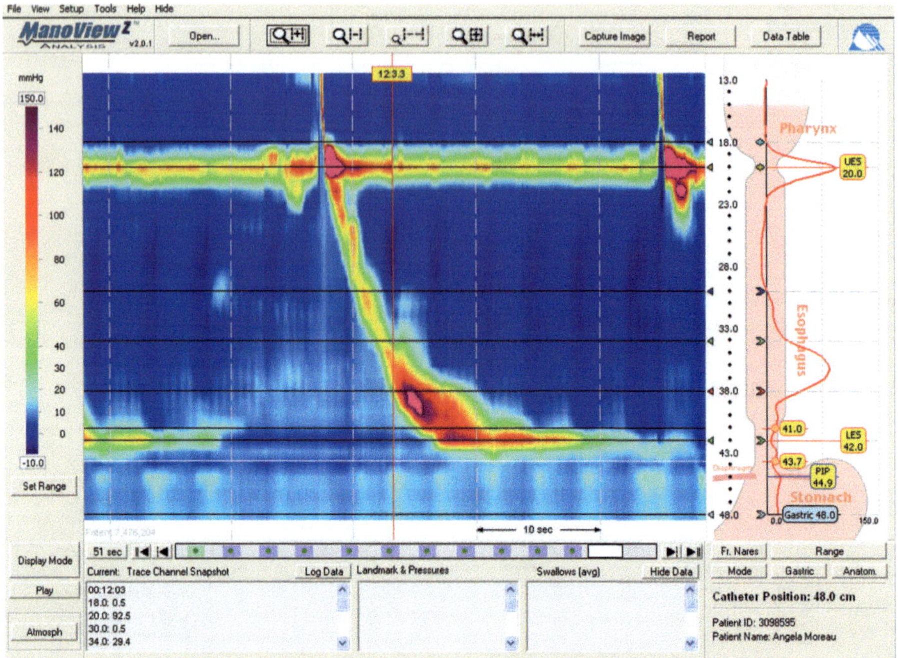

Fig. 4.2 Normal esophageal peristalsis by high-resolution manometry

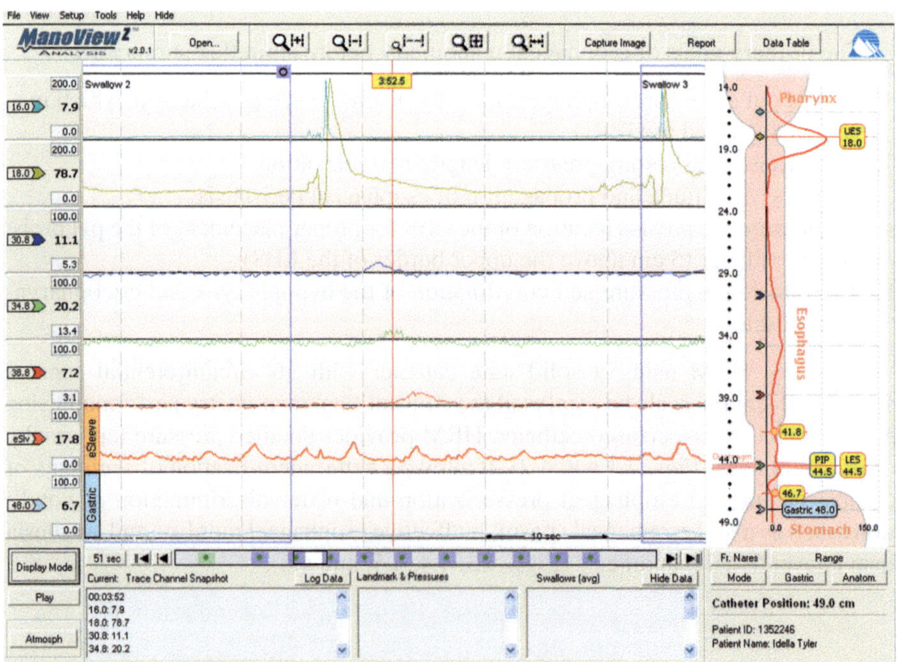

Fig. 4.3 Ineffective esophageal motility by conventional manometry

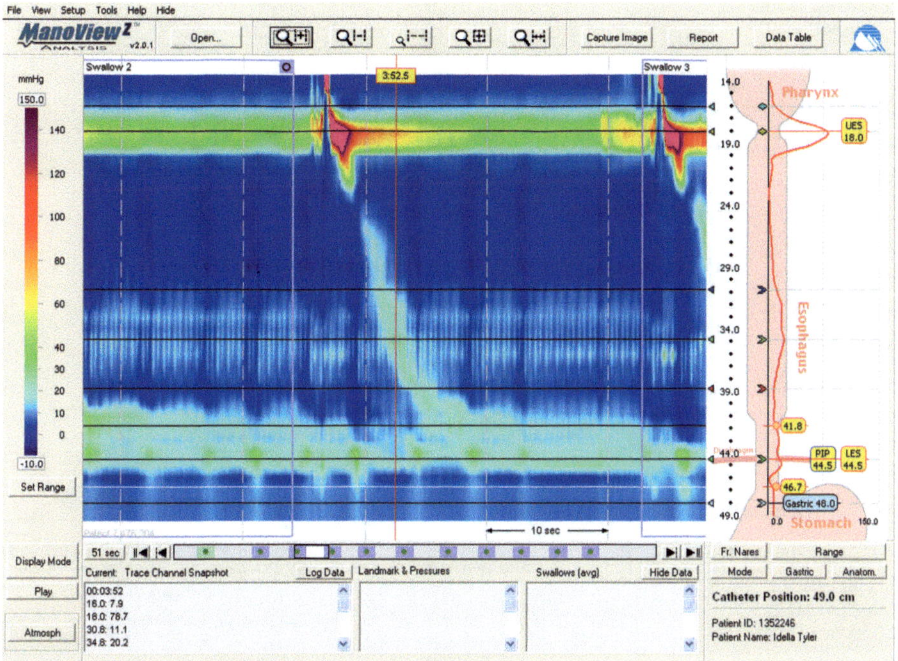

Fig. 4.4 Ineffective esophageal motility by high-resolution manometry

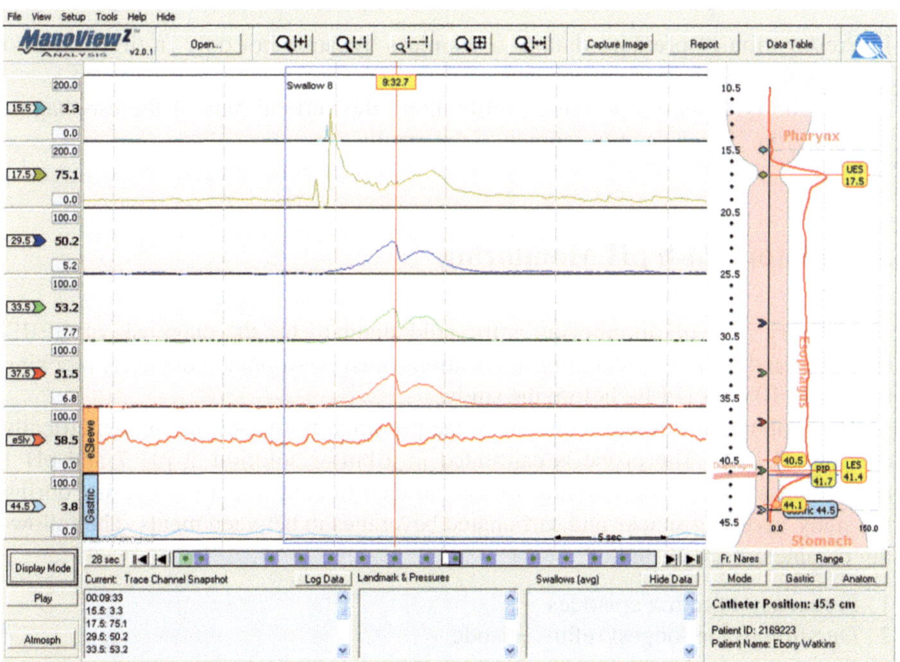

Fig. 4.5 Esophageal achalasia by conventional manometry

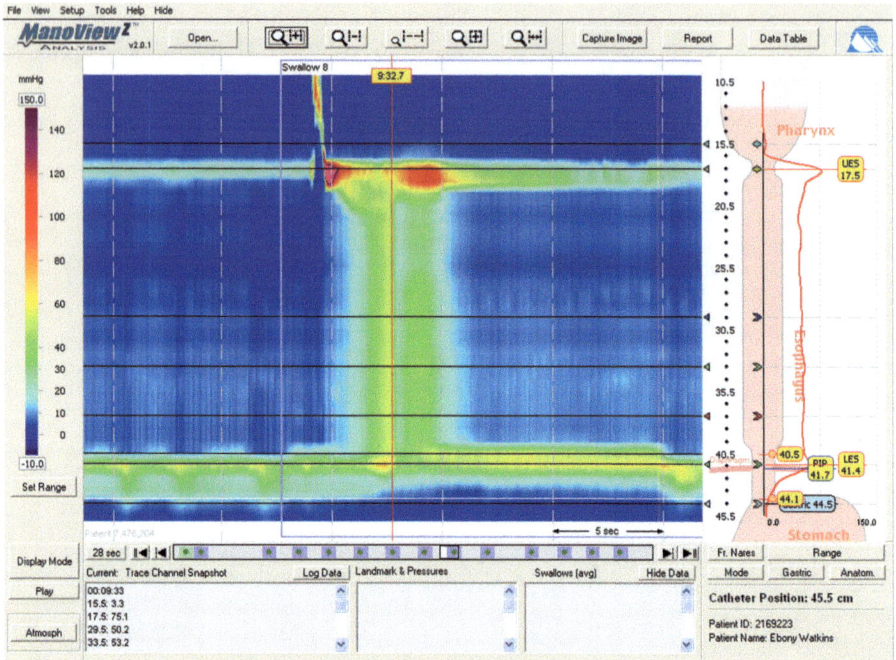

Fig. 4.6 Esophageal achalasia by high-resolution manometry

Other advantages of HRM include:

1. Presentation of pressure data as a seamless dynamic not only in time but also along the length of the esophagus
2. The ability to assess pressure profile along the vertical axis of the esophagus, improving therefore the accuracy of the results

Ambulatory 24-h pH Monitoring

Ambulatory 24-h pH monitoring is the gold standard for the diagnosis of GERD (Figs. 4.7 and 4.8). Antisecretory medications must be stopped 3 days (H_2-blocking agents) to 10 days (PPIs) before the study.

The probe is positioned 5 cm above the proximal border of the manometrically determined LES. The probe is calibrated in a buffer solution at pH 7 and pH 1 before and after the test. Patients are encouraged to consume a normal diet during the study, avoiding snacks and carbonated beverages in between meals. The following parameters are evaluated:

1. Frequency of reflux episodes
2. Duration of the longest reflux episode

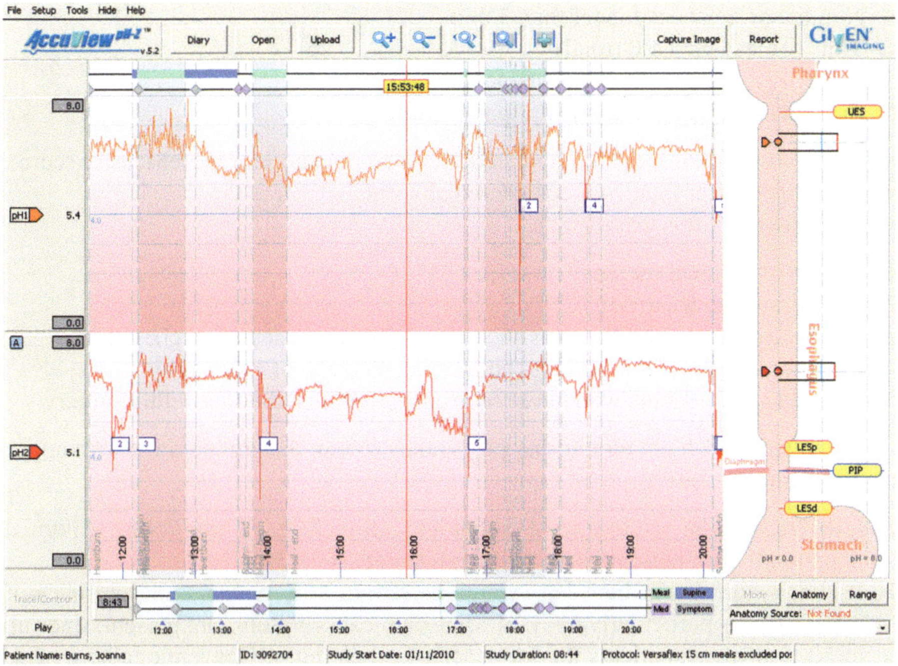

Fig. 4.7 Normal 24-h pH monitoring

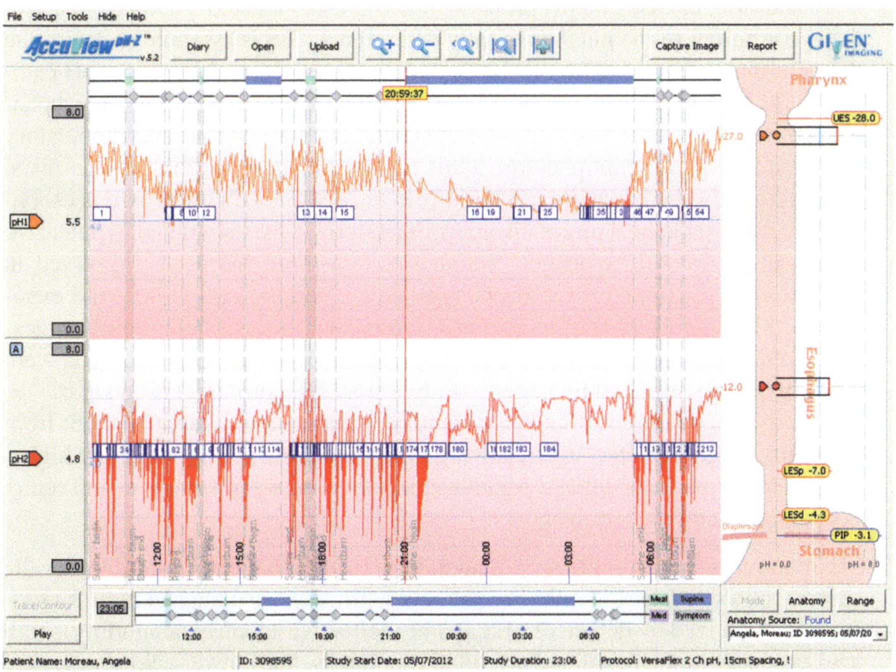

Fig. 4.8 Abnormal 24-h pH monitoring

3. Number of episodes longer than 5 min
4. Time pH less than 4.0 (total)
5. Time pH less than 4.0 in the supine position
6. Time pH less than 4.0 in the upright position

These six components are integrated into a composite score (DeMeester score), with a value greater than 14.7 considered abnormal.

Indications for this test include:

1. Failure of medical therapy
2. Preoperative evaluation
3. Presence of atypical symptoms such as cough, hoarseness, and chest pain
4. Presence of symptoms without endoscopic evidence of esophagitis
5. Evaluation of patients who have recurrent symptoms after antireflux surgery

Ambulatory 24-h pH monitoring plays a key role in the preoperative workup for the following reasons:

1. It determines the occurrence of pathologic reflux. The pH monitoring is normal in up to 30 % of patients with a clinical diagnosis of GERD.
2. It allows correlation between symptoms reported by patients and episodes of reflux. This is particularly relevant when atypical symptoms are present, since up to 50 % of these patients do not experience heartburn. Conventionally, an episode of cough is considered related to reflux if it occurs within 2 or 3 min of a reflux episode in the distal or both distal and proximal esophagus.

   In addition, the use of a pH probe with two sensors located 5 and 20 cm above the upper border of the manometrically determined LES is essential to determine the proximal extent of reflux. In 1993, Patti et al. used a double-sensor pH catheter in 70 GERD patients referred for evaluation of symptoms of gastroesophageal reflux. They compared clinical presentation, manometric and ambulatory pH monitoring data in patients with gastroesophageal reflux in the distal esophagus only and in patients with reflux in the distal and in the proximal esophagus. A pan-esophageal motor disorder, characterized by a short and hypotensive LES and ineffective esophageal peristalsis, was more frequently observed in patients with proximal reflux. Esophageal acid clearance was slower and exposure of the upper esophagus to acid was significantly longer. Symptoms suggestive of aspiration such as cough and wheezing and episodes of pneumonia were more frequently reported by patients with reflux in the proximal esophagus.

   Finally, the pH monitoring helps identify patients more likely to benefit from antireflux surgery, with cough resolving postoperatively in a significantly higher percentage of patients when a positive correlation between symptom and reflux is demonstrated preoperatively.

3. pH monitoring and esophageal manometry stratify patients according to the severity of the disease, identifying patients with worse esophageal motility profile (characterized by defective LES and/or ineffective esophageal motility), high acid exposure in the distal and proximal esophagus, and slower acid clearance.

An abnormal score not only confirms the diagnosis of GERD but also is an important outcome predictor after antireflux surgery. For instance, the 24-h pH monitoring score was the strongest predictor of good or excellent outcome in a multivariate analysis performed on 199 patients undergoing a laparoscopic Nissen fundoplication for the treatment of GERD. The same study showed that the outcome after surgery was fair or poor in 25 % of patients with typical symptoms and responsive to acid suppression therapy but with normal preoperative pH score. Others published similar results, reporting persistence of typical symptoms of GERD in 40 % of patients with normal reflux score on preoperative pH monitoring but only in 8 % of patients with pathologic score.

Lastly, ambulatory 24-h pH monitoring should be performed early in the evaluation of patients who have persisting or recurrent symptoms after antireflux surgery. Symptoms are not a reliable indicator of the presence of reflux since they are due to reflux in 30–40 % of patients only. Furthermore, up to 70 % of patients who are taking acid-reducing medications postoperatively have a normal pH monitoring.

An alternative diagnostic tool to measure gastroesophageal reflux is the 48-h wireless esophageal pH monitoring probe (Bravo™; Medtronic, Shoreview, MN). The capsule is pinned to the esophageal mucosa through a delivery system that is passed trans-orally: it is used to position properly the capsule, apply suction in order to draw the mucosa inside a tiny well located in the capsule, and deploy a fixing pin. Information is beamed via radiofrequency to a receiver that must be close to the patient.

This system was developed to avoid the shortcomings of catheter-based pH monitoring, including the discomfort of the pH catheter, social embarrassment, reduced daily activities, and changes in diet. This technology presents some advantages as it is not connected with a wire to the recorder and allows increasing recording duration up to 96 h.

However, wireless pH monitoring has several limitations:

1. It records the pH in the lower esophagus only.
2. It can only report acid reflux.
3. It causes chest discomfort in about 50 % of patients.
4. It can detach early from the esophageal wall causing false-positive results.

Multichannel Intraluminal Impedance pH Monitoring

Multichannel intraluminal impedance (MII) is a technique that measures flow of liquids and gas across the gastroesophageal junction, regardless of the pH of the gastric refluxate, by identifying differences in electrical conductivity induced by the presence of a bolus in the esophagus. Two consecutive sensors are in contact with the esophageal mucosa that has specific impedance value. When the esophageal lumen is filled with any substance that bridges the two sensors, the device detects this variance. Gas, liquid, and a mixture of them can be distinguished according to their different conductivity, regardless of the pH. The direction of flow is determined according to the order in which the sensors detect the material. As a consequence, a reflux episode from the stomach into the esophagus occurs when gastric contents are detected in the esophageal lumen first in distal sensors, then measured propagating aborally in at least two proximal sensors. MII consists of a catheter comparable with that of the conventional pH monitoring in which antimony sensors are used to measure the pH, while impedance sensors are dispatched in the catheter. Simultaneous detection of a reflux episode by the pH sensor and by the impedance sensors denotes reflux and allows characterization of a reflux episode as acidic, weakly acidic, or alkaline.

MII in association with pH monitoring is able to determine:

1. The physical characteristics (liquid, gas, or mixed) of the refluxate
2. The pH of the refluxate (acid, weakly acid, and alkaline)
3. The height of the reflux episode

Main indications for MII-pH are:

1. Patients with symptoms refractory to PPIs. Symptoms could be refractory to medical therapy in some patients because acid-suppressing medications only increase the pH of the gastric refluxate, without stopping reflux.
2. Patients with cough of unknown origin. When MII-pH monitoring is obtained in patients with atypical symptoms of GERD, it has been demonstrated that cough could be temporally associated with reflux episodes whose pH ranged between 4 and 7. Successful results after antireflux surgery have been reported in patients with persistent symptoms on acid-suppressive therapy that had a positive correlation with reflux episodes, regardless of the pH.

Radiolabeled Gastric Emptying Study

In some GERD patients, delayed gastric emptying is documented. In these patients, delayed gastric emptying may be associated with a progressive dilatation of the proximal stomach. As a consequence there is a progressive reduction in length of the LES that eventually becomes incompetent. The most common symptoms reported by these patients are dyspepsia, postprandial abdominal distention, bloating, and abdominal discomfort, along with the symptoms of gastroesophageal reflux. However, symptoms alone are not sensitive and specific for the diagnosis of delayed gastric emptying, and the emptying rate does not necessarily correlate with the symptoms thought to be secondary to delayed gastric emptying.

Recently, several studies have investigated the impact of delayed gastric emptying on the outcomes after antireflux surgery. For instance, Bais et al. demonstrated a decreased lag time between ingestion of food and the initiation of gastric emptying and increased rate of gastric emptying in 36 patients (26 with normal and 10 with delayed gastric emptying) undergoing a Nissen fundoplication for GERD. In addition, patients with preoperative delayed gastric emptying had normal values after surgery. More importantly, similar symptom control and side effects were reported in this series of GERD patients regardless of the gastric emptying rate. Others have not observed a relationship between gastric emptying and outcome of fundoplication in 372 (31 % with preoperative delayed gastric emptying) patients undergoing fundoplication for GERD.

It is thought that a Nissen fundoplication might improve gastric emptying by reducing the capacity of the fundic reservoir.

In conclusion, the gastric emptying study is not routinely performed in GERD patients before antireflux surgery. It should be considered in patients with significant nausea and bloating, and in those with endoscopic findings of retained food in the stomach after an overnight fast.

Summary

- The preoperative evaluation aims to establish the presence of abnormal esophageal acid exposure, to correlate reflux events with symptoms, and to identify anatomical and functional abnormalities secondary to reflux.
- A thorough workup should include a symptomatic evaluation, upper endoscopy, barium esophagram, esophageal manometry, ambulatory 24-h pH monitoring, and, in selected cases, multichannel intraluminal impedance and radiolabeled gastric emptying study.
- Typical symptoms of GERD such as heartburn and regurgitation have low sensitivity and specificity, leading to a wrong diagnosis of GERD in about 30 % of patients.
- The clinical response to PPIs is a good predictor of abnormal reflux and is an independent predictor of successful outcome after antireflux surgery, along with the presence of typical symptoms and abnormal ambulatory 24-h pH monitoring.
- The main goal of a barium esophagram is to define the anatomy of the esophagus, the gastroesophageal junction, and the stomach and not to establish the diagnosis of GERD.
- Upper endoscopy aims to detect Barrett's esophagus and erosive esophagitis and to rule out gastric and duodenal diseases.
- The primary purposes of esophageal manometry before antireflux surgery are to rule out primary esophageal motility disorders; to measure LES resting pressure, length, and relaxation; to assess amplitude and propagation of esophageal peristalsis; to precisely localize the LES for proper placement of the pH probe or MII catheter (5 cm above the upper border of the LES); and to evaluate the pressure and coordination of the UES.
- Main indications for ambulatory pH monitoring are failure of medical therapy; preoperative evaluation; presence of atypical symptoms such as cough, hoarseness, and chest pain; presence of symptoms without endoscopic evidence of

esophagitis; and evaluation of patients who have recurrent symptoms after antireflux surgery.
- Main indications for MII-pH are patients with symptoms refractory to PPIs and patients with cough of unknown origin.
- A radiolabeled gastric emptying study should be considered in patients with significant nausea and bloating and in those with endoscopic findings of retained food in the stomach after an overnight fast.

Selected Reading

1. Amano Y, Ishimura N, Furuta K, Okita K, Masaharu M, Azumi T, Ose T, Koshino K, Ishihara S, Adachi K, Kinoshita Y. Interobserver agreement on classifying endoscopic diagnoses of non erosive esophagitis. Endoscopy. 2006;38:1032–5.
2. Bais JE, Samsom M, Boudesteijn EA, van Rijk PP, Akkermans LM, Gooszen HG. Impact of delayed gastric emptying on the outcome of antireflux surgery. Ann Surg. 2001;234:139–46.
3. Bello B, Zoccali M, Gullo R, Allaix ME, Herbella FA, Gasparaitis A, Patti MG. Gastroesophageal reflux disease and antireflux surgery-what is the proper preoperative work-up? J Gastrointest Surg. 2013;17:14–20.
4. Blonski W, Vela MF, Castell DO. Comparison of reflux frequency during prolonged multichannel intraluminal impedance and pH monitoring on and off acid suppression therapy. J Clin Gastroenterol. 2009;43(9):816–20.
5. Campos GM, Peters JH, DeMeester TR, Oberg S, Crookes PF, Tan S, DeMeester SR, Hagen JA, Bremner CG. Multivariate analysis of factors predicting outcome after laparoscopic Nissen fundoplication. J Gastrointest Surg. 1999;3:292–300.
6. Chen MY, Ott DJ, Sinclair JW, Wu WC, Gelfand DW. Gastroesophageal reflux disease: correlation of esophageal pH testing and radiographic findings. Radiology. 1992;185:483–6.
7. Dallemagne B, Weerts J, Markiewicz S, Dewandre JM, Wahlen C, Monami B, Jehaes C. Clinical results of laparoscopic fundoplication at ten years after surgery. Surg Endosc. 2006;20:159–65.
8. Diener U, Patti MG, Molena D, Fisichella PM, Way LV. Esophageal dysmotility and gastroesophageal reflux disease. J Gastrointest Surg. 2001;5:260–5.
9. Galvani C, Fisichella PM, Gorodner MV, Perretta S, Patti MG. Symptoms are a poor indicator of reflux status after fundoplication for gastroesophageal reflux disease: role of esophageal function tests. Arch Surg. 2003;138:514–8.
10. Håkanson BS, Berggren P, Granqvist S, Ljungqvist O, Thorell A. Comparison of wireless 48-h (Bravo) versus traditional ambulatory 24-h esophageal pH monitoring. Scand J Gastroenterol. 2009;44(3):276–83.
11. Hirano I, Richter JE. Practice Parameters Committee of the American College of Gastroenterology. ACG practice guidelines: esophageal reflux testing. Am J Gastroenterol. 2007;102:668–85.
12. Jamieson JR, Stein HJ, DeMeester TR, Bonavina L, Schwizer W, Hinder RA, Albertucci M. Ambulatory 24-h esophageal pH monitoring: normal values, optimal thresholds, specificity, sensitivity and reproducibility. Am J Gastroenterol. 1992;87:1102–11.
13. Johnson F, Joelsson B, Gudmundsson K, Greiff L. Symptoms and endoscopic findings in the diagnosis of gastroesophageal reflux disease. Scan J Gastroenterol. 1987;22:714–8.
14. Kahrilas PJ, Ghosh SK, Pandolfino JE. Esophageal motility disorders in terms of pressure topography: the Chicago classification. J Clin Gastroenterol. 2008;42:627–35.
15. Khajanchee YS, Hong D, Hansen PD, Swanstrom LL. Outcomes of antireflux surgery in patients with normal preoperative 24-hour pH test results. Am J Surg. 2004;187:599–603.

16. Lord RV, Kaminski A, Oberg S, Bowrey DJ, Hagen JA, DeMeester SR, Sillin LF, Peters JH, Crookes PF, DeMeester TR. Absence of gastroesophageal reflux disease in a majority of patients taking acid suppression medications after Nissen fundoplication. J Gastrointest Surg. 2002;6:3–9.
17. Mainie I, Tutuian R, Agrawal A, Adams D, Castell DO. Combined multichannel intraluminal impedance-pH monitoring to select patients with persistent gastro-esophageal reflux for laparoscopic Nissen fundoplication. Br J Surg. 2006;93:1483–7.
18. Ott DJ. Gastroesophageal reflux. What is the role of barium studies? Am J Roentgenol. 1994;162:627–9.
19. Patti MG, Debas HT, Pellegrini CA. Clinical and functional characterization of high gastroesophageal reflux. Am J Surg. 1993;165:163–6.
20. Patti MG, Arcerito M, Tong J, de Pinto M, de Bellis M, Wang A, Feo CV, Mulvihill SJ, Way LW. Importance of preoperative and postoperative pH monitoring in patients with esophageal achalasia. J Gastrointest Surg. 1997;1:505–10.
21. Patti MG, Arcerito M, Feo CV, Worth S, De Pinto M, Gibbs VC, Gantert W, Tyrrell D, Ferrell LF, Way LW. Barrett's esophagus: a surgical disease. J Gastrointest Surg. 1999;3:397–403.
22. Patti MG, Arcerito M, Tamburini A, Diener U, Feo CV, Safadi B, Fisichella P, Way LW. Effect of laparoscopic fundoplication on gastroesophageal reflux disease-induced respiratory symptoms. J Gastrointest Surg. 2000;4:143–9.
23. Patti MG, Diener U, Tamburini A, Molena D, Way LW. Role of esophageal function tests in the diagnosis of gastroesophageal reflux disease. Dig Dis Sci. 2001;46:597–602.
24. Patti MG, Molena D, Fisichella PM, Perretta S, Way LW. Gastroesophageal reflux disease and chest pain. Results of laparoscopic antireflux surgery. Surg Endosc. 2002;16:563–6.
25. Pellegrini CA. Delayed gastric emptying in patients with abnormal gastroesophageal reflux. Ann Surg. 2001;234:147–8.
26. Pellegrini CA, Broderick WC, Van Dyke D, Way LW. Diagnosis and treatment of gastric emptying disorders. Clinical usefulness of radionuclide measurements of gastric emptying. Am J Surg. 1983;145:143–51.
27. Richter JE. Typical and atypical presentations of gastroesophageal reflux disease. The role of esophageal testing in diagnosis and management. Gastroenterol Clin North Am. 1996;25:75–102.
28. Streets CG, DeMeester TR. Ambulatory 24-hour pH monitoring: why, when, and what to do. J Clin Gastroenterol. 2003;37:14–22.
29. Tamhankar AP, Peters JH, Portale G, Hsieh CC, Hagen JA, Bremner CG, DeMeester TR. Omeprazole does not reduce gastroesophageal reflux: new insights using multichannel intraluminal impedance technology. J Gastrointest Surg. 2004;8:890–7.
30. Tutuian R, Mainie I, Agrawal A, Adams D, Castell DO. Nonacid reflux in patients with chronic cough on acid-suppressive therapy. Chest. 2006;130:386–91.
31. Viljakka M, Saali K, Koskinen M, et al. Antireflux surgery enhances gastric emptying. Arch Surg. 1999;134:18–21.
32. Wayman J, Myers JC, Jamieson GG. Preoperative gastric emptying and patterns of reflux as predictors of outcome after laparoscopic fundoplication. Br J Surg. 2007;94:592–8.

Chapter 5
Gastroesophageal Reflux Disease: Treatment

Marco E. Allaix, Bernardo A. Borraez, and Marco G. Patti

Abstract A laparoscopic total fundoplication has become the gold standard for the surgical treatment of gastroesophageal reflux disease. Short-term outcomes are excellent, with lower perioperative morbidity and faster recovery than conventional open total fundoplication. Long-term follow-up studies have shown similar symptom control between the two approaches. A laparoscopic partial fundoplication is performed in selected patients to reduce the incidence of postoperative dysphagia and gas-related symptoms. The sphincter augmentation device, a new minimally invasive antireflux procedure, has been recently proposed as an alternative to laparoscopic fundoplication.

Keywords Gastroesophageal reflux disease • Total fundoplication • Partial anterior fundoplication • Partial posterior fundoplication • Sphincter augmentation device

---

Conflict of Interest
The authors have no conflicts of interest to declare.

M.E. Allaix, MD
Department of Surgical Sciences, University of Torino,
Corso A.M. Dogliotti 14, 10126 Torino, Italy

B.A. Borraez, MD • M.G. Patti, MD, FACS (✉)
Department of Surgery, Center for Esophageal Diseases,
University of Chicago Pritzker School of Medicine,
5841 S. Maryland Ave, MC 5095, Room G-207, Chicago, IL 60637, USA
e-mail: mpatti@surgery.bsd.uchicago.edu

P.M. Fisichella et al. (eds.), *Esophageal Diseases*,
DOI 10.1007/978-3-319-04337-1_5, © Springer International Publishing Switzerland 2014

Introduction

Treatment options for GERD include medical therapy, such as proton pump inhibitors (PPIs) and H_2-blockers, and laparoscopic fundoplication. However, antisecretory medications improve or eliminate heartburn by changing the pH of the gastric refluxate, but they do not stop reflux. Laparoscopic fundoplication stops any type of reflux by restoring the competence of the lower esophageal sphincter (LES), decreasing the number of transient LES relaxations, and improving quality of esophageal peristalsis.

The last 20 years have witnessed a shift in the treatment of gastroesophageal reflux disease (GERD). While in the past the main indication for antireflux surgery was the absence of a good response to antisecretory medications, currently the best indication for surgery is instead a good control of symptoms with PPIs.

A laparoscopic total fundoplication (LTF) is considered today the gold standard for the surgical treatment of GERD, with better short-term outcomes and similar reflux control compared to open fundoplication. Control of reflux is not influenced by both pattern of reflux (i.e., upright versus supine) and patient's age. However, a small but significant incidence of postoperative dysphagia and gas-related symptoms is reported after this procedure. A laparoscopic partial fundoplication (LPF) has been proposed to minimize these side effects. However, the long-term outcomes are controversial, since some randomized clinical trials, mainly from Australia, found similar reflux control but higher incidence of dysphagia and gas-related symptoms after LTF, while several studies from the United States reported similar dysphagia rates after the two procedures, but a better reflux control after LTF.

The sphincter augmentation device (MSA) with the LINX Reflux Management System (Torax Medical) is a new minimally invasive antireflux procedure that has been recently proposed as alternative to laparoscopic fundoplication.

This chapter will review the current status of treatment of GERD, describing our surgical technique and focusing on surgical outcomes of both laparoscopic fundoplication and MSA.

Medical Therapy

PPIs are the main stem of medical therapy. These medications have been proved to be the most effective medical treatment for GERD in terms of esophagitis healing and symptom relief. However, esophagitis and symptoms tend to recur after discontinuation of therapy, and increasing doses to maintain healing of esophagitis are required in about 50 % of patients on maintenance PPIs.

Wileman et al. have recently published a meta-analysis of randomized or quasi-randomized controlled trials comparing medical management to laparoscopic fundoplication for GERD in adults. They found that laparoscopic fundoplication is more effective than medical therapy in improving symptoms and quality of life in the short to medium term.

While surgery aims to restore the competence of the LES, acid-suppressing medications can only modify the pH of the gastric refluxate. However, reflux still occurs because of an incompetent LES and ineffective esophageal peristalsis. In addition, medical therapy is largely ineffective for the treatment of the extra-esophageal manifestations of GERD due to the upward extension of the refluxate. Finally, PPIs can interfere with calcium absorption causing osteoporosis and fractures and cause C. difficile infection and abnormal cardiac activity due to decreased magnesium levels.

Surgical Treatment

Indications for Antireflux Surgery

(a) Pathologic gastroesophageal reflux documented by 24-h ambulatory pH monitoring and/or combined multichannel intraluminal impedance and pH testing (MII-pH)
(b) Heartburn and regurgitation not completely controlled by medications
(c) Respiratory symptoms thought to be induced by gastroesophageal reflux
(d) Desire of the patient to stop chronic use of PPI
(e) Poor patient's compliance with medical treatment
(f) Cost of medical therapy
(g) Development of osteoporosis
(h) C. difficile infections, pneumonia, or hypomagnesemia
(i) Young patients in whom life-long medical treatment is not advisable

Laparoscopic Total Fundoplication

Positioning of the Patient on the Operating Table

- The patient lies supine on the operating table in low lithotomy position with the lower extremities extended on stirrups with knees flexed 20–30°.
- A bean bag is inflated to avoid sliding of the patient as a consequence of the steep reverse Trendelenburg position used during the entire procedure.
- Pneumatic compression stockings are used to reduce the risk of deep venous thrombosis that is associated with both increased abdominal pressure secondary to pneumoperitoneum and the decreased venous return secondary to the steep reverse Trendelenburg position.
- An orogastric tube is placed to decompress the stomach, and it is removed at the end of the procedure.
- The surgeon stands between the patient's legs, while the first and second assistant stand on the right and left side of operative table, respectively (Fig. 5.1).

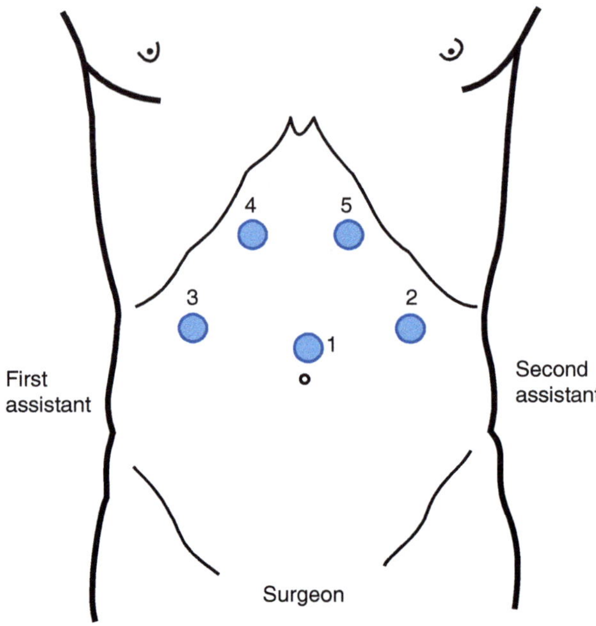

Fig. 5.1 Trocars' placement. Trocar *1* 30° camera, Trocar *2* Babcock clamp, Trocar *3* liver retractor, Trocar *4* and *5* dissection and suturing instruments

Table 5.1 Instrumentation for laparoscopic fundoplication

Five 10-mm ports
0° and 30° scope
Graspers and needle holder
Babcock clamp
L-shaped hook cautery with suction-irrigation capacity
Scissors
Laparoscopic clip applier
Electrothermal bipolar vessel sealing system
Liver retractor
Suturing device
2-0 silk sutures
Penrose drain
56 French esophageal bougie

Instrumentation for Laparoscopic Fundoplication

The instruments that are required for the procedure are listed in Table 5.1.

Step 1: Placement of trocars

- A five-trocar technique is used for the procedure (Fig. 5.1).
- Trocar 1 is placed 14 cm inferior to the xiphoid process, in the midline or 1–2 cm to the left of the midline to be in line with the esophagus. Extreme care must be taken when positioning this trocar, since the insertion site is just above the aorta and its bifurcation. In order to increase the distance between the abdominal wall

and the aorta, therefore reducing the risk of vessel injuries, the abdomen is initially inflated by using a Veress needle to a pressure of 15 mmHg. Then, an optical port with a 0° scope is placed under direct vision. Once this port is placed, the 0° scope is replaced with a 30° scope, and the other trocars are inserted under laparoscopic vision.

- Trocar 2 is placed in the left midclavicular line at the same level with trocar 1, and it is used for insertion of a Babcock clamp, for a grasper to hold the Penrose drain placed around the esophagus, or for devices used to divide the short gastric vessels.
- Trocar 3 is placed in the right midclavicular line at the same level of the other two trocars, and it is used for the insertion of a retractor to lift the left lateral segment of the liver.
- Trocars 4 and 5 are placed under the right and left costal margins, so that their axes form an angle of about 120° with the camera. They are used for the dissecting and suturing instruments.

Step 2: Division of gastrohepatic ligament; identification of right crus of the diaphragm and posterior vagus nerve

- The gastrohepatic ligament is divided, beginning above the caudate lobe of the liver, where the ligament is usually very thin, until the right crus of the diaphragm is identified. An accessory left hepatic artery originating from the left gastric artery is frequently present in the gastrohepatic ligament. It may be divided with no clinical consequences if this vessel limits the exposure.
- The right crus is separated from the right side of the esophagus by blunt dissection, the posterior vagus nerve is identified, and the right crus is dissected inferiorly toward the junction with the left crus. The use of a bipolar instrument allows to perform a safer right crus dissection than the electrocautery, with a reduced risk of injury to the posterior vagus nerve due to the lateral spread of the monopolar current.

Step 3: Division of peritoneum and phreno-esophageal membrane above the esophagus; identification of the left crus of diaphragm and anterior vagus nerve

The peritoneum and the phreno-esophageal membrane above the esophagus are transected with the electrocautery, with identification of the anterior vagus nerve. To avoid injury to the anterior vagus nerve or the esophageal wall, the nerve should be left attached to the esophageal wall, and the peritoneum and the phreno-esophageal membrane should be lifted from the wall by blunt dissection before they are divided.

- The left crus of the diaphragm is dissected bluntly downward toward the junction with the right crus.

Step 4: Division of short gastric vessels

The short gastric vessels are taken down all the way to the left pillar of the crus, starting at the level of the middle portion of the gastric body and continuing upward until the most proximal short gastric vessel is divided.

Possible complications during this step of the procedure are bleeding, either from the short gastric vessels or from the spleen, and damage to the gastric wall.

Step 5: Creation of a window between gastric fundus, esophagus, and diaphragmatic crura; placement of Penrose drain around the esophagus

- A Babcock clamp is applied at the level of the esophagogastric junction and the esophagus is retracted upward.
- A window is opened by a blunt and sharp dissection under the esophagus, between the gastric fundus, the esophagus, and the left pillar of the crus.
- The window is then enlarged, and a Penrose drain is passed around the esophagus, incorporating both the anterior and the posterior vagus nerves.

The two main complications that can occur during this part of the procedure are:

1. Creation of a left pneumothorax
2. Perforation of the gastric fundus

Step 6: Closure of crura

- Interrupted 2-0 silk sutures are tied intracorporeally to close the diaphragmatic crura.
- Retraction of the esophagus upward and toward the patient's left with the Penrose drain is essential to provide proper exposure.
- The first stitch should be placed just above the junction of the two pillars.
- Additional stitches are placed 1 cm apart, and a space of about 1 cm is left between the uppermost stitch and the esophagus.

Step 7: Insertion of the bougie into esophagus and across the esophageal junction

- After removal of the orogastric tube, a lubricated 56 French bougie is inserted down the esophagus through the esophagogastric junction by the anesthesiologist. Lubrication of the bougie and slow advancement of the bougie reduce the risk of esophageal perforation.
- The crura must be snug around the esophagus but not too tight: a closed grasper should slide easily between the esophagus and the crura.

Step 8: Wrapping of gastric fundus around the lower esophagus

- The surgeon gently pulls the gastric fundus under the esophagus with two graspers. The use of atraumatic graspers during this step of the procedure reduces the risk of damage to the gastric wall. Delivering the fundus under the esophagus and checking for the origins of the transected short gastric vessels help evaluate whether the wrap is going to be floppy. If the wrap remains to the right side of the esophagus and does not retract back to the left, then it is floppy and suturing can be performed. If not, the surgeon must make sure that the upper short gastric vessels have been transected and the posterior dissection completed.
- The left and right sides of the fundus are wrapped above the esophagogastric junction. A Babcock clamp introduced through trocar 2 is used to hold the two flaps together during placement of the first stitch.
- The two edges of the wrap are secured to each other by three 2-0 silk placed at 1 cm of distance from each other (Fig. 5.2).

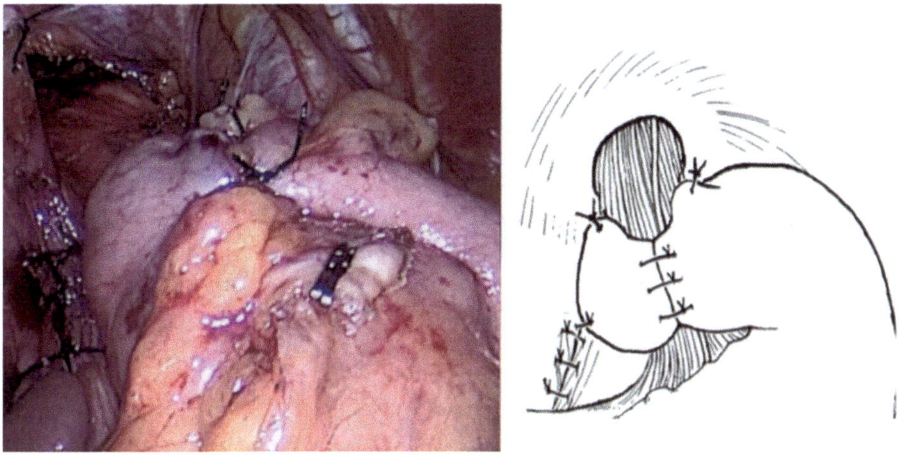

Fig. 5.2 Total fundoplication

- The wrap should be long no more than 2–2.5 cm.

Step 9: Final inspection, removal of instruments and trocars from the abdomen, and closure of the port sites

The instruments and the trocars are removed from the abdomen under direct vision, and the trocars sites are closed.

Laparoscopic Partial Fundoplication

The first six steps are identical to those of a LTF.

(a) *Partial posterior fundoplication*

- The delivered gastric fundus is gently pulled under the esophagus using two graspers.
- Three 2-0 silk sutures are placed on each side of the wrap between the muscular layers of the esophageal wall and the gastric fundus, leaving 80–120° of the anterior esophageal wall uncovered.
- Two coronal stitches are placed between the top of the wrap, the esophagus, and the right or left pillar of the crus.
- One additional stitch is placed between the right side of the wrap and the closed crura.
- The resulting wrap measures about 240–280° (Fig. 5.3).

(b) *Partial anterior fundoplication*

- It is a 180° anterior fundoplication.
- Two rows of sutures (2-0 silk) are used. The first row is on the left side of the esophagus and consists of three stitches. The top stitch incorporates the

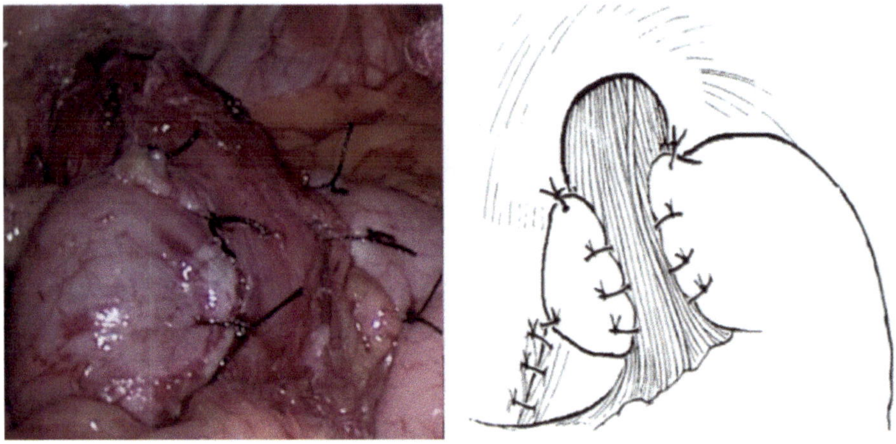

Fig. 5.3 Partial posterior fundoplication

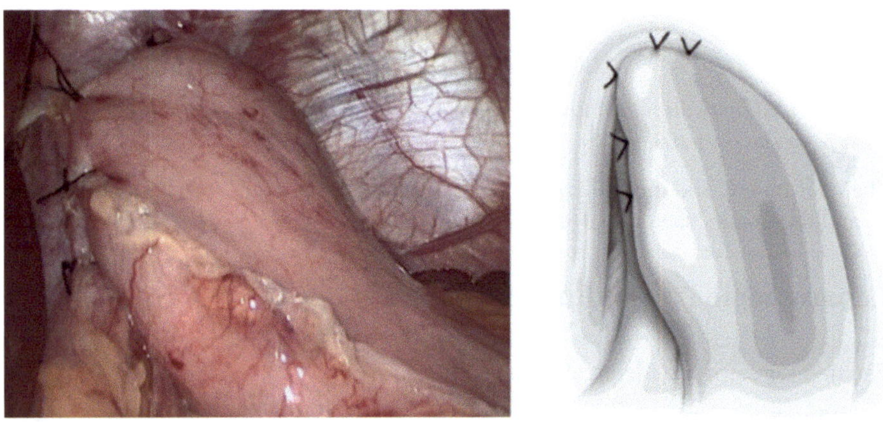

Fig. 5.4 Partial anterior fundoplication

fundus of the stomach, the left side of the esophageal wall, and the left pillar of the crus. The second and third stitches incorporate the gastric fundus and the muscular layer of the left side of the esophagus.

- The fundus is then folded over the esophagus so that the greater curvature of the stomach is next to the right pillar of the crus.
- The second row of sutures on the right side of the esophagus consists of three stitches between the fundus and the right pillar of the crus.
- Finally, two additional stitches are placed between the fundus and the rim of the esophageal hiatus to eliminate any tension from the fundoplication (Fig. 5.4).

Postoperative Course

- Patients start a soft diet the morning of the first postoperative day.
- Patients are instructed to avoid meat, bread, and carbonated beverages for the following 2 weeks.
- About 85 % of patients are discharged within 23 h, and 95 % of patients are discharged within 48 h.
- Most patients resume their regular activity within 2 weeks.

Postoperative Complications

- Esophageal or gastric perforation may occur during any step of the dissection and is secondary to traction or inadvertent electrocautery burns.
- Clinical signs of a leak usually appear during the first 48 h with peritoneal signs in case of spillage limited to the abdomen or shortness of breath and a pleural effusion if spillage also occurs in the chest.
- A contrast study with a water-soluble contrast agent is necessary to detect the site of the leak.
- A reoperation with direct repair is the optimal management of the leak.

Short-Term Outcomes

Some degree of transient dysphagia is very common after LTF. If dysphagia persists beyond 6–10 weeks, one or more of the following causes should be considered:

1. A too tight or too long (i.e., >2.5 cm) wrap. In case of a too tight wrap, the treatment modality of choice is endoscopic dilatation; redo surgery should be considered in case of failure of endoscopic treatment.
2. Lateral torsion of the wrap to the right with corkscrew effect secondary to tension from intact short gastric vessels or to a small gastric fundus.
3. A wrap made with the body of the stomach rather than the fundus.
4. Choice of the wrong procedure. A partial wrap is preferable in case of severely impaired or absent esophageal peristalsis, reducing the incidence of postoperative dysphagia and gas bloat syndrome.

Long-Term Outcomes: Laparoscopic Total or Partial Fundoplication?

An LPF (posterior, 180° anterior, and 90° anterior) has been proposed as an alternative to LTF to minimize or prevent postoperative dysphagia and gas-related symptoms.

Anterior (180° and 90°) LPF vs. LTF

Some randomized controlled trials (RCTs) have compared LTF to an anterior 180° or 90° LPF. Based on the evidence currently available, there are no differences in incidence of heartburn and use of PPIs after anterior 180° LPF and LTF, while they are higher after 90° anterior LPF than LTF at 5-year follow-up. Dysphagia is less common after LPF (180° and 90° anterior) than LTF at 5 years after surgery. The long-term outcomes at 10-year follow-up are similar.

These results should be interpreted with caution, since 24-h pH monitoring was not used in these studies to objectively assess the incidence of gastroesophageal reflux at long-term follow-up. It is known that ambulatory 24-h pH monitoring is positive for pathological gastroesophageal reflux in less than 40 % of patients with recurrent heartburn. On the other hand, 5-year follow-up studies have shown that LPF achieves a less effective control of reflux than LTF, with recurrent reflux detected by pH monitoring in more than 50 % of patients after LPF.

Posterior LPF vs. LTF

The effect of a posterior LPF as an alternative to LTF has been investigated in terms of incidence of postoperative dysphagia and wind-related symptoms. Based on the results of several RCTs, similar control of reflux and overall patient satisfaction are achieved after the two procedures. Postoperative dysphagia, inability to belch, gas bloating, need for endoscopic dilatations, or surgical reoperations are more common after LTF. However, these initial mechanical advantages seem to disappear over time.

The interpretation of these data may be biased by the short-follow-up, small sample sizes of the studies and lack of postoperative objective evaluation of reflux with 24-h pH monitoring. Indeed, the results of large comparative studies suggest poorer long-term control of reflux after partial LPF.

LPF: Anterior or Posterior?

Based on the similar reflux control and reduced postoperative dysphagia after LPF, Hagedorn et al. randomized 47 patients to an anterior 120° LPF and 48 patients to a posterior (Toupet) LPF. Reflux control was significantly better at 24-h pH monitoring after posterior LPF. Postoperative dysphagia and ability to belch were similar between the two groups.

In conclusion, an LTF is the procedure of choice for the surgical treatment of GERD, while an LPF (either anterior 180° or posterior) should be performed only in patients with severe impairment of peristalsis and in patients with achalasia.

Laparoscopic Magnetic Sphincter Augmentation (MSA)

Recently, magnetic sphincter augmentation (MSA) with the LINX Reflux Management System (Torax Medical) is a minimally invasive operation that increases the sphincter barrier with a standardized, reproducible, and reversible laparoscopic procedure, without altering the gastric anatomy. The device consists of a series of magnetic beads interlinked with independent titanium wires that create a dynamic flexible and expandable ring mimicking the physiological movement of the esophagus. Main indications are GERD confirmed by 24-h ambulatory pH monitoring and incomplete symptom relief despite maximum medical therapy.

The results of two single-institution studies show that the laparoscopic implantation of MSA is easy and safe. Postoperatively, the esophageal acid exposure decreases, reflux symptoms improve, and the majority of patients stop PPIs. However, only large RCTs with long follow-up comparing MSA and laparoscopic fundoplication will clarify the role of this device in the treatment of GERD.

Summary

- PPIs are the main stem of medical therapy.
- Acid-suppressing medications can only modify the pH of the gastric refluxate, while surgery restores the competence of the LES.
- A laparoscopic total fundoplication is considered today the gold standard for the surgical treatment of GERD, with better short-term outcomes and similar reflux control compared to open fundoplication.
- A small but significant incidence of postoperative dysphagia and gas-related symptoms is reported after LTF.
- A LPF (either anterior 180° or posterior) should be performed only in patients with GERD with severe impairment of peristalsis and in patients with achalasia.
- Magnetic sphincter augmentation (MSA) is a new minimally invasive operation that increases the sphincter barrier without altering the gastric anatomy.

Selected Reading

1. Baigrie RJ, Cullis SNR, Ndhluni AJ, Cariem A. Randomized double-blind trial of laparoscopic Nissen fundoplication versus anterior partial fundoplication. Br J Surg. 2005;92:819–23.
2. Bonavina L, Saino G, Lipham JC, Demeester TR. LINX(®) Reflux Management System in chronic gastroesophageal reflux: a novel effective technology for restoring the natural barrier to reflux. Therap Adv Gastroenterol. 2013;6:261–8.
3. Bonavina L, Saino G, Bona D, Sironi A, Lazzari V. One hundred consecutive patients treated with magnetic sphincter augmentation for gastroesophageal reflux disease: 6 years of clinical experience from a single center. J Am Coll Surg. 2013;217:577–85.

4. Broeders JA, Rijnhart-de Jong HG, Draaisma WA, Bredenoord AJ, Smout AJ, Gooszen HG. Ten-year outcome of laparoscopic and conventional nissen fundoplication: randomized clinical trial. Ann Surg. 2009;250:698–706.
5. Broeders JAJL, Mauritz FA, Ahmed Ali U, Draaisma WA, Ruurda JP, Gooszen HG, Smout AJ, Broeders IA, Hazebroek EJ. Systematic review and meta-analysis of laparoscopic Nissen (posterior total) versus Toupet (posterior partial) fundoplication for gastro-oesophageal reflux disease. Br J Surg. 2010;97:1318–30.
6. Broeders JA, Broeders EA, Watson DI, Devitt PG, Holloway RH, Jamieson GG. Objective outcomes 14 years after laparoscopic anterior 180-degree partial versus Nissen fundoplication: results from a randomized trial. Ann Surg. 2013;258:233–9.
7. Cai W, Watson DI, Lally CJ, Devitt PG, Game PA, Jamieson GG. Ten-year clinical outcomes of a prospective randomized clinical trial of laparoscopic Nissen versus anterior 180° partial fundoplication. Br J Surg. 2008;95:1501–5.
8. Dallemagne B, Weerts J, Markiewicz S, Dewandre JM, Wahlen C, Monami B, Jehaes C. Clinical results of laparoscopic fundoplication at ten years after surgery. Surg Endosc. 2006; 20:159–65.
9. Engström C, Lönroth H, Mardani J, Lundell L. An anterior or posterior approach to partial fundoplication? Long-term results of a randomized trial. World J Surg. 2007;31:1221–5.
10. Galvani C, Fisichella PM, Gorodner MV, Perretta S, Patti MG. Symptoms are a poor indicator of reflux status after fundoplication for gastroesophageal reflux disease: role of esophageal functions tests. Arch Surg. 2003;138:514–8.
11. Ganz RA, Peters JH, Horgan S, Bemelman WA, Dunst CM, Edmundowicz SA, Lipham JC, Luketich JD, Melvin WS, Oelschlager BK, Schlack-Haerer SC, Smith CD, Smith CC, Dunn D, Taiganides PA. Esophageal sphincter device for gastroesophageal reflux disease. N Engl J Med. 2013;368:719–27.
12. Hagedorn C, Jönson C, Lönroth H, Ruth M, Thune A, Lundell L. Efficacy of an anterior as compared with a posterior laparoscopic partial fundoplication: results of a randomized, controlled clinical trial. Ann Surg. 2003;238:189–96.
13. Herbella FA, Tedesco P, Nipomnick I, Fisichella PM, Patti MG. Effect of partial and total laparoscopic fundoplication on esophageal body motility. Surg Endosc. 2007;21:285–8.
14. Horgan S, Pohl D, Bogetti D, Eubanks T, Pellegrini CA. Failed antireflux surgery. What have we learned from reoperations? Arch Surg. 1999;134:809–17.
15. Horvath KD, Jobe BA, Herron DM, Swanstrom LL. Laparoscopic Toupet fundoplication is an inadequate procedure for patients with severe reflux disease. J Gastrointest Surg. 1999;3: 583–91.
16. Khajanchee YS, O'Rourke RW, Lockhart B, Patterson EJ, Hansen PD, Swanstrom LL. Postoperative symptoms and failure after antireflux surgery. Arch Surg. 2002;137:1008–14.
17. Lord RV, Kaminski A, Oberg S, Bowrey DJ, Hagen JA, DeMeester SR, Sillin LF, Peters JH, Crookes PF, DeMeester TR. Absence of gastroesophageal reflux disease in a majority of patients taking acid suppression medications after Nissen fundoplication. J Gastrointest Surg. 2002;6:3–9.
18. Ludemann R, Watson DI, Jamieson GG, Game PA, Devitt PG. Five-year follow-up of a randomized clinical trial of laparoscopic total versus anterior 180° fundoplication. Br J Surg. 2005;92:240–3.
19. Makris KI, Cassera MA, Kastenmeier AS, Dunst CM, Swanström LL. Postoperative dysphagia is not predictive of long-term failure after laparoscopic antireflux surgery. Surg Endosc. 2012;26:451–7.
20. Meneghetti AT, Tedesco P, Galvani C, Gorodner MV, Patti MG. Outcomes after laparoscopic Nissen fundoplication are not influenced by the pattern of reflux. Dis Esophagus. 2008;21:165–9.
21. Morgenthal CB, Shane MD, Stival A, Gletsu N, Milam G, Swafford V, Hunter JG, Smith CD. The durability of laparoscopic Nissen fundoplication: 11-year outcomes. J Gastrointest Surg. 2007;11:693–700.
22. Nijjar RS, Watson DI, Jamieson GG, Archer S, Bessell JR, Booth M, Cade R, Cullingford GL, Devitt PG, Fletcher DR, Hurley J, Kiroff G, Martin IJ, Nathanson LK, Windsor JA. International

Society for the Diseases of the Esophagus-Australasian Section. Five-year follow-up of a multicenter, double-blind randomized clinical trial of laparoscopic Nissen vs anterior 90 degrees partial fundoplication. Arch Surg. 2010;145:552–7.
23. Oleynikov D, Eubanks TR, Oelschlager BK, Pellegrini CA. Total fundoplication is the operation of choice for patients with gastroesophageal reflux and defective peristalsis. Surg Endosc. 2002;16:909–13.
24. Patterson EJ, Herron DM, Hansen PD, Ramzi N, Standage BA, Swanström LL. Effect of an esophageal bougie on the incidence of dysphagia following Nissen fundoplication: a prospective, blinded, randomized clinical trial. Arch Surg. 2000;135:1055–61.
25. Patti MG, Arcerito M, Feo CV, De Pinto M, Tong J, Gantert W, Tyrrell D, Way LW. An analysis of operations for gastroesophageal reflux disease. Identifying the important technical elements. Arch Surg. 1998;133:600–6.
26. Patti MG, Robinson T, Galvani C, Gorodner MV, Fisichella PM, Way LW. Total fundoplication is superior to partial fundoplication even when esophageal peristalsis is weak. J Am Coll Surg. 2004;198:863–9.
27. Patti MG, Gasper WJ, Fisichella PM, Nipomnick I, Palazzo F. Gastroesophageal reflux disease and connective tissue disorders: pathophysiology and implications for treatment. J Gastrointest Surg. 2008;12:1900–6.
28. Spence GM, Watson DI, Jamiesion GG, Lally CJ, Devitt PG. Single center prospective randomized trial of laparoscopic Nissen versus anterior 90 degrees fundoplication. J Gastrointest Surg. 2006;10:698–705.
29. Tedesco P, Lobo E, Fisichella PM, Way LW, Patti MG. Laparoscopic fundoplication in elderly patients with gastroesophageal reflux disease. Arch Surg. 2006;141:289–92.
30. Thompson SK, Jamieson GG, Myers JC, Chin KF, Watson DI, Devitt PG. Recurrent heartburn after laparoscopic fundoplication is not always recurrent reflux. J Gastrointest Surg. 2007;11:642–7.
31. Watson DI, Jamieson GG, Pike GK, Davies N, Richardson M, Devitt PG. Prospective randomized double-blind trial between laparoscopic Nissen fundoplication and anterior partial fundoplication. Br J Surg. 1999;86:123–30.
32. Watson DI, Jamieson GG, Lally C, Archer S, Bessell JR, Booth M, Cade R, Cullingford G, Devitt PG, Fletcher DR, Hurley J, Kiroff G, Martin CJ, Martin IJ, Nathanson LK, Windsor JK. International Society for Diseases of the Esophagus–Australasian Section. Multicenter, prospective, double-blind, randomized trial of laparoscopic Nissen vs. anterior 90 degrees partial fundoplication. Arch Surg. 2004;139:1160–7.
33. Watson DI, Devitt PG, Smith L, Jamieson GG. Anterior 90° partial vs Nissen fundoplication–5 year follow-up of a single-centre randomised trial. J Gastrointest Surg. 2012;16:1653–8.

Chapter 6
Treatment of Paraesophageal Hernias

Anahita Jalilvand, Justin B. Dimick, and P. Marco Fisichella

Abstract The goal of this chapter is to describe the pathophysiology and classification, clinical presentation, and indications for treatment and an overview of the surgical management of patients with paraesophageal hernias. A description of the technical principles of the repair will be described.

Keywords Paraesophageal hernias • Gastroesophageal reflux disease • Laparoscopic antireflux surgery • Esophageal function testing • Laparoscopic repair • Thoracoscopic repair

A paraesophageal hernia occurs when part of the gastric fundus herniates through the esophageal hiatus of the diaphragm and lies alongside the esophagus. In contrast to sliding hiatal hernias, paraesophageal hernias have a "true hernia sac," made up of peritoneum. Paraesophageal hernia represents approximately 5 % of all hiatal hernias and is more common in the elderly.

A. Jalilvand, MD
Department of Surgery, Loyola University Medical Center and Loyola Stritch School of Medicine, 2160 South 1st Ave, Maywood, IL 60153, USA

J.B. Dimick, MD, MPH, FACS
Department of Surgery, University of Michigan Health System, 2124 Taubman Health Care Center, Ann Arbor, MI 48109-5343, USA

P.M. Fisichella, MD, MBA, FACS (✉)
Department of Surgery, Boston Veteran Administration Healthcare System, 1400 VFW Parkway, West Roxbury, MA 02132, USA

Department of Surgery, Brigham and Women's Hospital, Harvard Medical School, Boston, MA, USA
e-mail: piero.fisichella@va.gov

P.M. Fisichella et al. (eds.), *Esophageal Diseases*,
DOI 10.1007/978-3-319-04337-1_6,

Classification of Hiatal Hernias

Paraesophageal hernias are a subclass of hiatal hernias (type II and III). In general, hiatal hernias are classified in four types (Fig. 6.1): type I, commonly known as a sliding hiatal hernia, is the most common (95 %) and occurs when the gastroesophageal junction is displaced superiorly into the thoracic cavity; type II occurs when the stomach migrates into the chest and "rolls" over the esophagus with the gastroesophageal junction still laying down into the abdomen; type III occurs when the stomach migrates into the chest and "rolls" over the esophagus with a concomitant migration of the gastroesophageal junction into the chest (this type of hernia or "mixed," or "true paraesophageal" is a combination of the "sliding" and "rolling" types) (Figs. 6.2 and 6.3); type IV occurs when, together with the stomach, there is herniation of other intra-abdominal contents through the hiatus (e.g., small bowel, colon, duodenum, or pancreas) (Figs. 6.4 and 6.5).

This anatomical classification is useful because it helps us understand the symptoms experienced by patients with different types of hernias. In general, patients with a type I hiatal hernia experience typical symptoms of gastroesophageal reflux disease (GERD), such as heartburn and regurgitation. As the gastroesophageal is displaced into the chest, the lower esophageal sphincter (LES) becomes incompetent as it is subjected to the negative pressure of the thoracic cavity and the pinchcock action of the "external sphincter" of the diaphragm is lost. The angle of His is also lost as the hernia becomes compartmentalized in the chest. Patients with a type II hernia also experience dysphagia due to external compression of the intra-abdominally located gastroesophageal junction by the paraesophageal hernia rather than typical symptoms of GERD. Patients with type III and IV hernias in general complain of a combination of symptoms of gastroesophageal reflux disease and dysphagia (synonym of obstruction).

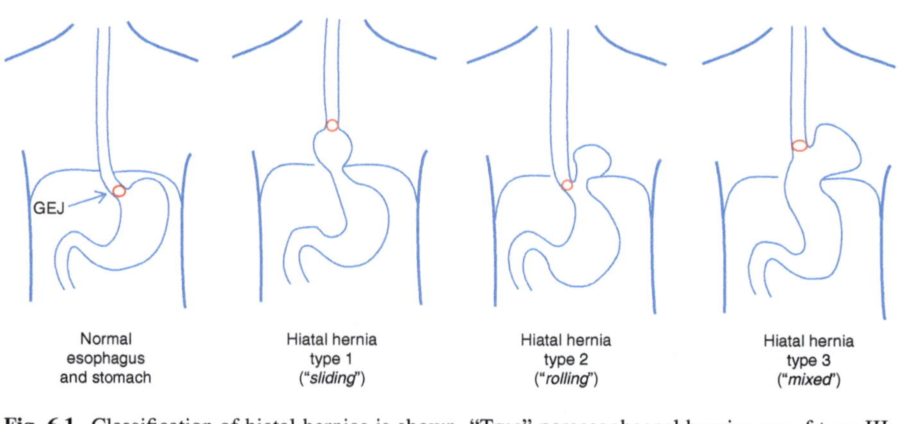

Fig. 6.1 Classification of hiatal hernias is shown. "True" paraesophageal hernias are of type III. Note the location of the gastroesophageal junction (GEJ) in the different types of hernias

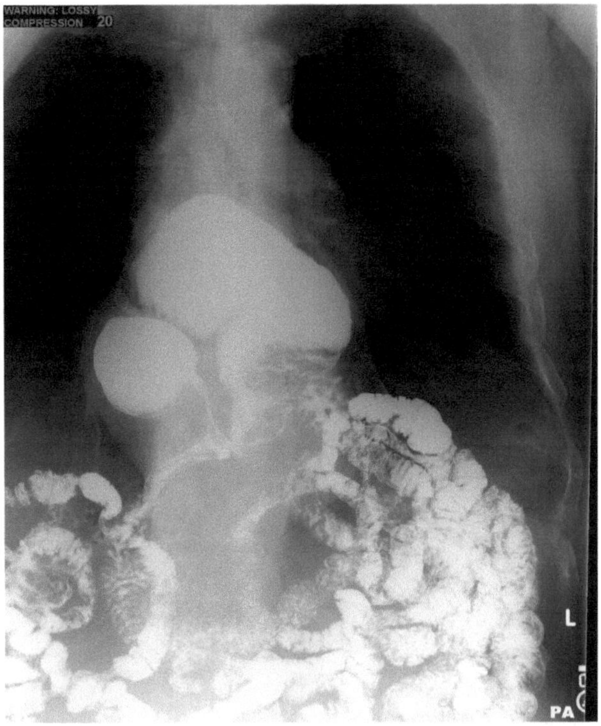

Fig. 6.2 A barium swallow (anteroposterior view) is shown of a patient who presented with a type III paraesophageal hernia with "hour glass" stomach, which is an anteriorly herniated fundus, oriented "upside down" with respect to the rest of the stomach

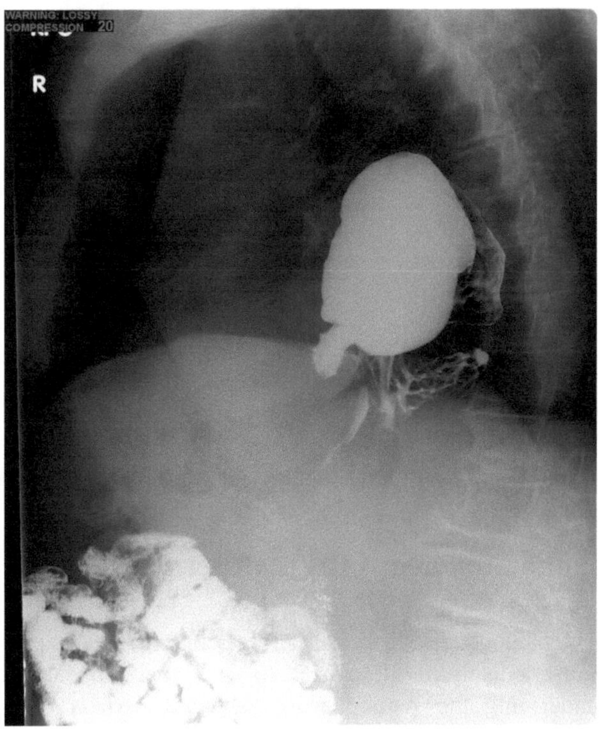

Fig. 6.3 A barium swallow (lateral view) is shown of a patient who presented with a type III paraesophageal hernia with "hour glass" stomach. The lateral view clearly shows the anteriorly herniated fundus lying alongside the esophagus in its "para"-esophageal location

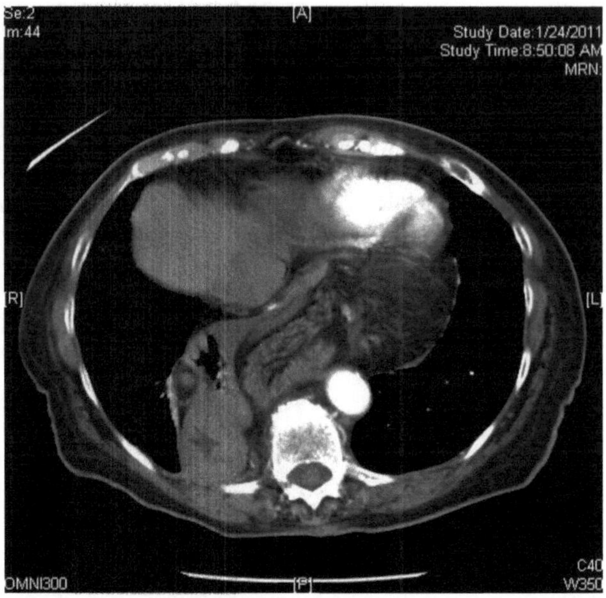

Fig. 6.4 A CT scan is shown of a patient who presented with herniation of pancreas into the posterior mediastinum (coronal view)

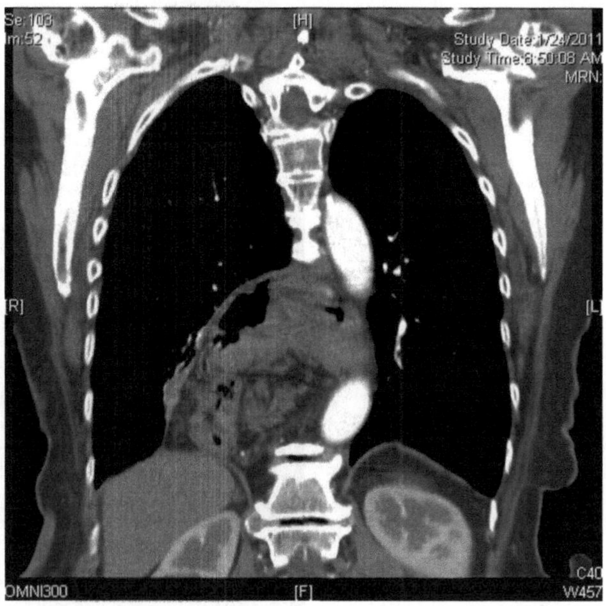

Fig. 6.5 A CT scan is shown of a patient who presented with herniation of pancreas into the posterior mediastinum (axial view)

Pathophysiology of Hiatal Hernias

The pathogenesis of hiatal hernias continues to be poorly described and their true cause is likely multifactorial. As such, there appears to be three dominant theories underlying the pathogenesis of hiatal hernias: (1) increased intra-abdominal pressure that displaces the gastroesophageal junction upward into the thorax; (2) esophageal shortening from congenital causes or acquired secondary to fibrosis; and (3) widening of the hiatus from congenital or acquired molecular and cellular changes in the crural muscles or in the connective tissue of the diaphragm.

Because of the increased incidence of other abdominal hernias in association with type II hiatal, these theories suggest an intrinsic defect in collagen formation. Similarly, obesity, which is associated with an increased intra-abdominal pressure, has also shown to be a risk factor for the development of hiatal hernias; furthermore, obesity is also a risk factor for recurrence after surgical repair.

Clinical Presentation

Paraesophageal hernias differ in symptomology from type I hiatal hernias. While sliding hiatal hernias are associated with an incompetent LES leading to worsening gastroesophageal reflux disease, paraesophageal hernias traditionally do not affect the competency of the LES. In contrast, paraesophageal hernias involve an anteriorly herniated fundus oriented "upside down" with respect to the rest of the stomach, predisposing it to twist on itself (Fig. 6.3). Therefore, symptoms due to paraesophageal hernias are mostly mechanical and include gastric obstruction, strangulation, incarceration, and ulceration. Pulmonary symptoms either from chronic aspiration due to gastric obstruction or from the thoracic displacement secondary to the herniation can also be observed. Chronic venous congestion of the herniated gastric mucosa along with ulceration (Cameron's ulcers) can also result in occult bleeding and anemia. Since type III paraesophageal hernias are essentially a combination of types I and II, their symptomology involves worsening of both GERD and esophagitis as well as mechanical symptoms. Type IV paraesophageal hernias present similarly to other hiatal hernias, although their symptomology will also depend on what abdominal contents have herniated through the hiatus. A common presentation is a small bowel obstruction from herniation and incarceration of small bowel and duodenum (Figs. 6.6, 6.7, and 6.8). Since type III paraesophageal hernias are much more common than types II or IV, most patients with paraesophageal hernias will present with concomitant worsening GERD.

Diagnostic Testing

Although most patients with paraesophageal hernias are symptomatic, there is still a significant group of patients who are diagnosed incidentally. It is important to note that a thorough history is necessary to determine if patients are truly asymptomatic, as many may only appear to have nonspecific complaints unrelated to hernia. Although standard work-up typically begins with a barium swallow, followed by upper endoscopy and esophageal manometry, many patients, especially those who

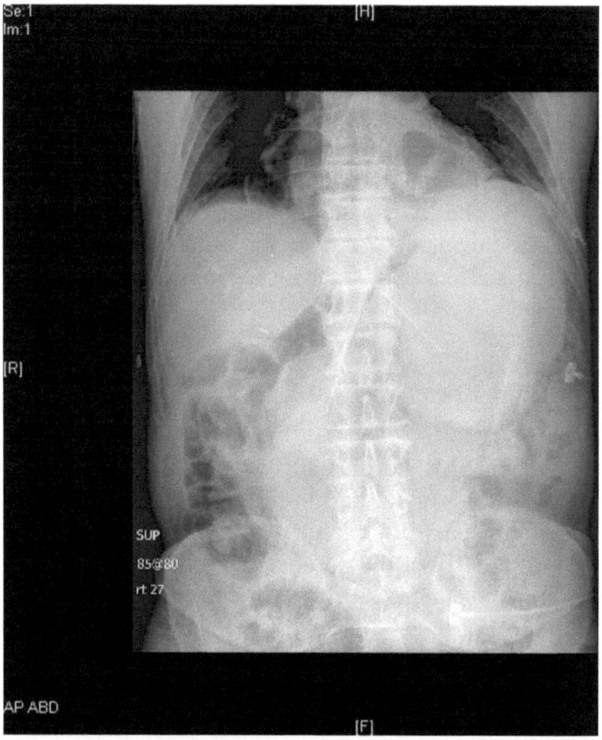

Fig. 6.6 An abdominal X-ray is shown of a patient who presented with symptoms of small bowel obstruction. Loops of small bowel are present in the chest centrally, and the stomach is distended, whereas air is present throughout the colon

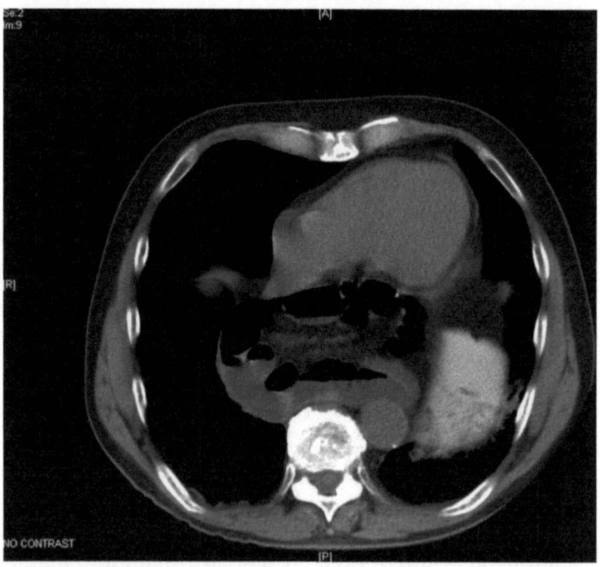

Fig. 6.7 A CT scan is shown of a patient with a type IV hernia with herniation of the small bowel. Loops of the small bowel are present in the posterior mediastinum

are asymptomatic or minimally symptomatic, have their hernias discovered during tests performed for other conditions. Figures 6.9 and 6.10 demonstrate the presence of a paraesophageal hernia on a routine chest X-ray.

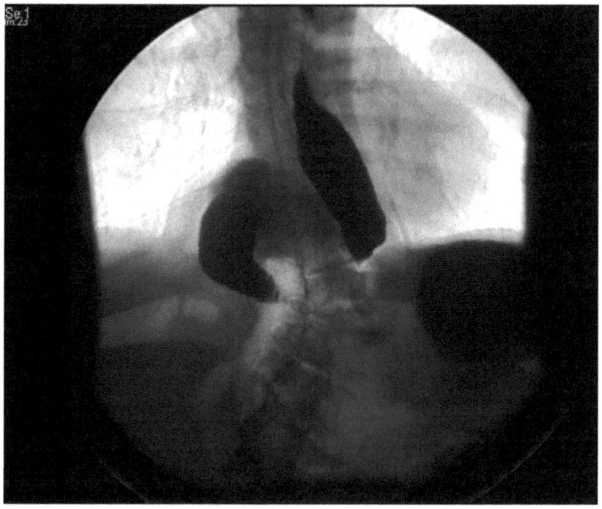

Fig. 6.8 A barium swallow is shown of a patient with a type IV hernia with herniation of the duodenum. The gastroesophageal junction is located in the abdomen and externally compressed by the hernia. In this case, the remembrance of the distal esophagus to the "bird's beak" esophagus characteristic of achalasia mandated esophageal manometry to exclude achalasia and correctly plan a total fundoplication

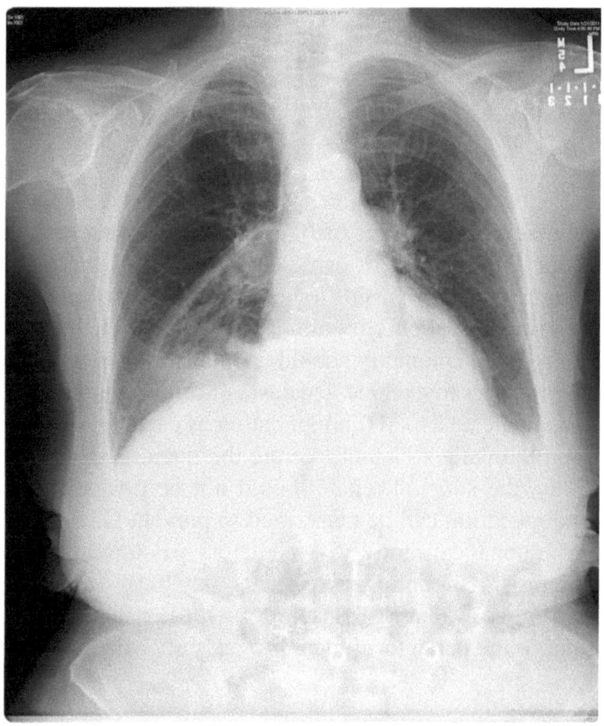

Fig. 6.9 A chest X-ray (anteroposterior view) is shown of a patient suggestive of a hiatal hernia. A barium swallow showed a type III paraesophageal hernia

Barium swallow is perhaps the most important study, giving valuable information as to the size of the stomach herniated and the location of the gastroesophageal junction (intra-abdominal or intrathoracic).

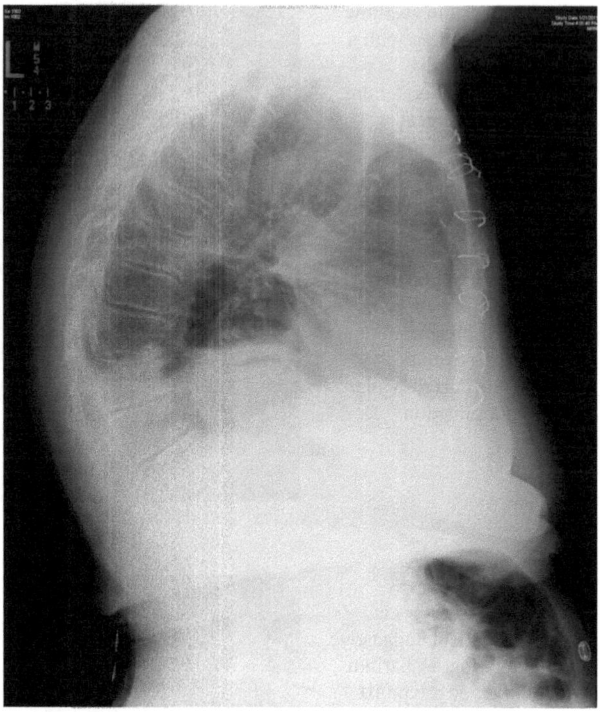

Fig. 6.10 A chest X-ray (lateral view) is shown of a patient suggestive of a hiatal hernia. The esophagus filled with air is demonstrated together with an air-fluid level (likely the stomach) behind the heart. A barium swallow showed a type III paraesophageal hernia

Endoscopy is useful for visualization of the esophageal and gastric mucosa, as it can detect the presence of Barrett's esophagus, erosive esophagitis, and Cameron's ulcers. Furthermore, it can also determine if there are any lesions suspicious for malignancy, which needs to be documented prior to surgical management.

Since all patients require a fundoplication in addition to a hernia repair, an esophageal manometry should be included in diagnostic approach for surgical planning in order to exclude achalasia or an esophageal motility disorder, which would contraindicate a total fundoplication as part of the repair. Of note, in those few cases when the patient cannot tolerate the manometry catheter, or if they present emergently, the surgical repair should not be postponed, and in these cases, a partial fundoplication can be performed to prevent GERD without documentation of normal esophageal motility. Ambulatory pH monitoring is typically not required for diagnosis, although many patients may have worsening GERD symptoms prompting further evaluation. Baseline 24 h pH values may also prove useful in order to monitor the patient's clinical progress after the hernia repair.

Indications for Surgery

The management of paraesophageal hernias is still widely debated today. The indications for surgical treatment as well as the techniques utilized have been a source of much debate. Due to the risks of strangulation and incarceration and the perioperative mortality of emergent surgeries (especially in elderly patients with complex comorbidities), traditionally, most surgeons opted to repair paraesophageal hernias regardless of whether the patient was symptomatic or not. Current strategies have moved away from this approach to a more conservative algorithm. Recent studies have shown that elective and emergent hernia repairs are equally effective. Therefore, for patients who are minimally symptomatic and in whom the hernia has been discovered incidentally, careful observation with a "watchful waiting" strategy can be a reasonable alternative, as long as there is both patient and physician education on symptoms concerning for strangulation and incarceration. Worrisome symptoms that may prompt elective repair include severe regurgitation, aspiration, cough, anemia, or dysphagia. Gastric volvulus is an indication for emergent surgical intervention and is classically described by the Borchardt triad, which includes the inability to pass a nasogastric tube, retching without actual food regurgitation, and chest or epigastric pain. On the other hand, patients who are younger (<50 years old) and healthier may be more likely to encounter complications from their hernia given their life expectancy. For these patients, elective repair may be a more appropriate solution, provided that a comprehensive review of the risks, benefits, and alternatives available is thoroughly discussed with the patients as well as incidence of recurrence and complications and expected quality of life. To summarize, in general, elective surgical management is reserved for young patients or for those who are symptomatic.

Overview of Surgical Management

The surgical approaches used to repair paraesophageal hernias are widely debated. The repair is very technically demanding and requires a thorough understanding of esophageal and gastric anatomy and physiology.

Paraesophageal hernia repair generally includes four steps: hernia sac dissection and resection, esophageal mobilization, crural repair, and fundoplication. Traditionally, these steps have been accomplished using an open transthoracic approach, which includes a left thoracotomy, direct visualization of the hernia, mobilization of the esophagus to the aortic arch, and dissection and resection of the hernia sac. The main advantage of the transthoracic approach is the direct visualization and accessibility of the esophagus, which is essential in this procedure. Proper mobilization of the esophagus is highly correlated to the success rate of the procedure (recurrence rates are low after open repairs), as it ensures a tension-free repair. Postoperative pain at the thoracotomy incision is the most commonly reported symptom, and this can be quite debilitating for the patient, as some experience this as a chronic, long-term complication.

The advent of laparoscopy has introduced an alternative to open procedures, provided that the essential steps of the procedure can be adequately accomplished. Although the recurrence rate with laparoscopic approach has been shown to be somewhat higher, a laparoscopic repair can be equally effective with significant reduction in morbidity and mortality in experienced hands. Recurrences in fact are usually small and asymptomatic and are mostly linked to the presence of short esophagus and tension at the diaphragmatic crura during their closure.

Techniques to overcome the presence of axial tension due to the presence of short esophagus include aggressively mobilizing the esophagus and extensive dissection of the hernia sac in the posterior mediastinum. An esophageal lengthening procedure, such as a Collis gastroplasty, can be used to further reduce this tension and decrease the risk of recurrence. This procedure consists in stapling vertically and laterally alongside the esophagus onto the angle of His, thus effectively creating a "neo-esophagus." This procedure lengthens the esophagus inferior to the diaphragm and allows for more a successful fundoplication without tension.

Techniques to overcome the presence of tension due to a large hiatus include relaxation of the diaphragmatic crura, along with the use of mesh. The goal of mesh repair is to oppose the radial tension by strengthening the hiatal orifice. While most surgeons use mesh, this continues to be debated, as many have shown that if improperly positioned, the mesh can cause severe complications, such as erosions requiring gastric resection. As of today, most surgeons have adopted a selective approach to the use of mesh. In general, mesh is placed to buttress the hiatus after closure in those patients with thin crura unable to withstand the tension of the primary closure.

The need for antireflux surgery in addition to paraesophageal hernia repair has also been debated. However, most surgeons prefer to perform a total fundoplication as this corrects gastroesophageal reflux if present preoperatively. It also prevents the development of reflux due to the extensive dissection and destruction of some of the continence mechanisms of the gastroesophageal junction; and it is a very good form of gastropexy, anchoring the stomach below the diaphragm, thereby reducing recurrences. A fundoplication reduces the need for a tube gastrostomy, which is seldom performed in the modern era.

Although a Nissen fundoplication is the procedure of choice, a partial posterior (Toupet) or anterior (Dor) fundoplication rather than a Nissen, or total, fundoplication may be considered when a patient presents with signs and symptoms of incarceration or strangulation (which do not allow to perform an esophageal manometry preoperatively) and when an underlying esophageal motility disorder is present (which would reduce the risk of postoperative dysphagia) (Fig. 6.8).

Obese patients with paraesophageal hernias present a different challenge. First, the recurrence rate after paraesophageal hernia repairs in obese patients is significantly increased. Second, simply addressing the paraesophageal hernia does not necessarily address obesity. As such, in obese patients who qualify for bariatric surgery, a sleeve gastrectomy or gastric bypass should be considered along with paraesophageal hernia repair. An important consideration should be made for patients who are obese and have worsening GERD symptoms; for these patients, a sleeve gastrectomy may not be an appropriate antireflux surgery, as it does not appropriately address reflux and may even make it worse. In these patients, a Roux-en-Y gastric bypass is a more suitable option, targeting obesity, lowering paraesophageal recurrence, and allowing for better reflux control. In fact, a Roux-en-Y gastric bypass offers protection against all forms of reflux: acid (because the small gastric pouch is devoid of parietal cells) and alkaline (because the Roux-en-Y limb avoids reflux of bile).

Postoperative Management

Hospital stay for patients is largely determined by what approach is used for the paraesophageal hernia repair. Patients undergoing laparoscopic repair have been reported to stay an average of one night, while open procedures usually require patients to stay between 3 and 12 days. If the operation is done laparoscopically, the Foley is removed in the operating room and the patient is discharged home the next day after tolerating a soft-mechanical diet, which is then advanced at the first follow-up visit in the clinic. Immediately in the postoperative period, routine precautions including precautions for deep venous thrombosis, incentive spirometry, along with adequate pain control, are implemented (open and thoracic cases will require epidural catheter for pain control and continuation of Foley catheter). Moreover, there is no consensus as to whether barium swallow should be obtained. Most authors agree that if the patient does not undergo any esophageal lengthening procedure, such as a Collis gastroplasty, there is no need for a contrast study. Conversely, if a Collis gastroplasty is performed, a barium swallow may be needed to document the absence of a leak and gastroesophageal patency before the nasogastric tube is removed (this is placed intraoperatively and usually kept for 48 h postoperatively). Barium swallow is usually obtained between 6 and 12 months postoperatively to assess for any recurrence.

Summary

- In general, elective surgical management is reserved for young patients (<50) or for those who are symptomatic.
- The risk of strangulation is small; therefore, older patients and those symptomatic or minimally symptomatic can be watched.
- Morbid obese patients should undergo surgery for morbid obesity.
- Best diagnostic tests are upper endoscopy and barium swallow. Manometry must be done to identify an underlying esophageal motility disorder that may require a partial fundoplication instead of the conventional total fundoplication.
- Short esophagus is rare; when present, an esophageal lengthening procedure (Collis gastroplasty) should be performed.
- Hiatal closure: mesh or no mesh policy is adopted selectively. Relaxing diaphragmatic incisions are done by some authors.
- Which fundoplication? Partial or total depends on esophageal motility. During emergencies, when an esophageal manometry cannot be done, a partial fundoplication should be performed to reduce the incidence of postoperative dysphagia in those with unknown esophageal motility.
- A fundoplication is the best form of gastropexy that eliminates the need for a tube gastrostomy.

Selected Reading

1. Casabella F, Sinanan M, Horgan S, et al. Systematic use of gastric fundoplication in laparoscopic repair of paraesophageal hernias. Am J Surg. 1996;171:485–9.
2. Dallemagne B, Kohnen L, Perretta S, et al. Laparoscopic repair of paraesophageal hernia. Long-term follow-up reveals good clinical outcome despite high radiological recurrence rate. Ann Surg. 2011;253:291–6.
3. Fisichella PM. A synopsis of techniques for paraesophageal hernia repair: different approaches to current controversies. Surg Laparosc Endosc Percutan Tech. 2013;23(5):423–4.
4. Gantert WA, Patti MG, Arcerito M, et al. Laparoscopic repair of paraesophageal hiatal hernias. J Am Coll Surg. 1998;186:428–32.
5. Hashemi M, Peters JH, DeMeester TR, Huprich JE, Quek M, Hagen JA, Crookes PF, Theisen J, DeMeester SR, Silin LF, Bremner CG. Laparoscopic repair of large type III hiatal hernia: objective follow-up reveals high recurrence rate. J Am Coll Surg. 2000;190:553–61.
6. Horvath KD, Swanstrom LL, Jobe BA. The short esophagus: pathophysiology, incidence, presentation, and treatment in the era of laparoscopic antireflux surgery. Ann Surg. 2000;232:630–40.
7. Luketich JD, Nason KS, Christie NA, et al. Outcomes after a decade of laparoscopic giant paraesophageal hernia repair. J Thorac Cardiovasc Surg. 2010;139:395–404.
8. Merchant AM, Cook MV, Srinivasan J, et al. Comparison between laparoscopic paraesophageal hernia repair with sleeve gastrectomy and paraesophageal hernia repair alone in morbidly obese patients. Am Surg. 2009;75:620–5.
9. Oelschlager BK, Yamamoto K, Woltman T, et al. Vagotomy during hiatal hernia repair: a benign esophageal lengthening procedure. J Gastrointest Surg. 2008;12:1155–62.
10. Oelschlager BK, Pellegrini CA, Hunter JG, et al. Biologic prosthesis to prevent recurrence after laparoscopic paraesophageal hernia repair: long-term follow-up from a multicenter, prospective, randomized trial. J Am Coll Surg. 2011;213:461–8.
11. Paul S, Nasar A, Port JL, et al. Comparative analysis of diaphragmatic hernia repair outcomes using the Nationwide Inpatient Sample Database. Arch Surg. 2012;147:607–12.
12. Pfluke JM, Parker M, Bowers SP, et al. Use of mesh for hiatal hernia repair: a survey of SAGES members. Surg Endosc. 2012;26:1843–8.
13. Salvador-Sanchis JL, Martinez-Ramos D, Herfarth A, et al. Treatment of morbid obesity and hiatal paraesophageal hernia by laparoscopic Roux-en-Y gastric bypass. Obes Surg. 2010; 20:801–3.
14. Stylopoulos N, Gazelle GS, Rattner DW. Paraesophageal hernias: operation or observation? Ann Surg. 2002;236:492–501.
15. Weber C, Davis CS, Shankaran V, Fisichella PM. Hiatal hernias: a review of the pathophysiologic theories and implication for research. Surg Endosc. 2011;25(10):3149–53.
16. Zehetner J, DeMeester SR, Ayazi S, et al. Laparoscopic versus open repair of paraesophageal hernia: the second decade. J Am Coll Surg. 2011;212:813–20.

Chapter 7
Extraesophageal Manifestation of Gastroesophageal Reflux Disease

Fernando A.M. Herbella and Attila Dubecz

Abstract Gastroesophageal reflux disease (GERD) is defined by the Montreal Consensus as "a condition which develops when the reflux of stomach contents causes troublesome symptoms and/or complications." The Brazilian Consensus is more precise and acknowledges the plethora of GERD symptoms defining GERD as "a chronic disorder related to the retrograde flow of gastro-duodenal contents *into the esophagus and/or adjacent organs, resulting in a spectrum of symptoms*, with or without tissue damage." This make clear that GERD has a myriad of clinical presentations encompassing esophageal and extraesophageal symptoms making the diagnosis of the disease difficult in some cases. Virtually all adjacent organs to the esophagus may be affected by the gastric contents and new discoveries are made on a regular basis showing that even distant organs may be affected by GERD as well. Extraesophageal presentations can have multifactorial, often non-GERD, causes, and causality between reflux and these clinical entities is sometimes difficult to prove.

Keywords Esophageal manometry • Ambulatory pH monitoring • Cough • Microaspiration • Hoarseness • Pulmonary fibrosis

F.A.M. Herbella, MD (✉)
Department of Surgery, Federal University of São Paulo,
Rus Diogo de Faria 1087 cj 301, São Paulo 04037-003, Brazil
e-mail: herbella.dcir@epm.br

A. Dubecz, MD
Department of General and Thoracic Surgery, Klinikum Nürnberg Nord, Nürnberg, Germany
e-mail: attila.dubecz@klinikum-nuernberg.de

P.M. Fisichella et al. (eds.), *Esophageal Diseases*,
DOI 10.1007/978-3-319-04337-1_7, © Springer International Publishing Switzerland 2014

Introduction

Gastroesophageal reflux disease (GERD) is defined by the Montreal Consensus as "a condition which develops when the reflux of stomach contents causes troublesome symptoms and/or complications." The Brazilian Consensus is more precise and acknowledges the plethora of GERD symptoms defining GERD as "a chronic disorder related to the retrograde flow of gastro-duodenal contents *into the esophagus and/or adjacent organs, resulting in a spectrum of symptoms*, with or without tissue damage." This make clear that GERD has a myriad of clinical presentations encompassing esophageal and extraesophageal symptoms making the diagnosis of the disease difficult in some cases. Virtually all adjacent organs to the esophagus may be affected by the gastric contents and new discoveries are made on a regular basis showing that even distant organs may be affected by GERD as well (Fig. 7.1). Extraesophageal presentations can have multifactorial, often non-GERD, causes, and causality between reflux and these clinical entities is sometimes difficult to prove (Fig. 7.2).

This chapter reviews extraesophageal (previously called atypical) manifestation of GERD.

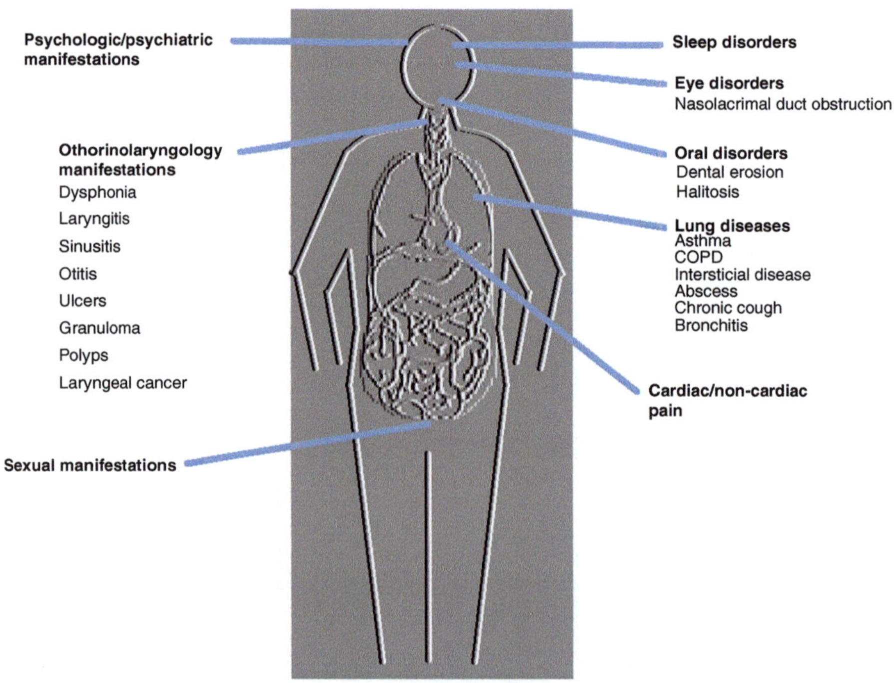

Fig. 7.1 Extraesophageal manifestations of the gastroesophageal reflux disease (GERD)

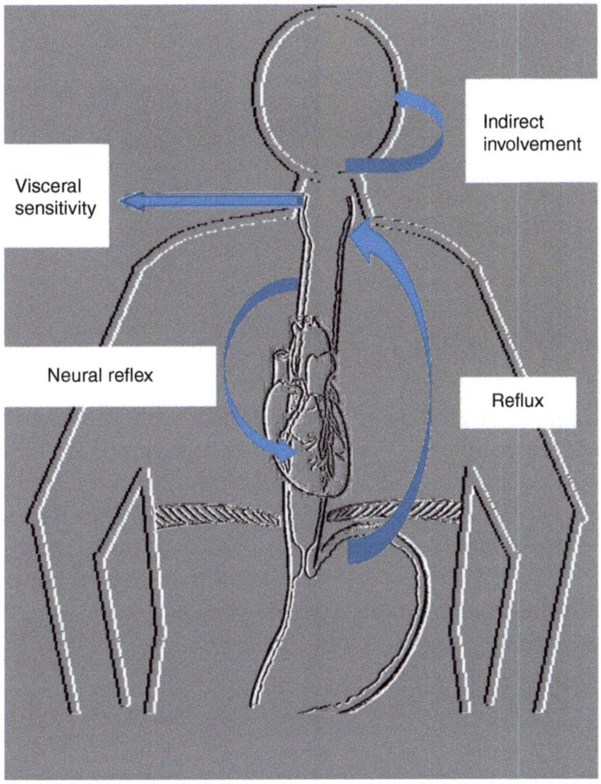

Fig. 7.2 Extraesophageal gastroesophageal reflux disease (GERD) symptoms pathophysiology

Pathophysiology

GERD pathophysiology has been reviewed in Chap. 3. However, extraesophageal symptoms have some peculiarities.

First and most important, there is not a broadly accepted threshold for normal versus pathologic proximal reflux, different from the distal reflux which is considered abnormal based on an elevated DeMeester score, or a percentage of time the pH is below 4.0 during pH monitoring, or the presence of distal erosive esophagitis.

Second, studies of impedance–pH in patients on acid-reducing medications showed that nonacid proximal reflux may cause extraesophageal symptoms and, thus, these symptoms may not respond to medical therapy.

Four theories, isolated or synergistically, may explain the genesis of extraesophageal symptoms.

Reflux Theory

Gastric contents (acid and nonacid) may reflux to upper-level esophagus and pharynx and lead to direct damage to adjacent organs. Ambulatory pH monitoring and impedance studies showed that reflux may occur all the way to the pharynx. Furthermore, pepsin, bile salts, and other digestive substances have been found in bronchioalveolar lavage.

Reflex Theory

Extraesophageal symptoms may occur without proximal acid exposure or in organs not susceptible to reflux. Very interestingly, some studies showed that distal GERD may be detected in almost half of the patients evaluated for chronic cough or asthma; however, less than half of these patients have proximal reflux. These symptoms may be explained by neural reflexes.

Esophageal mucosal stimulation may lead to vagal triggering. Chloridric acid instillation into the distal esophagus via a nasogastric tube may lead to esophageal as well as extraesophageal manifestations, such as bronchial and even coronary spasm, an obsolete test called Bernstein test.

Sensitivity

Different individuals show distinct responses to visceral stimulation with gastric contents. This different sensitivity may explain symptoms in patients with physiologic reflux and the difficulty to identify a threshold for pathologic proximal reflux.

A direct evaluation of esophageal sensitivity may be obtained by acid infusion in the esophagus (Bernstein test), intraesophageal balloon distention, electrical stimulation, and pharmacologic provocative tests, even though they are rarely used. Temporal correlation of reflux and symptoms during pH monitoring is a better indirect evaluation of visceral sensitivity as it will be discussed below.

Indirect Involvement

Gastroduodenal contents may reflux to sensitive organs and provoke damage that may extend to adjacent organs. A good example is the origin of GERD-related otitis due to Eustachian tube dysfunction based on edema on the rhinopharyngeal region.

Diagnostic Workup

Upper Digestive Endoscopy

Upper digestive endoscopy may establish a diagnosis of GERD in the presence of erosive esophagitis, Barrett's esophagus, or nonmalignant stenosis. Other indirect contributors to GERD, such as hiatal hernia, may also be found.

In the absence of erosive esophagitis or Barrett's esophagus, endoscopy has poor specificity and sensitivity. Almost half of the patients with pH monitoring-proven GERD may have a normal endoscopy. This is in part due to the widespread and liberal use of acid-reducing medications that may mask the real endoscopic findings. Furthermore, there are no specific findings for proximal reflux, such as proximal esophagitis.

Esophageal Function Tests

Manometry evaluates changes in the esophageal motility that may be associated with GERD physiopathology, such as lower esophageal sphincter (LES) competence and esophageal body peristalsis; however, manometry cannot confirm a suspected diagnosis of GERD. In the case of extraesophageal symptoms, the analysis of the upper esophageal sphincter (UES) is controversial. While some authors believe a hypotonic UES is part of a panesophageal motor dysfunction that affects all 3 barriers to aspiration – the lower esophageal sphincter, the esophageal peristalsis, and the UES – others believe that a hypertonic UES in some patients is a natural mechanism to protect against aspiration.

Ambulatory pH monitoring is the gold standard test for the diagnosis of GERD. Although the threshold for distal reflux is very well defined and widely accepted, the normative value for proximal acid reflux is a controversial topic. There is no widely accepted reference value for proximal acid or nonacid exposure.

Apart from acid exposure, pH monitoring may evaluate temporal correlation between symptoms and episodes of reflux. A positive correlation is probably the best method to incriminate GERD as the pathogenesis for symptoms. Furthermore, a positive correlation also predicts response to treatment. Obviously, some symptoms are not temporally correlated to reflux but the result of chronic inflammation, such as hoarseness, and, thus, not amenable to temporal symptom–reflux correlation. Different methods have been described to interpret the correlation between reflux and symptoms. The most important are:

(a) Symptom Index (SI): it is defined as the percentage of symptom episodes that are related to reflux. Although very simple to understand and use, it does not consider the number of reflux and the number of symptoms. Thus a patient with 200 episodes of reflux and 20 of them correlated to symptoms will have a SI of 10 % as much as a patient with 10 episodes of reflux, one of them correlated to symptoms. Similarly, a SI of 50 % will be found in a patient that referred 2 episodes of symptom with 1 of them correlated to reflux and another patient with 100 episodes of symptom with 50 of them correlated to reflux. SI is more likely to be positive when the number of reflux episodes is high. There is no consensus on which percentage represents a significant correlation with number ranging from 50 to 80 %.

(b) Symptom Sensitivity Index (SSI): it is defined as the percentage of the number of symptom associated reflux episodes over the total number of reflux episodes. SSI is more likely to be positive when the number of symptom episodes is high. Values over 10 % are considered significant.

(c) Symptom-Association Probability (SAP): it is a complex mathematical equation that represents the likelihood that the patient's symptoms are related to reflux. Although it is considered the best method by some authors, the number obtained is often a fraction and not intuitive. An SAP >95 % is statistically significant.

Studies of impedance–pH measurements in patients on acid-reducing medications showed that nonacid proximal reflux may cause extraesophageal symptoms; however, clinical use of impedance–pH may be controversial due to studies with controversial results, the rarity of isolated nonacid reflux because it seems that it parallels acid reflux, and a lack of clinical implication regarding prognosis, therapeutic decisions, or postoperative evaluation.

Laryngoscopy

Laryngoscopy is an office procedure frequently performed by ENT surgeons in patients with suspected GERD. The findings suggestive of GER are erythema, edema, ventricular obliteration, post-cricoid hyperplasia, and pseudosulcus. These findings, however, are suboptimal predictors for GERD because they have low sensitivity and specificity.

Belafsky developed a complex scoring in order to improve accuracy. It is based on 8 findings: subglottic edema, ventricular edema, erythema, vocal cord edema, diffuse laryngeal edema, hypertrophy of the posterior commissure, granuloma or granulation tissue, and thick endolaryngeal mucus. The total score can range from 0 (best) to 26 (worst) (Table 7.1).

Other Tests

Barium esophagram may show gastric reflux to the upper esophagus or even pharynx; however, the sensitivity of the test is poor and no objective parameters can be measured.

Table 7.1 Belafsky reflux score system for laryngoscopy

Finding	Score
Subglottic edema	Absent – 0/Present – 2
Ventricular obliteration	Absent – 0/Partial – 2/Complete – 4
Erythema/hyperemia	Absent – 0/Arytenoids – 2/Diffuse – 4
Vocal fold edema	Absent – 0/Mild – 1/Moderate – 2/Severe – 3 /Polypoid – 4
Diffuse laryngeal edema	Absent – 0/Mild – 1/Moderate – 2/Severe – 3/Obstructing – 4
Post. commissure hypertrophy	Absent – 0/ Mild – 1 /Moderate – 2/Severe – 3/Obstructing – 4
Granuloma	Absent – 0/Present – 2
Thick endolaryngeal mucus	Absent – 0/Present – 2

Detection of pepsin, bile salts, and other digestive substances in bronchioalveolar lavage is feasible but rarely used in clinical practice.

The Bernstein test consists in the dripping of acid into the esophagus through a nasogastric tube in order to incite symptoms. This test is no longer used.

Oropharyngeal pH testing detects liquid and aerosolized acid in the oropharynx with some technical advantages over conventional pH meters. The real clinical use of the device is still under scrutiny.

Target Organs

Otorhinolaryngology Manifestations

Common reflux-related otorhinolaryngology disorders are chronic laryngitis and, according to recent evidence, potentially also chronic sinusitis and otitis media. Less common are contact ulceration and granuloma, laryngeal and subglottic stenosis, and laryngeal carcinoma. A large case control study examining over 100,000 patients with erosive esophagitis or esophageal stricture found significant associations between these findings and several otorhinolaryngology disorders when compared to healthy controls. Other studies, however, did not find more reflux by pH monitoring in patients in comparison to volunteers. The similarity of proximal acid exposure in healthy individuals and patients may show that laryngopharyngeal sensitivity to acid may play a role in the genesis of symptoms.

Belafsky developed a clinical scoring system to suggest that laryngopharyngeal reflux is the cause of laryngitis or pharyngitis. A number above 13 is considered positive (Table 7.2).

The exact relationship between proximal reflux and laryngeal malignancy is unclear, but the available data suggest that most patients who develop laryngeal cancer both smoke and have laryngopharyngeal reflux. In a study reporting 31 consecutive cases of laryngeal carcinoma, less than 60 % of these patients were active smokers but 84 % had LPR verified by pH-metry.

Table 7.2 Belafsky clinical scoring system to laryngopharyngeal reflux

Within the last month, how did the following problems affect you?
(Grade symptoms from 0 (no problem) to 5 (severe problem))
1. Hoarseness or a problem with your voice
2. Clearing your throat
3. Excess throat mucus or postnasal drip
4. Difficulty swallowing food, liquids, or pills
5. Coughing after you ate or after lying down
6. Breathing difficulties or choking episodes
7. Troublesome or annoying cough
8. Sensation of something sticking in your throat or a lump in your throat
9. Heartburn, chest pain, indigestion, or stomach acid coming up

Lung Manifestations

The association of GERD and pulmonary diseases is well known. Many studies have shown a higher incidence of GERD in patients with asthma, fibrosis, lung abscess, chronic cough, bronchitis, and chronic obstructive pulmonary disease (COPD). The pathophysiology of these diseases may be linked to the reflux and the reflex theories; thus, proximal reflux and aspiration may not necessary be found during workup. Extraesophageal GERD complaints are frequently common to the symptomatic manifestation of the lung disease and thus a confounding factor. Therefore clinical questionnaires are insufficient and objective determination of GERD is mandatory for the correct management of these patients.

Asthma is a heterogeneous clinical syndrome characterized by nonspecific airway hyperresponsiveness and inflammation. GERD is a trigger and/or comorbid disorder in approximately 75 % of asthmatics with adult onset of the disease, and it is recognized as a risk factor for asthma exacerbations as well as a key factor in difficult-to-treat asthma. It must be remembered that most asthma medications affect esophageal motility, especially the lower esophageal sphincter tonus, thus accentuating GERD.

Chronic cough is defined as a cough with >8 weeks' duration. GERD account for near 10 % of the cases. Other causes to be excluded are the use of medications (especially angiotensin inhibitors), smoking, postnasal drip syndrome, and asthma.

Idiopathic pulmonary fibrosis (IPF) is an interstitial lung disease characterized by aberrant fibroblast proliferation which is felt to be secondary to recurrent epithelial injury. Recently, different studies showed a higher prevalence of GERD in these patients, and surgical antireflux therapy showed to improve significantly the outcomes of these patients, even taking some patients out of the waiting list for lung transplantation.

Table 7.3 Smith and Knight Classification for dental erosion (tooth wear)

0 – no loss of enamel surface characteristics, no cervical loss of contour
1 – loss of enamel surface characteristics or cervical minimal loss of contour
2 – loss of enamel exposing dentine for less than one third of surface or cervical defect less than 1 mm deep
3 – loss of enamel exposing dentine for more than one third of surface, loss of enamel and substantial loss of dentine, or cervical defect less than 1–2 mm deep
4 – complete enamel loss–pulp exposure–secondary dentine exposure or cervical defect more than 2 mm deep–pulp exposure–secondary dentine exposure

COPD is probably the main pulmonary disease that lacks a satisfactory number of studies dealing with esophageal function tests and objective evaluation of acid exposure and esophageal motility. However, some series shows a high prevalence of GERD. The response to treatment is still elusive.

In general, most of the pulmonary diseases associated to GERD show only a modest response to medical therapy with acid-reducing medications, since available drugs do not prevent reflux and the aspiration of gastric contents is nocive to the lungs irrespective of pH.

Oral Manifestations

Dental

Dental erosions have been reported in up to 65 % of GERD patients. However, the topic is controversial due to conflicting results and other possible causes for dental erosions, such as alteration in the saliva composition and ingestion of caustic food. Nevertheless, most authors believe gastric acid is able to reach the teeth and dissolve the hydroxyapatite crystals in enamel. Tooth erosion is highly unlikely to be caused by alkaline bile juices.

The diagnostic criteria for dental erosions are loss of tooth structure of noncarious etiology, outside the areas of contact or occlusal guidance, and a glossy, smooth, rounded shape. The severity of the erosion areas may be quantified using different indices. The most common is the one proposed by Smith and Knight (Table 7.3).

Halitosis

Halitosis affects a large proportion of the population. The exact pathophysiological mechanism of halitosis is unclear, although it has been attributed mainly to oral maladies. The association between halitosis and digestive diseases is very controversial. While some studies point out a strong correlation between halitosis and altered upper endoscopy or GERD symptoms, others do not show this correlation, but most authors agree that halitosis may be an extraesophageal symptom of GERD.

GERD is found in about 15 % of the patients in series of patients with halitosis. Also, the presence of volatile sulfur-containing compounds in the exhaled air measured at the halimeter correlates with esophagitis.

Cardiac and Noncardiac Chest Pain

GERD may lead to episodes of reflux referred as chest pain or induce esophageal dysmotility also reported as pain. Moreover, GERD may induce a vagal reflex culminating in coronary vasoconstriction and transitory heart ischemia. Other confounding factors muddy the waters during the evaluation of patients with chest pain, such as the sharing of risk factors for both GERD and heart diseases (obesity, smoking), triggers for symptoms (copious meals, exercise, strong emotions), symptoms (pain may be described as squeezing or burning in the substernal location with possible radiation to the neck, arms, or back), and amelioration with smooth muscle relaxants.

Cardiac pain may have an origin due to a cardioesophageal reflex mediated by the vagi nerve. Physiological studies showed that balloon distention of the esophagus and the instillation of chloridric acid into the esophagus may lead to bradycardia, tachycardia, or coronary spasm.

Noncardiac chest pain was considered by the Montreal Consensus on GERD an esophageal manifestation; however, the topic will be treated in this chapter as most authors still consider the symptom an extraesophageal manifestation of the disease. The pain may occur due to esophageal mucosal stimulation with gastroduodenal contents or, more commonly, due to dysmotility. Esophageal motility disorders may be considered primary (when no other cause is diagnosed) or secondary (when a cause is detected, such as GERD). Primary disorders must be treated with smooth muscle relaxants such as nitrates or calcium channel blockers. Dysmotility secondary to GERD must have the treatment directed toward reflux control, either medically or surgically.

Obviously, these patients must be checked for coronary artery disease. Esophageal function tests are also required since esophageal manometry may demonstrate a dysmotility pattern that may explain the symptoms and pH monitoring may confirm pathologic reflux and prevent unnecessary time loss and costs with inadequate treatments or even avoid disastrous consequence such as the prescription of smooth muscle relaxants that will lead to relaxation of the lower esophageal sphincter in patients with GERD.

Sleep Manifestations

Nighttime GERD symptoms are reported by 2/3 of the GERD patients. One study showed that 75 % of GERD patients reported that these symptoms affected their sleep, 63 % believed that heartburn negatively affected their ability to sleep well,

40 % believed that sleep difficulties caused by nighttime heartburn impaired their ability to function the following day, 42 % stated that they accepted they could not sleep through the night, 39 % reported that they took naps whenever possible, 34 % reported sleeping in a chair or in a seated position, and 27 % reported that their heartburn-induced sleep disturbances kept their spouses from having a good night's sleep.

Nocturnal episodes of reflux arise and may be more severe than daytime reflux due to delayed gastric emptying, decreased pressure of the upper esophageal sphincter, diminished esophageal peristalsis, and decreased saliva secretion that occur during sleep. Awakening from sleep because of GERD symptoms (heartburn, regurgitation, or cough mainly) results in initiation of swallowing and increase in esophageal clearance to prevent aspiration. Studies with simultaneous pH and polysomnogram also showed that GERD episodes during the night may be symptomatic or not; thus even patients without GERD night symptoms may have sleep problems related to GERD. Accordingly, suspected cases must undergo a pH monitoring.

Few studies have shown improvement in night symptoms and subjective impression on sleep quality after clinical therapy for GERD with proton pump inhibitors; however, amelioration in objective parameters measured during a polysomnogram has not been demonstrated.

The literature is scarce in regard to the outcomes of antireflux operations and sleep problems.

Sexual Manifestations

Chronic diseases may affect sexual behavior due to the onset of symptoms during intercourse, the reduced sense of well-being, and the awareness of being chronically ill. This may significantly affect quality of life. GERD may course with all these conditions.

Heartburn can occur during sexual intercourse, a condition called "reflux dyspareunia," as coined by Kirk in 1986. This author found a prevalence of 77 % of this condition when women are actively interrogated about the symptom. Very interestingly, 80 % of them improved after GERD treatment. Other study found similar results with difficulty in attaining orgasm and painful intercourse as the main complaints and significant improvement with treatment, either medical or surgical.

Psychologic/Psychiatric Manifestation

GERD symptoms are reported by almost half of the psychiatric patients. On the other hand, GERD patients demonstrate significantly higher anxiety and depression scores as compared with normal subjects. This strong association of the diseases may be multifactorial. Psychiatric diseases, from complex illness to as simple as acute stress, may reduce esophageal perception thresholds for pain resulting in low-intensity stimuli perceived as being painful or lead to hypervigilance and overreporting of stimulus intensity. This is marked in patients with GERD and symptoms linked to esophageal hypersensitivity such as noncardiac chest pain. Parallel to the psychiatric diseases, the use of psychotropic medication that may affect esophageal clearance or LES pressure, smoking, and alcohol drinking are common in this population.

The outcome of either medical or surgical therapy for GERD is severely affected by psychiatric disorders. One study showed that the satisfaction with antireflux operations drops from 95 to 11 % if a psychiatric disorder is detected. Psychological intervention improves results.

Conclusions

GERD may affect directly or indirectly several organs apart from the esophagus.

Diagnosing extraesophageal symptoms of GERD can be difficult due to the lack of concomitant typical symptoms of GERD, which can be absent in 40–60 % of asthmatics, 57–94 % of patients with otolaryngology complaints, and 43–75 % of patients with chronic cough. The diagnosis of GERD as a cause of extraesophageal symptoms needs a high degree of suspicion and very careful evaluation of patients. It must also be in mind that the diagnosis of pathologic proximal reflux and microaspiration must be based on a sum of clinical parameters, not from a single piece of information, since the accuracy of diagnostic tests (laryngoscopy, endoscopy, and pH or impedance–pH monitoring) for patients with suspected extraesophageal manifestations of gastroesophageal reflux disease is suboptimal.

Response of extraesophageal symptoms to treatment is inferior to the response of esophageal GERD symptoms. The key for treating these patients is based on clinical evaluation, proper testing, and tailored treatment.

Summary

- GERD may affect directly or indirectly several organs apart from the esophagus.
- GERD may cause extraesophageal symptoms due to reflux of gastric contents into adjacent organs, neural reflex due to esophageal stimulation, increased visceral sensitivity to physiologic reflux, or indirect involvement.
- The diagnosis of extraesophageal manifestations of GERD may be difficult, since symptoms mimic other diseases, causes may be multifactorial, and the accuracy of diagnostic tests is suboptimal.
- Objective evaluation for GERD may save time, money, and unnecessary treatment.

- A careful evaluation of patients with extraesophageal manifestations of GERD and the correct understanding of the pathophysiology of the disease are necessary to enhance outcomes since therapy may not bring excellent results.

Selected Reading

1. Belafsky PC, Postma GN, Koufman JA. The validity and reliability of the reflux finding score (RFS). Laryngoscope. 2001;111:1313–7. The paper describes a scoring system for laryngoscopic findings in GERD.
2. Belafsky PC, Postma GN, Koufman JA. Validity and reliability of the reflux symptom index (RSI). J Voice. 2002;16:274–7. A clinical score system for suspected pharyngo-laryngeal reflux.
3. Bredenoord AJ, Weusten BL, Smout AJ. Symptom association analysis in ambulatory gastrooesophageal reflux monitoring. Gut. 2005;54:1810–7. A good review on the methods for the evaluation of symptom-reflux correlation at the pH monitoring.
4. Fujiwara Y, Arakawa T, Fass R. Gastroesophageal reflux disease and sleep. Gastroenterol Clin North Am. 2013;42:57–70. An extensive review on sleep disturbances and GERD.
5. Heatley M, Rose K, Weston C. The heart and the oesophagus: intimate relations. Postgrad Med J. 2005;81:515–8. A comprehensive review on the link between GERD and the heart.
6. Herbella FA, Patti MG. Gastroesophageal reflux disease: from pathophysiology to treatment. World J Gastroenterol. 2010;16:3745–9. A review on GERD pathophysiology.
7. Iovino P, Pascariello A, Limongelli P, Tremolaterra F, Consalvo D, Sabbatini F, Amato G, Ciacci C. The prevalence of sexual behavior disorders in patients with treated and untreated gastroesophageal reflux disease. Surg Endosc. 2007;21:1104–10. Epub 2007 Mar 13. This study analyzed sexual manifestation in patients with GERD compared to healthy volunteers.
8. Jobe BA, Richter JE, Hoppo T, Peters JH, Bell R, Dengler WC, DeVault K, Fass R, Gyawali CP, Kahrilas PJ, Lacy BE, Pandolfino JE, Patti MG, Swanstrom LL, Kurian AA, Vela MF, Vaezi M, DeMeester TR. Preoperative diagnostic workup before antireflux surgery: an evidence and experience-based consensus of the Esophageal Diagnostic Advisory Panel. J Am Coll Surg. 2013;217:586–97. doi:10.1016/j.jamcollsurg.2013.05.023. Epub 2013 Aug 21. A consensus from experts from the field on diagnostic workup for GERD.
9. Kirk AJ. Reflux dyspareunia. Thorax. 1986;41:215–6. The first description and a significant series of sexual manifestation of GERD.
10. Madanick RD. Extraesophageal presentations of GERD: where is the science? Gastroenterol Clin North Am. 2014;43:105–20. A comprehensive review on different extra-esophageal symptoms of GERD.
11. Marsicano JA, de Moura-Grec PG, Bonato RC, Sales-Peres Mde C, Sales-Peres A, Sales-Peres SH. Gastroesophageal reflux, dental erosion, and halitosis in epidemiological surveys: a systematic review. Eur J Gastroenterol Hepatol. 2013;25:135–41. A systematic review showing controversies in the association of GERD and halitosis, but a significant number of publications pointing to a casual effect.
12. Mizyed I, Fass SS, Fass R. Review article: gastro-oesophageal reflux disease and psychological comorbidity. Aliment Pharmacol Ther. 2009;29:351–8. doi:10.1111/j.1365-2036.2008.03883.x. Epub 2008 Nov 8. A systematic review on the association of GERD and psychologic/psychiatric manifestations.
13. Neto SC, Herbella FA, Silva LC, Patti MG. Ratio between proximal/distal gastroesophageal reflux does not discriminate abnormal proximal reflux. World J Surg. 2014;38(4):890–6. doi: 10.1007/s00268-013-2341-x.
14. Oranu AC, Vaezi MF. Noncardiac chest pain: gastroesophageal reflux disease. Med Clin North Am. 2010;94:233–42. An excellent review on GERD as a cause of chest pain.

15. Pearson JP, Parikh S, Orlando RC, Johnston N, Allen J, Tinling SP, Johnston N, Belafsky P, Arevalo LF, Sharma N, Castell DO, Fox M, Harding SM, Morice AH, Watson MG, Shields MD, Bateman N, McCallion WA, van Wijk MP, Wenzl TG, Karkos PD, Belafsky PC. Review article: reflux and its consequence--he laryngeal, pulmonary and oesophageal manifestations. Conference held in conjunction with the 9th International Symposium on Human Pepsin (ISHP) Kingston-upon-Hull, UK, 21-23 April 2010. Aliment Pharmacol Ther. 2011;33 Suppl 1:1–71. A series of 11 articles dealing with the pathophysiology of GERD and extra-esophageal manifestation.
16. Picos A, Chisnoiu A, Dumitrasc DL. Dental erosion in patients with gastroesophageal reflux disease. Adv Clin Exp Med. 2013;22:303–7. A review on dental erosion and GERD.
17. Sweet MP, Patti MG, Hoopes C, Hays SR, Golden JA. Gastro-oesophageal reflux and aspiration in patients with advanced lung disease. Thorax. 2009;64:167–73. A review on GERD and pulmonary diseases.
18. Velanovich V, Karmy-Jones R. Psychiatric disorders affect outcomes of antireflux operations for gastroesophageal reflux disease. Surg Endosc. 2001;15:171–5. This study shows that the outcomes of antireflux operations are severely affected by psychiatric comorbidity.

Chapter 8
Epiphrenic Diverticulum

Anahita Jalilvand and P. Marco Fisichella

Abstract The goal of this chapter is to describe the pathophysiology, clinical presentation, and proper methods of diagnosis and treatment of patients with epiphrenic diverticula. Finally, an overview of the surgical management will be provided and the indications for surgery and the description of the laparoscopic repair and the thoracic approach will be described.

Keywords Epiphrenic diverticula • Gastroesophageal reflux disease • Laparoscopic antireflux surgery • Esophageal function testing • Laparoscopic repair • Thoracoscopic repair

Epiphrenic diverticula are a rare disease that is commonly associated with an underlying motility disorder of the esophagus. Treatment of this underlying motility disorders must be included in the management of epiphrenic diverticula to prevent postoperative complications and recurrences.

A. Jalilvand, MD
Department of Surgery, Loyola University Medical Center and Loyola Stritch School of Medicine, 2160 South 1st Ave, Maywood, IL, USA

P.M. Fisichella, MD, MBA, FACS (✉)
Department of Surgery, Boston Veteran Administration Healthcare System, 1400 VFW Parkway, West Roxbury, MA 02132, USA

Department of Surgery, Brigham and Women's Hospital, Harvard Medical, Boston, MA USA
e-mail: piero.fisichella@va.gov

P.M. Fisichella et al. (eds.), *Esophageal Diseases*,
DOI 10.1007/978-3-319-04337-1_8, © Springer International Publishing Switzerland 2014

Pathophysiology

Esophageal diverticula are generally categorized using two characteristics: their anatomic location along the esophagus and whether they are pulsion or traction diverticula. The most common anatomic presentations are at the pharyngoesophageal junction, the mid-esophagus, and the epiphrenic region. Pharyngoesophageal or Zenker's diverticula are by far the most common presentation, while epiphrenic are the least common. The distinction between pulsion and traction diverticula relates to the mechanism of the diverticulum. Pulsion diverticula occur due to an increase in intraluminal pressure, which over time can create a false diverticulum. This type of diverticulum consists only of mucosal and submucosal layers. In contrast to this, traction diverticula, which are seen typically in the mid-esophageal region, are caused by external traction on the esophageal wall, such as might be seen in chronic mediastinal inflammation from tuberculosis or histoplasmosis. By exerting force on the outside of the esophagus rather than from within, as in the case of increased intraluminal pressure, this kind of external traction can lead to a true diverticulum, which involves all three mucosal, submucosal, and muscular layers of the esophageal wall.

Epiphrenic diverticula are classified as pulsion or false diverticula. As their name implies, they are located in the distal esophagus and typically arise below the lower esophageal sphincter. They are commonly found on the right side of the esophagus. There has been a very well documented pathophysiologic link between the presence of esophageal motility disorders and the incidence of epiphrenic diverticula. In fact, anywhere from 35 to 100 % of patients with epiphrenic diverticula can have comorbid motility disorders, which include achalasia, diffuse esophageal spasm, nonspecific esophageal motility disorders, and nutcracker esophagus. Given such high prevalence of esophageal dysmotility in these patients, it is currently thought that epiphrenic diverticula are caused by an underlying motility pathology, which involves a lack of coordination between the distal esophagus and the lower esophageal sphincter. Over time, this discoordination can lead to increased intraluminal pressure and the development of an outpouching of esophageal mucosal and submucosal layers. Although the motility disorder is thought to be initiating the pathology, it is often diagnosed secondary to the presence of the diverticulum when symptoms usually prompt diagnostic investigations. It is speculated that the episodic nature of motility disorders at the very early stages may account for the delay in diagnosis.

Epidemiology

Of all esophageal diverticula, epiphrenic diverticula are the least common. Since many patients with this pathology are asymptomatic, particularly when the diverticula are small, their true incidence is not well documented. Most commonly, epiphrenic diverticula are observed in either middle-aged or elderly populations, which is consistent with a gradual weakness in the esophageal wall observed in the pathophysiology of pulsion diverticula. Malignant conversion of epiphrenic diverticula has been reported in the literature and can occur in 0.3–3.3 % of patients. Most often, these are patients who were asymptomatic and therefore were never diagnosed with an epiphrenic diverticulum. For this reason, when these patients do present clinically, the malignancy is typically at an advanced stage. The most common malignant type of cancer that arises in epiphrenic diverticula is of the squamous type, and the malignant transformation is thought to arise secondary to chronic stasis and fermentation of food within the diverticula.

Clinical Presentation

The majority of epiphrenic diverticula are found incidentally. In fact, less than 40 % of patients with epiphrenic diverticula complain of any symptoms. However, when patients are symptomatic, commonly reported symptoms include dysphagia, regurgitation of undigested food, chest pain, heartburn, nocturnal aspiration, aspiration pneumonia, and, if severe, weight loss. Because the etiology of the diverticulum is often the underlying motility disorder of the esophagus, most symptoms such as dysphagia, regurgitation, chest pain, and heartburn may be due to the motility disorder rather than the diverticulum itself. This is why the size of the diverticulum does not correlate to the severity of symptoms experienced by the patient. Regurgitation of undigested food, nocturnal aspiration, and aspiration pneumonia, however, are more suggestive of a symptomatic diverticulum, but again, little correlation between the size of the diverticulum and the severity of these symptoms has been found. Lastly, when the diverticulum becomes large enough, it may cause odynophagia and weight loss by compressing the esophagus.

Diagnostic Testing

Evaluation of epiphrenic diverticula begins by assessing the severity of the patient's symptoms; dysphagia, regurgitation, and aspiration are considered indications for further clinical assessment. Importantly, dysphagia should always prompt in ruling out esophageal cancer. Further diagnostic workup includes the following: barium esophagogram, upper endoscopy, and esophageal manometry, with or without ambulatory pH monitoring.

Barium esophagogram is typically the first diagnostic test to be performed. Not only are the findings diagnostic, but a contrast esophagogram can provide useful information for surgical planning, including the location of the diverticulum (left or right chest and distance from the diaphragmatic hiatus), the diameter of its pouch, as well as the length and width of its neck (Fig. 8.1). Barium esophagogram can also depict any abnormalities of the gastroesophageal junction, such as hiatal hernias or

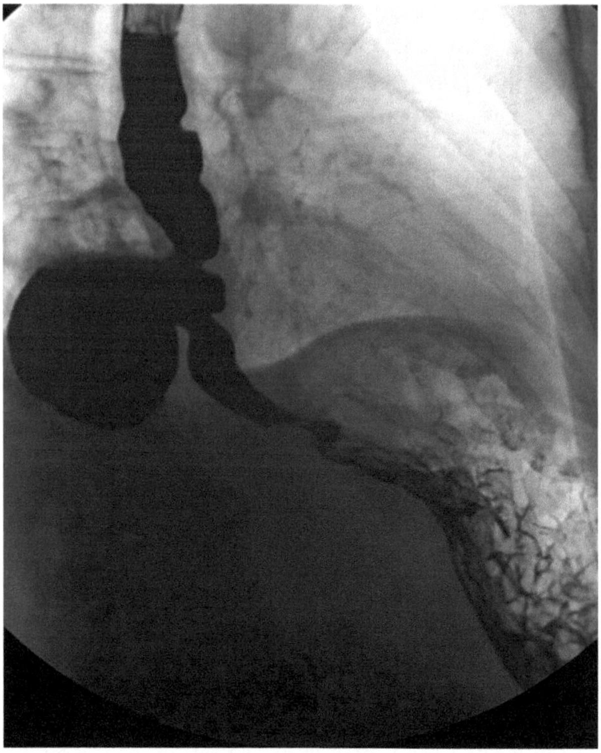

Fig. 8.1 The barium esophagogram shows a 6×7 cm epiphrenic diverticulum with an underlying esophageal motility disorder (corkscrew esophagus). In this 88-year-old male, the diverticulum was located high in the mediastinum and the barium swallow allowed planning a thoracoscopic resection

lesions suspicious for a malignant process. Furthermore, disordered contractions of the distal esophagus, corkscrew esophagus from diffuse esophageal spasm, or tertiary contractions can also be seen on esophagograms, which can prove useful in providing information on esophageal motility. Hiatal hernias are sometimes identified in conjunction with epiphrenic diverticula as well.

Upper endoscopy is used to evaluate for mucosal lesions within the diverticulum and to search for any additional pathology in the upper gastrointestinal tract, such as esophageal and gastric ulcers, Barrett's esophagus, or esophagitis, which may contribute the patient's clinical presentation. As with any esophageal pathology, any masses suspicious for malignancy should be documented and taken into consideration before any surgical management is attempted. Another advantage of performing an upper endoscopy after the contrast study of the esophagus is that the presence of the esophageal diverticulum detected on barium esophagogram may alert the provider performing the endoscopy to avoid intubating and perforating the diverticulum.

Esophageal manometry is usually performed to identify and classify definitively any underlying motility disorders. Some may argue, however, that manometry has only an academic role, as its results would not modify the patients' surgical treatment, should one assume that almost if not all epiphrenic diverticula are caused by an underlying esophageal motility disorder. Conversely, most argue that the documentation of any existing esophageal dysmotility is fundamental to determining with certainty any underlying motility disorders. Commonly identified motility disorders of the esophagus most likely associated with esophageal diverticula include achalasia, diffuse esophageal spasm, nutcracker esophagus, and hypertensive esophagus. While identification of the esophageal dysmotility is very important, normal manometry results should not be used to influence the surgical management. In fact, in a few cases, due to the episodic nature of most motility disorders, normal manometry results do not necessarily exclude the presence of dysmotility.

Finally, ambulatory pH monitoring may also be obtained to further characterize patients who are presenting with symptoms such as heartburn and regurgitation in order to rule out GERD. This step may be unnecessary in most cases but is important in selected patients as the treatment of GERD is diametrically opposite to that of the epiphrenic diverticulum and/or an esophageal motility disorder.

Indications for Surgery

Proper treatment and management strategies for patients with esophageal diverticula have been a source of controversy. To begin with, the surgical options for definitive treatment are typically very challenging and can only be performed by experienced foregut surgeons. Furthermore, even in expert hands, these surgeries have the potential for very serious complications, such as esophageal perforation, leak, or empyema. On the other hand, because of the potentially life-threatening complications from epiphrenic diverticula, such as aspiration pneumonia, some have argued that all epiphrenic diverticula should be resected regardless of the symptoms. There is additional concern that larger diverticula have an increased, albeit small, risk for malignant transformation of the diverticular mucosa due to long-standing inflammation. Most of the current literature, however, suggests that the risks of surgical management outweigh the incidence of these rare complications. Therefore, treatment of epiphrenic diverticula is thus usually reserved for symptomatic patients who are considered good surgical candidates.

Overview of Surgical Management

Management of epiphrenic diverticula requires three steps: addressing the underlying motility disorder, removal of the diverticulum, and prevention of postoperative GERD. The steps of the operation (performed with the laparoscopic approach) are illustrated in Figs. 8.2, 8.3, 8.4, 8.5, and 8.6. These steps are usually accomplished by performing an esophageal myotomy to address underlying motility disorders, a diverticulectomy when appropriate (when the diverticulum is big enough to be resected safely), and a partial fundoplication to address postoperative reflux symptoms. The performance of a partial posterior or a partial anterior fundoplication does not have a preferential effect in preventing GERD postoperatively: both work

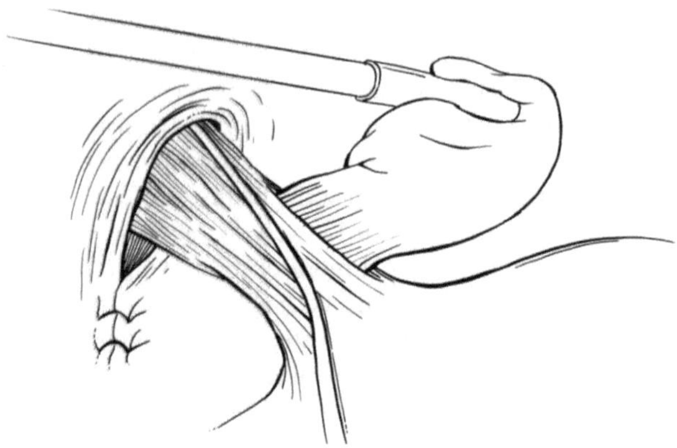

Fig. 8.2 The surgical management of a patient with a diverticulum includes the three steps illustrated in Figs. 8.2, 8.3, 8.4, 8.5, and 8.6: diverticulectomy, myotomy, and partial fundoplication. An epiphrenic diverticulum is shown delivered below the diaphragm into the abdominal cavity and with its neck completely mobilized. Its relationship with the anterior vagus nerve is demonstrated. The hiatus has been closed with two stitches without tension

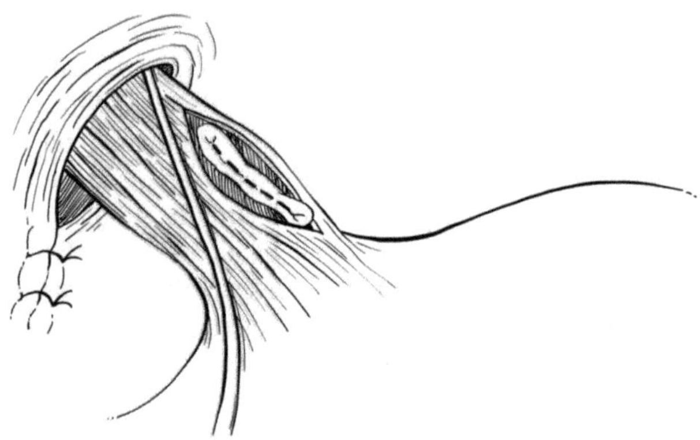

Fig. 8.3 The stump of the neck of the diverticulum with the longitudinal staple line across the esophageal submucosa is shown

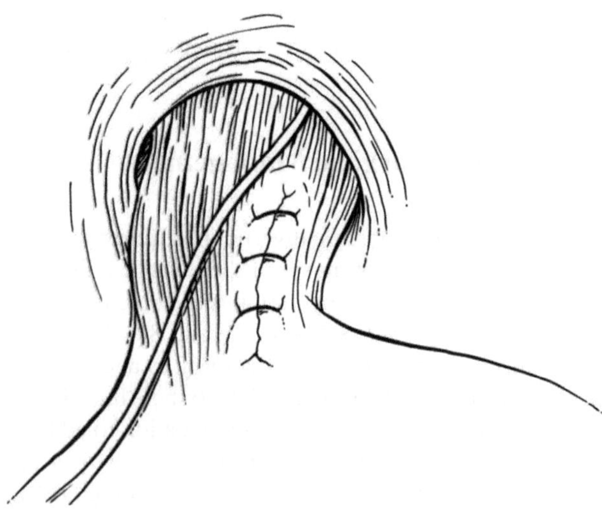

Fig. 8.4 The defect of the esophageal musculature is closed with interrupted sutures to imbricate the staple line

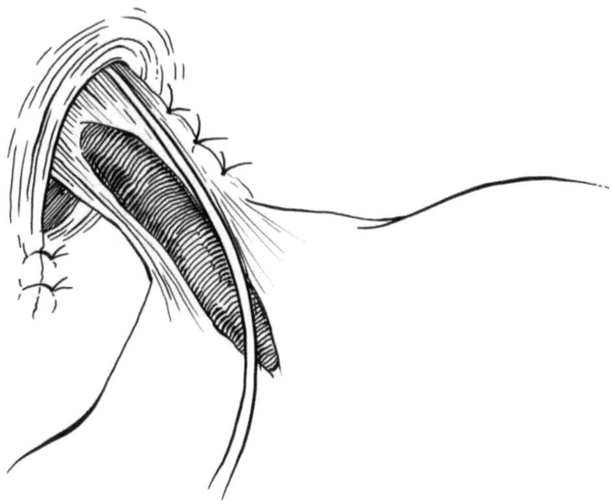

Fig. 8.5 A contralateral cardiomyotomy is shown extending onto the body of the esophagus and for 3 cm onto the anterior wall of the stomach. The cardiomyotomy is 10 cm long and it is located contralateral to the original location of the diverticulum

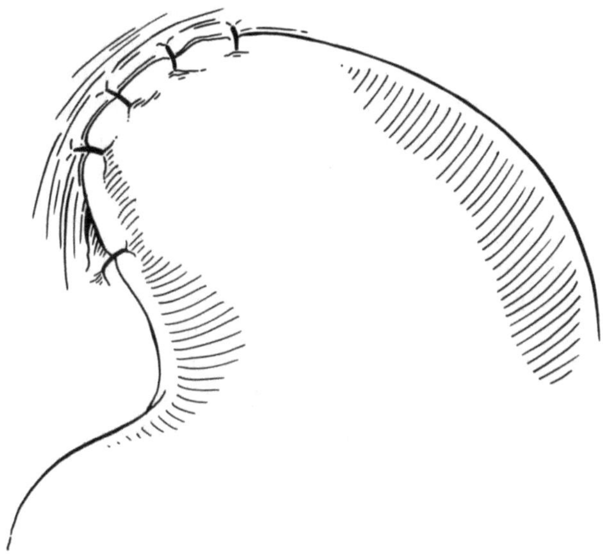

Fig. 8.6 A completed partial anterior 180° fundoplication is fashioned by folding the gastric fundus over the myotomy and the staple line and suturing it superiorly onto the apex of the left and right pillars of the crus diaphragm and then medially onto the right edge of the myotomy as described originally by André Dor in 1962

equally well. However, in those patients who receive an esophageal myotomy, the myotomy incision can result in an incompetent LES, and in order to prevent the resultant GERD, an anterior partial fundoplication is usually done to protect the myotomy in case of inadvertent perforation or to protect the staple line of the diverticulectomy against a potential disruption and subsequent leak.

Historically, a transthoracic approach through a right thoracotomy incision has been the standard of care. Since most diverticula are found on the right side of the esophagus, a right-sided incision theoretically allows for better accessibility. In turn, this ensures optimal visualization and access to the distal esophagus and provides the best exposure for the resection of the diverticulum, oversewing of the esophageal musculature over the staple line for diverticulectomy, and contralateral distal esophageal myotomy. Importantly, the right lung is deflated during an open transthoracic approach, and a chest tube is always required postoperatively.

With advances in minimally invasive operative techniques, laparoscopy has also become a reasonable alternative, and it is now considered the approach of choice in most cases. The same steps as described with thoracic approaches are carried out using a laparoscopic approach. The advantages of laparoscopic approach include an avoidance of performing surgery through the chest, which can be a source of significant pain postoperatively and discomfort associated with the chest tube. A thoracoscopic approach can also prolong hospital stay and requires intubation with a double-lumen endotracheal tube or bronchial block by the anesthesiologist. Other advantages of laparoscopic approach include an easier application of endostapler to transect the diverticula (which needs to be applied longitudinally, along the major axis of the esophagus) and greater ease in performing the cardiomyotomy (which needs to be extended at least 3 cm below the gastroesophageal junction onto the anterior wall of the stomach), the partial fundoplication, and the closure of the diaphragmatic hiatus. However, these advantages may be limited in cases with larger diverticula, long distances between the neck of the diverticulum and the hiatus (usually about 10 cm), and the presence of dense adhesions between the diverticulum and adjacent mediastinal structures, making the dissection, application of the stapler, and approximation of the muscle layers more difficult laparoscopically. In these circumstances, video-assisted thoracoscopic surgery (VATS) may be more the appropriate approach of choice.

The most common complication from either surgical approach is leakage from the staple line after diverticulectomy, with other severe complications including sepsis, pneumonia, empyema, and abscess formation. Performing an appropriate myotomy is crucial to obtain symptom resolution when an esophageal motor disorder is identified and to eliminate the risk of a leak. When the diverticulectomy is performed without a myotomy, the staple line is subject to the same high pressures distally that caused the pulsion diverticula initially. To be effective, the esophageal myotomy should be made contralateral to the diverticulum and should extend 5–8 cm above the gastroesophageal junction and not less than 3 cm below the gastroesophageal junction, onto the anterior stomach wall. Vagal nerve injury or transection can also be a complication, particularly with aggressive mediastinal and gastroesophageal dissection.

At present, there are no studies comparing the outcomes of laparoscopic and thoracoscopic approaches, and given the limited number of cases and the variety of surgical techniques and measured outcomes, it is difficult to make a quantitative conclusion about the superiority of one procedure over another. Having said that, both treatment strategies have been shown to be very effective surgical modalities, each approach having its own advantages and disadvantages.

Postoperative Management

When a laparoscopic approach is used, patients typically will be admitted overnight while they remain NPO. The following day, some advocate obtaining a contrast esophagogram to rule out the possibility of a leak at the staple line, at which point, the patient can be slowly transferred to a soft diet. Patients are sent home on a soft diet for approximately a week. Follow-up is usually scheduled for one week postoperatively. Most patients are able to tolerate a full diet at this time.

Patients who underwent a thoracoscopic repair may have a similar hospital course, although they are likely to be admitted for a longer period of time. Most common postoperative complaints are related to pain at the thoracotomy incision site and the discomfort of a chest tube.

Summary

- Epiphrenic diverticula are commonly associated with an underlying motility disorder of the esophagus.
- Retained food within the diverticulum can lead to chronic inflammation, which in turn is associated with a small, albeit rare, chance of malignant degeneration into a squamous cell esophageal cancer.
- Treatment of the underlying motility disorders must be included in the management of epiphrenic diverticula to prevent postoperative leaks (outflow obstruction) and recurrences.
- Symptoms related to epiphrenic diverticula may be due to the underlying motility disorder rather than the diverticulum itself, underlining the importance of addressing motility disorders when considering a treatment option.
- A laparoscopic approach is the approach of choice in most cases.
- A laparoscopic approach consists of the following: diverticulectomy, myotomy, and partial fundoplication.
- A thoracoscopic approach is indicated when the diverticulum is big and located high in the mediastinum.
- The advantages of laparoscopic approach include easier application of endostapler to transect the diverticulum and greater ease in performing the myotomy, the partial fundoplication, and the closure of the diaphragmatic hiatus.
- A thoracoscopic approach can cause considerable postoperative pain and discomfort associated with the chest tube. A thoracoscopic approach can also prolong hospital stay and requires intubation with a double-lumen endotracheal tube or bronchial block by the anesthesiologist.

Selected Reading

1. Del Genio A, Rossetti G, Maffettone V, Renzi A, Brusciano L, Limongelli P, et al. Laparoscopic approach in the treatment of epiphrenic diverticula: long-term results. Surg Endosc. 2004;18:741–5.
2. Fernando HC, Luketich JD, Samphire J, Alvelo-Rivera M, Christie NA, Buenaventura PO, et al. Minimally invasive operation for esophageal diverticula. Ann Thorac Surg. 2005;80(6):2076–80.
3. Fisichella PM. Laparascopic repair of epiphrenic diverticulum. Semin Thorac Cardiovasc Surg. 2012;24:223–8.
4. Fraiji Jr E, Bloomston M, Carey L, Zervos E, Goldin S, Banasiak M, et al. Laparoscopic management of symptomatic achalasia associated with epiphrenic diverticulum. Surg Endosc. 2003;17:1600–3.
5. Lai ST, Hsu CP. Carcinoma arising from an epiphrenic diverticulum: a frequently misdiagnosed disease. Ann Thorac Cardiovasc Surg. 2007;13:110–3.
6. Matthews BD, Nelms CD, Lohr CE, Harold KL, Kercher KW, Heniford BT. Minimally invasive management of epiphrenic esophageal diverticula. Am Surg. 2003;69(6):465–70.
7. Melman L, Quinlan J, Robertson B, Brunt LM, Halpin VJ, Eagon JC, Frisella MM, Matthews BD. Esophageal manometric characteristics and outcomes for laparoscopic esophageal diverticulectomy, myotomy, and partial fundoplication for epiphrenic diverticula. Surg Endosc. 2009;23:1337–41.
8. Nehra D, Lord RV, DeMeester TR, Theisen J, Peters JH, Crookes PF, Bremner CG. Physiologic basis for the treatment of epiphrenic diverticulum. Ann Surg. 2002;235(3):346–54.
9. Rosati R, Fumagalli U, Elmore U, de Pascale S, Massaron S, Peracchia A. Long-term results of minimally invasive surgery for symptomatic epiphrenic diverticulum. Am J Surg. 2011;201(1):132–5.
10. Soares R, Herbella FA, Prachand VN, Ferguson MK, Patti MG. Epiphrenic diverticulum of the esophagus. From pathophysiology to treatment. J Gastrointest Surg. 2010;14:2009–15.
11. Soares RV, Montenovo M, Pellegrini CA, Oelschlager BK. Laparoscopy as the initial approach for epiphrenic diverticula. Surg Endosc. 2011;25(12):3740–6.
12. Tedesco P, Fisichella PM, Way LW, Patti MG. Cause and treatment of epiphrenic diverticula. Am J Surg. 2005;190:902–5.
13. Zaninotto G, Parise P, Salvador R, Costantini M, Zanatta L, Rella A, Ancona E. Laparascopic repair of epiphrenic diverticulum. Semin Thorac Cardiovasc Surg. 2012;24:218–22.

Chapter 9
Evaluation and Treatment of Zenker's Diverticulum

Cheryl C. Nocon and Louis D. Portugal

Abstract The goal of this chapter is to describe the pathophysiology of Zenker's diverticulum, their clinical presentation, and indications for treatment and provide an overview of the surgical management of patients with this rare esophageal pathology. Treatment approaches discussed include open transcervical resection, endoscopic stapled diverticulotomy, endoscopic harmonic scalpel diverticulotomy, and flexible endoscopic diverticulotomy. Finally, a comparison of the open and endoscopic approaches will be provided.

Keywords Zenker's diverticulum • Open transcervical resection • Endoscopic stapled diverticulotomy

Epidemiology, Anatomy, and Pathophysiology

Zenker's diverticulum (ZD), the most common type of diverticulum in the upper gastrointestinal tract, is a mucosal outpouching along the posterior hypopharyngeal wall. More common in men than women, it usually presents after the age of 70 and rarely before the age of 40. Prevalence varies by geography, with ZD more common in northern Europe, the US, Canada, and Australia. Its prevalence in the general population ranges from 0.01 to 0.11 %. However, the true incidence is difficult to

C.C. Nocon, MD (✉) • L.D. Portugal, MD
Section of Otolaryngology-Head and Neck Surgery, The University of Chicago Medical Center, 5841 S. Maryland Avenue, MC 1035, Chicago, IL 60637, USA
e-mail: cheryl.nocon@uchospitals.edu

P.M. Fisichella et al. (eds.), *Esophageal Diseases*,
DOI 10.1007/978-3-319-04337-1_9,

determine given the unknown number of asymptomatic patients who harbor the anatomic abnormality.

ZD originates within Killian's triangle, an area of relative muscular weakness located between the inferior constrictor muscles and the cricopharyngeus muscle (CP). These muscles comprise the upper esophageal sphincter (UES). In ZD, mucosa herniates through the muscular wall, creating a bridge of the mucosa, submucosa, connective tissue, and muscle that separates the diverticular lumen from the esophagus. It tends to develop on the left side, likely due to the slight convexity of the cervical esophagus to the left. The carotid artery is also more laterally positioned on the left, making it less adherent to the adjacent prevertebral fascia and creating a potential space for the sac.

Although it is generally accepted that ZD is an acquired pulsion diverticulum, there is no consensus on the exact mechanism of formation. Theories of pathogenesis center around two main abnormalities: muscular wall weakness and CP/UES dysfunction. Whereas there are no published studies that demonstrate muscular deficiency of the pharyngoesophageal wall, many studies have examined the role of sphincter dysfunction and elevated intrasphincteric pressures. Possible causes include excessive contraction of UES, incomplete UES relaxation, incomplete UES opening, and incoordination of pharyngeal contractions and UES opening. Manometric studies have been inconclusive. Manofluorography, however, has demonstrated abnormally high intrabolus UES pressures resulting from CP spasm. Evidence implicating CP in ZD pathogenesis also comes from studies on the association between CP spasm and gastroesophageal reflux disease (GERD) and the association between GERD and ZD. This relationship is further supported by histologic studies of CP specimens in ZD patients, which have shown increased type I muscle fibers, suggesting tonically active muscle.

Presentation and Evaluation

The most common presenting symptom is dysphagia. Other complaints include regurgitation, choking, halitosis, globus pharyngeus, chronic cough, hoarseness, and recurrent aspiration pneumonia. Patients may report noisy deglutition or borborygmi. There are minimal findings on physical exam but may include hypopharyngeal pooling on laryngoscopy, weight loss, dehydration, and Boyce's sign – a neck mass that gurgles on palpation. Hypopharyngeal pooling of secretions and post-swallow hypopharyngeal reflux are predictive of larger diverticula. An increase in the severity of dysphagia or the development of red flag symptoms – odynophagia, hemoptysis, and hematemesis – should raise suspicion for squamous cell carcinoma within the pouch, which has an incidence of up to 1.1 % (Table 9.1).

Diagnosis is confirmed by barium swallow, which can identify the pouch and define its size (Fig. 9.1). As a dynamic study of the swallowing mechanism, contrast videofluoroscopy is useful in identifying small diverticula that may be missed on a static radiographic image. Endoscopy may also incidentally identify a ZD during a gastrointestinal evaluation. The actual size measured on preoperative barium

Table 9.1 Presentation, evaluation, and treatment of Zenker's diverticulum

Symptoms	Dysphagia, regurgitation, choking, halitosis, globus pharyngeus, chronic cough, borborygmi
Signs	Recurrent aspiration pneumonia, weight loss, dehydration, Boyce's sign, hypopharyngeal pooling on laryngoscopy
Diagnosis	Barium swallow radiography, contrast videofluoroscopy, endoscopy
Treatment	Open: cricopharyngeal myotomy, diverticulectomy, diverticulopexy, diverticular inversion
	Rigid endoscopic: CO_2 laser, stapler, harmonic scalpel
	Flexible endoscopic: needle-knife, argon plasma coagulation, monopolar coagulation

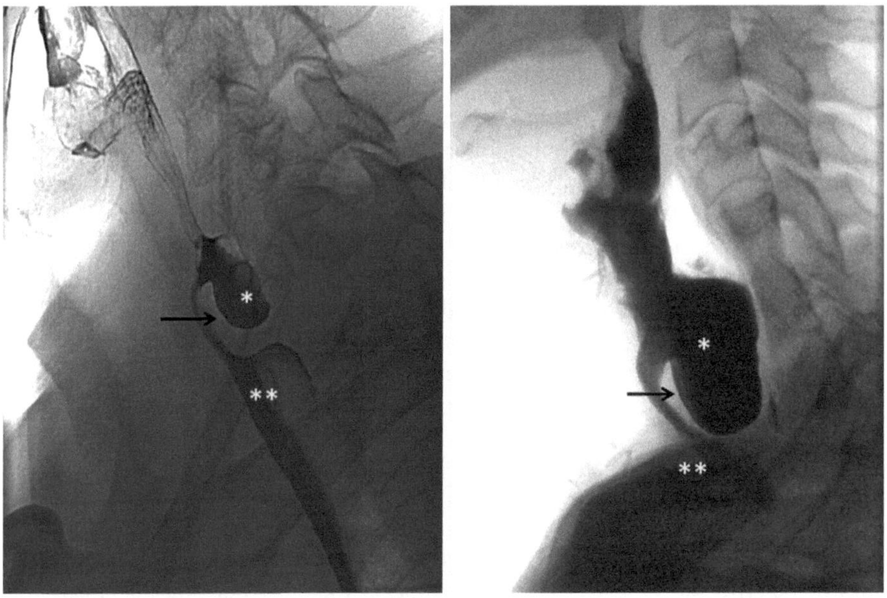

Fig. 9.1 Barium swallow demonstrating diverticula. *Arrow*: cricopharyngeal bar; * diverticulum; ** esophagus

radiography has been shown to correlate with the surgical measurements of the pouch, which can be useful in selecting a surgical approach.

Management of ZD

The main indication for treatment is symptomatic ZD. Complications of ZD that make treatment more urgent include aspiration pneumonia, significant weight loss, and warning signs that are suggestive of malignancy. Relative contraindications include minimal symptoms, small pouches, and comorbidities that preclude safe administration of general anesthesia. Specifically for endoscopic approaches, contraindications include limited neck extension and inadequate oral opening.

In the case of isolated CP dysfunction or asymptomatic small diverticula, nonsurgical options are available, including botulinum toxin injections and balloon dilatation of the UES. Treatment of larger or symptomatic ZD, however, should involve the surgical release of the CP muscle. Because of the role of CP in ZD formation, it is clear that CP myotomy should always be part of the treatment algorithm. Patient and surgeon factors dictate whether an open or endoscopic approach should be employed. If the patient is not a surgical candidate for ZD repair, a gastrostomy tube is ultimately the long-term solution for symptomatic ZD.

Open Transcervical Approach

The traditional approach to ZD has been open transcervical repair. This consists of CP myotomy alone or in combination with diverticulectomy, diverticulopexy, or diverticular inversion. Myotomy should always be included in the surgical management of ZD, given the high rate of long-term recurrence in its absence. Myotomy reduces both UES resting pressures and intrabolus pressures, as demonstrated by pharyngoesophageal manometry.

The patient is orotracheally intubated under general anesthesia. Perioperative antibiotics are routinely administered and usually continued until the start of oral intake. With the patient supine, neck hyperextended, and head turned away from the involved side, an incision is made in a skin crease anterior to the sternocleidomastoid (SCM) muscle at the level of the cricoid cartilage and carried down through platysma. Subplatysmal flaps are raised inferiorly and superiorly. The SCM and carotid sheath are retracted laterally, while the strap muscles, thyroid gland, and larynx are retracted medially. This exposes the pharynx and cervical esophagus. Blunt dissection and careful bipolar cautery of surrounding loose connective tissue help to identify the pouch. The oblique muscle fibers of the inferior constrictor muscle are differentiated from the transverse muscle fibers of the CP, between which sits the pouch.

Cricopharyngeal Myotomy

Using a small hemostat, the CP muscles are transected in layers and gently separated until the underlying hypopharyngeal mucosa is reached. Some surgeons advocate extension of the myotomy several centimeters inferiorly to include the proximal cervical esophagus in order to reduce recurrence. This maneuver should be performed as close to the midline as possible to avoid injury to the recurrent laryngeal nerve (RLN), which travels along the tracheoesophageal groove. Other nearby structures that should be preserved include the descending hypoglossal nerve and the superior laryngeal nerve. A bougie dilator may be placed in the esophagus prior

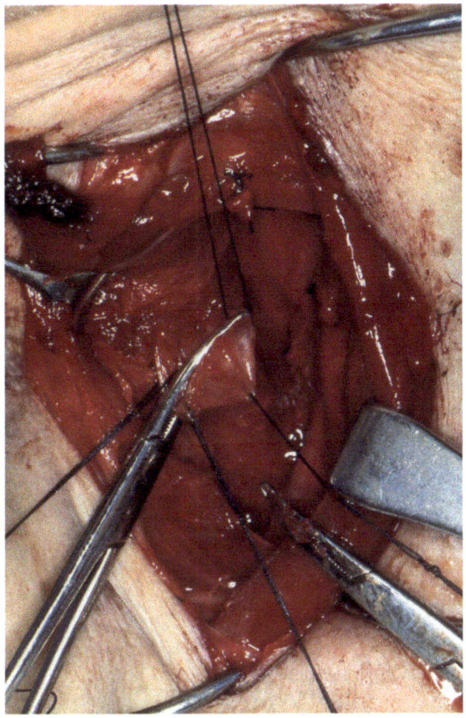

Fig. 9.2 Dissection of diverticulum through left transcervical incision. Larynx and strap muscles retracted medially, SCM and great vessels retracted laterally. Diverticulum clamped, suspended by traction sutures

to myotomy to enhance visualization of the muscles and mucosa following transection. Care is taken to avoid inadvertent entrance into the pharynx. If this occurs, a nasogastric tube should be placed under direct visualization, the mucosa repaired primarily in layers, and the patient kept NPO. The major risks of this open approach include RLN injury, pharyngocutaneous fistula, mediastinitis, hemorrhage, and pouch recurrence. For a small pouch, CP myotomy should result in its marsupialization. Large pouches, however, do not have a satisfactory outcome when treated with myotomy alone and should be addressed with a combined treatment approach.

Diverticulectomy

Diverticulectomy, as the most logical choice for sac elimination, used to be the initial surgical option (Fig. 9.2). However, leakage at the resection suture line was a major complication, resulting in unacceptably high rates of mediastinitis and sepsis. Diverticulectomy without concurrent myotomy has also resulted in high recurrence rates, underscoring the importance of addressing the CP at the time of surgery.

Diverticulectomy used to be performed with hand-sewn closure after pouch excision, which can be technically difficult in the retropharyngeal space of the neck. To avoid leakage and mediastinitis, the patient has a nasogastric tube and is kept NPO for approximately a week in the hospital on antibiotics (Fig. 9.3). The introduction

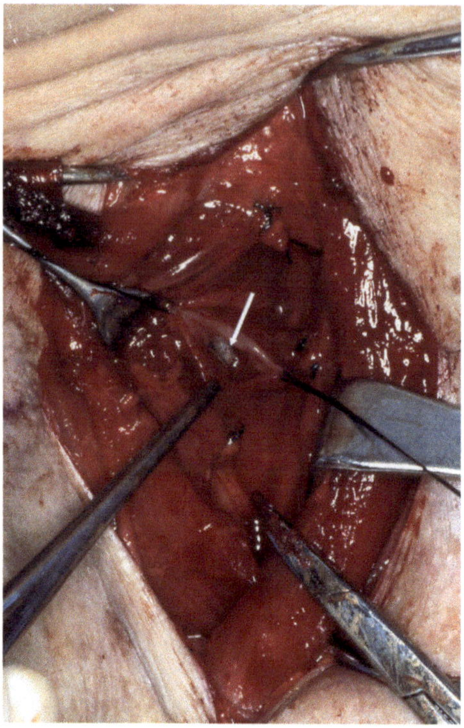

Fig. 9.3 Excised diverticulum revealing nasogastric tube in the esophagus (*arrow*)

of staple-assisted techniques has reduced this risk and led to more secure pharyngeal closures. Studies have demonstrated low rates of postoperative fistula (1.7 %), quick resumption of oral intake, and good long-term results. The decision of how and when to restart oral intake is largely surgeon-dependent. Many surgeons opt to wait several days with a nasogastric tube or rule out leakage on esophagram. Other risks of staple diverticulectomy are the same as for myotomy alone and remain low, including RLN palsy (0.8 %), recurrence (1.7 %), and wound hematoma (0.8 %).

Diverticulopexy

Diverticulopexy involves fixation of the base of the pouch superiorly to the prevertebral fascia or pharyngeal musculature. The pouch should be secured firmly cephalad such that the neck of the pouch is not in a dependent position and cannot accumulate debris. Failure to properly secure the pouch may result in the development of a caudally extending diverticulum. The advantage of diverticulopexy over diverticulectomy is that the hypopharyngeal mucosa is left intact, theoretically eliminating the risk of leakage or fistula formation. It has been shown to yield shorter hospital stays, earlier resumption to oral intake, shorter antibiotic treatment, and less overall cost. Interestingly, no difference in complications or symptomatic outcomes has been demonstrated.

Diverticular Inversion

An alternative technique is diverticular inversion, in which the sac is invaginated into the esophageal lumen and a purse-string suture is placed around the neck for closure. The hypopharyngeal mucosa is again not breached, and compared to diverticulectomy, inversion results in shorter hospital stays and fewer complications. Patients also resume an oral diet more quickly. The most recent comparative study did not demonstrate a significant difference in complication rates or patient satisfaction between the two groups, though most complications did occur in the diverticulectomy group.

Comparison of Open Techniques

There have been no randomized studies of the different open approaches for ZD. Most of the available studies are retrospective with a small number of patients, and few are comparative with nonstandardized selection criteria. In a 2013 systematic review, the majority of studies on open approaches in the last 20 years focused on CP myotomy and diverticulectomy, establishing the technique as a popular choice among surgeons. Nonetheless, a basic algorithm for the surgical treatment of ZD can be drawn from the available literature. Small (<1 cm) symptomatic diverticula can likely be treated effectively with CP myotomy alone. Medium-sized (1–4 cm) diverticula can be treated with CP myotomy and diverticulopexy or inversion, based on surgeon preference. Finally, large (>4 cm) diverticula are probably best suited for CP myotomy and diverticulectomy, given that suspension of a large sac may create a bulky compressive mass. Excision is also the only way to eliminate the small risk of carcinoma that may arise in the diverticulum.

Endoscopic Approach

An endoscopic approach to ZD was reported as early as 1917, when Mosher described sharply dividing the common wall, or cricopharyngeal bar, between the diverticulum and the esophageal lumen. Early adoption, however, was tempered by high rates of mediastinitis and death. The operating microscope and carbon dioxide (CO_2) laser were introduced in 1984 with good results and low morbidity. The use of a KTP/532 laser has also been described with comparable results. Because these "sutureless" methods rely only on coagulation and eschar formation to seal the edges of the cut mucosa and prevent leakage, they did not gain initial widespread acceptance. Technical refinements addressed these concerns, making endoscopic repair of ZD the first-line option for many surgeons.

The therapeutic goal of endoscopic repair of ZD is to create a common cavity between the diverticulum and esophageal lumen by dividing the septum, or common wall, that separates the two. Because the septum contains the cricopharyngeal

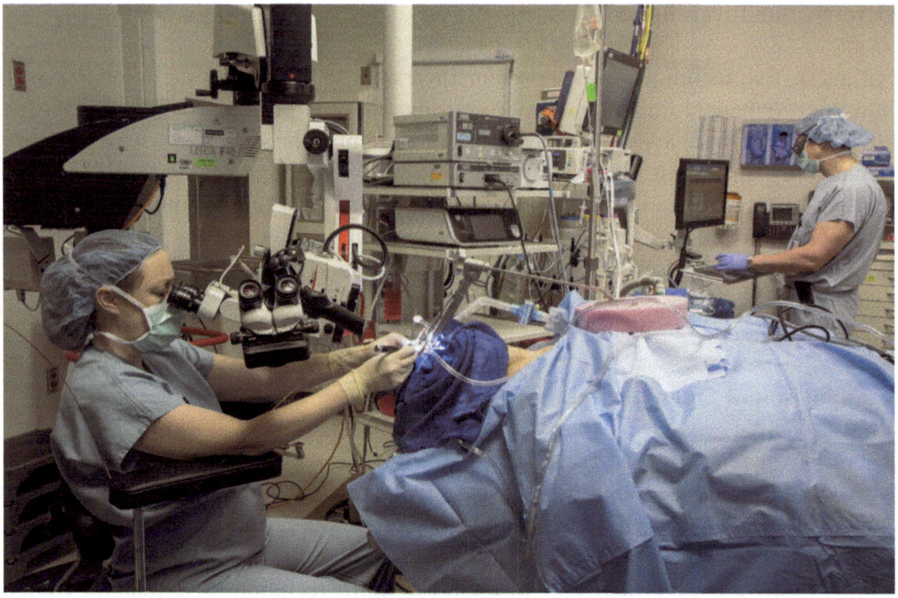

Fig. 9.4 Operating room setup: Diverticuloscope placed in suspension. Operating microscope stationed at head of bed. Operating chair with adjustable arm rests for improved instrument stabilization. Fire precautions observed

muscle, a CP myotomy is necessarily performed during endoscopic repair. This essentially eliminates the diverticular space, creates one large lumen, and restores normal outflow through the pharyngoesophageal segment.

Regardless of which device is utilized for division of the common wall, the setup is similar (Fig. 9.4). The appropriate patient has adequate oral opening, no neck mobility limitation, no obstructive macroglossia or micrognathia and lacks prominent teeth that can be easily chipped by the instruments. Predictors of poor endoscopic exposure include a short neck, short hyomental distance, and a high BMI. The patient is orotracheally intubated under general anesthesia and positioned supine with the neck fully extended. Perioperative antibiotics are routinely administered. A tooth guard is placed on the maxillary teeth. Several types of rigid diverticuloscopes have been developed to isolate the common wall. The popular bivalved Weerda diverticuloscope has long rigid valves, capable of opening in two separate and independent manners: the jaw can slide open with the blades parallel as well as hinge open at an angle. Both mechanisms are required to provide optimal exposure and passage of instruments (Fig. 9.5).

The endoscope is carefully introduced into the esophageal inlet, taking care not to damage the patient's teeth. Under direct visualization, it is advanced into the esophageal lumen. A zero-degree telescope confirms correct positioning. It is slowly withdrawn until the common wall sits between the valves. The endoscope is then

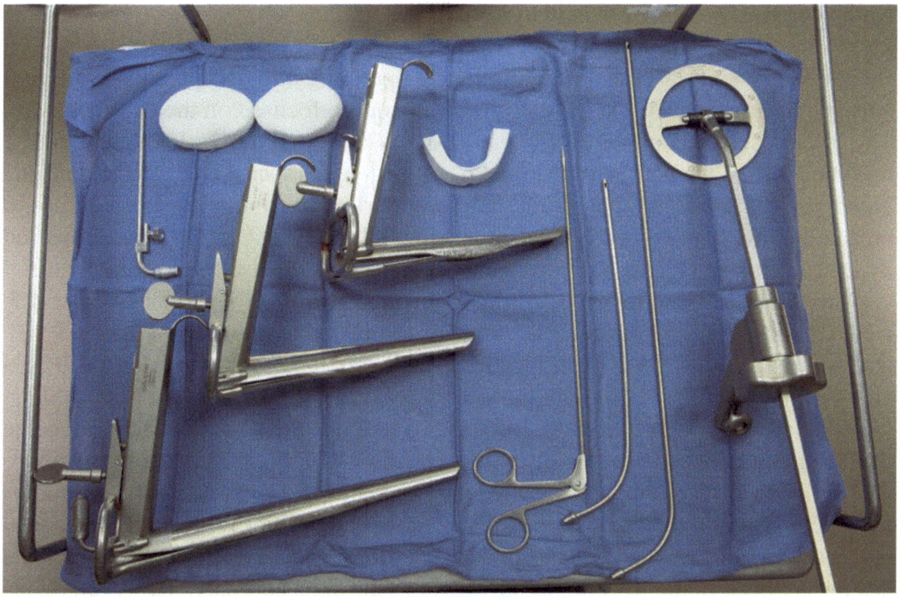

Fig. 9.5 Equipment for endoscopic repair: various sizes of Weerda diverticuloscopes, tooth guard, eye pads, suction tips, forceps, and suspension arm

Fig. 9.6 Endoscopic view of cricopharyngeal bar (Image courtesy of Alexander Langerman, MD)

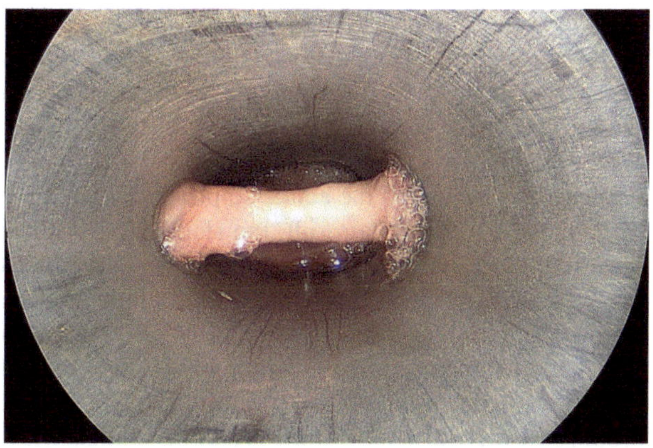

advanced so that the anterior valve is in the esophagus and the posterior valve is inside the diverticulum, showing the full depth of the pouch. The valves are then widened to expose the entire common wall, and the endoscope is placed in suspension (Fig. 9.6). A blunt-tipped instrument can probe the bottom of the diverticulum to elongate and straighten the septum. Residual food and debris is suctioned out of the pouch.

Endoscopic CO_2 Laser Diverticulotomy

In endoscopic CO_2 laser diverticulotomy, an operating microscope with a 400 mm lens and an attached CO_2 laser micromanipulator are focused on the common wall. The laser is set on continuous mode at 5–10 W and used to divide the wall at the midline down to the bottom of the pouch. A full-length mucosal incision reveals the underlying CP fibers as they retract laterally during division. Care is taken not to breach the investing fascial layer as it is approached. Visualization is not impaired by instruments and the laser micromanipulator affords precise laser beam control.

A recent systematic review identified 19 studies with 1,060 patients who underwent CO_2 laser procedures for ZD, reporting an overall complication rate of 9.3 % and mortality of 0.2 %. Complications included mediastinitis (1.3 %), fistula (1.1 %), and bleeding (1 %). The low risk of leakage for this "sutureless" technique is attributed to the high-energy high-focus beam of the laser. Some authors advocate the closure of the open mucosa of the transected CP bar, but the advantage of suture and fibrin glue to close the mucosal wound has not been clearly established. Studies have demonstrated the laser's efficacy and safety, with improved symptom scores, high rates of satisfaction, low rates of complications, and quick recovery times. This has mostly been found to compare favorably to the open approach. However, recurrence rates have been shown to favor the open approach in comparative studies.

Endoscopic Stapler Diverticulotomy

In endoscopic stapler diverticulotomy, a linear stapler is introduced into the endoscope and engages the CP bar such that the cartridge blade sits in the esophagus and the anvil blade is in the diverticulum. A telescope confirms correct placement of the stapler. When the stapler is fired, the CP muscle is cut and sealed simultaneously with a double row of staples along the incision line. Because the distal end of the stapler extends beyond the actual stapling segment, a residual pouch remains, typically about 1.5 cm. As a result, the stapler is considered contraindicated for small diverticula (<3 cm). However, technique modifications can increase the length of the septal tissue to be stapled. These include shortening the instrument tip and employing traction sutures to more fully deliver the septum into the blades.

There have been over 40 studies involving 1,800 patients, revealing an overall complication rate of 7.1 % and mortality of 0.3 %. Overall, endoscopic stapling has produced excellent short- and long-term results, with significant improvement in over 85 % of patients. However, when categorized by diverticulum size, patients with pouches <3 cm reported poorer outcomes, underscoring its limitation in smaller diverticula. Major complications such as perforation are rare. Similar to the laser, the stapler results in shorter operative times, shorter hospital stays, and quicker resumption of oral intake when compared to open approaches. Studies suggest that endoscopic stapling also compares favorably to the laser with regard to recovery times. With respect to recurrent pouches, both endoscopic laser and stapler revision surgery have been shown to be effective and allow the surgeon to avoid the pitfalls of working in a previously operated neck.

Variations in Endoscopic Approach

Endoscopic Harmonic Scalpel Diverticulotomy

Recently, the use of the harmonic scalpel has been described for endoscopic repair. The harmonic scalpel relies on ultrasonographic mechanical energy to simultaneously cut and coagulate tissue. There are few published studies on the topic, with most studies reporting good outcomes, low complication rates, and quick recovery times. Comparative studies on the harmonic scalpel and the stapler report conflicting complication rates between the two techniques. More studies are needed to validate these preliminary results and determine long-term outcomes.

Flexible Endoscopic Diverticulotomy

Flexible endoscopic diverticulotomy was first described in 1995. It has since gained traction among gastroenterologists who can perform the procedure in inpatient or outpatient endoscopy suites under conscious sedation or general anesthesia. It is an appealing alternative for high-risk elderly patients who cannot tolerate general anesthesia or patients with anatomy that make rigid endoscopy difficult. The principles are the same as in rigid endoscopic diverticulotomy: the common wall is divided, thereby creating a common cavity while performing a myotomy. The patient is placed in the left lateral decubitus position, and an initial endoscopic exam is performed to identify the pouch and remove any retained debris with a nasogastric tube. A guidewire is used to insert the tube, which is then left in the esophagus during the procedure to protect the anterior esophageal wall from injury. There are several techniques, including performing the procedure "freehand" or using accessory devices, such as a transparent hood, a cap, or soft diverticuloscope. These attachments improve septum exposure, stabilize the position of the scope, and protect the mucosal walls from thermal injury. There are three principal techniques to divide the septum: needle-knife incision, argon plasma coagulation, and monopolar coagulation using forceps.

Review of the literature reveals an overall complication rate of 15 % and mortality of 0 %. Complications include perforation (4 %) and bleeding (3 %). Perforations visualized on endoscope may be immediately addressed with endoclips, and intraprocedural bleeding can be controlled with an epinephrine injection. Recurrence is an issue, with rates as high as 20 %. However, repeat sessions are common and can be performed more safely than other techniques in high-risk patients. Flexible endoscopic diverticulotomy is currently in its early stages, as evidenced by the lack of a standardized approach or optimal technique. Additional studies are needed to determine which technique or accessory devices are best suited for which patient populations.

Comparison of Open Versus Endoscopic Approaches

To date, there have been no prospective, randomized studies comparing the different approaches to determine the superiority of one technique over the other. The large number of retrospective studies and the few comparative studies that vary in inclusion criteria, sample size, follow-up period, and definition of recurrence make it difficult to draw firm conclusions. In general, these studies conclude that endoscopic repair results in a lower complication rate, shorter hospital stay, faster time to oral intake, and shorter operative time. However, there are limits to endoscopic treatment. The reported conversion rate to an open procedure, or the surgical abortion rate due to poor endoscopic exposure, ranges from 0 to 30 %. The average conversion rate is 1.7 % with the laser and 5.6 % with the stapler. The most commonly cited reason is anatomic limitation. High conversion rates and recurrence rates with endoscopic treatment may be offset by the increased inpatient hospital charges and higher morbidity associated with open surgery. Nonetheless, both approaches appear to improve quality of life and achieve high patient satisfaction rates.

Conclusions

Symptomatic ZD is a relatively rare disease of the elderly that can cause significant morbidity. The treatment has evolved over the past century, a reflection of the better understanding of the underlying pathophysiology. There has also been a trend toward minimally invasive techniques. No consensus exists to guide management, and practice patterns are largely shaped by personal preferences and experiences with the various techniques. Nevertheless, some general guidelines have emerged. Given the important role of CP muscle pathology in ZD development, a CP myotomy must always be included in any treatment plan. Open CP myotomy alone is best suited for very small pouches. Diverticulopexy and diverticular inversion have less associated morbidity than diverticulectomy for moderately sized pouches. Larger pouches may benefit more from diverticulectomy, especially in healthy young patients or patients for whom carcinoma is a concern. Endoscopic approaches result in less overall complications and should be employed in patients with comorbidities who would not tolerate postoperative complications or a longer procedure under general anesthesia. The endoscopic stapler is a popular, safe, and effective technique but is contraindicated in smaller pouches. Flexible endoscopy is a good alternative to patients who cannot tolerate rigid endoscopy, although long-term studies and standardized techniques are lacking. Endoscopic procedures are safe and effective in revision surgeries.

Summary

- ZD is the most common type of diverticulum in the upper gastrointestinal tract.
- Cricopharyngeal muscle dysfunction is central to ZD formation, and its release is the cornerstone of surgical treatment.

- ZD is a disease of the elderly, commonly presents with dysphagia and regurgitation, and is diagnosed by barium swallow.
- Treatment depends on the surgical risk of the patient and diverticulum size.
- Open surgery is reserved for healthy patients with contraindications to endoscopy. Cricopharyngeal myotomy alone can be used to treat small pouches but should be combined with diverticulectomy, diverticulopexy, or diverticular inversion for larger pouches.
- Rigid endoscopic approaches result in fewer complications and are a good option for elderly or high-risk patients. Endoscopic laser and stapler diverticulotomies are both safe and effective, but the stapler is contraindicated in smaller pouches.
- Variations in endoscopic techniques lack long-term studies.

Selected Reading

1. Adam SI, Paskhover B, Sasaki CT. Laser versus stapler: outcomes in endoscopic repair of Zenker diverticulum. Laryngoscope. 2012;122:1961–6. Endoscopic CO2 laser and endoscopic stapling groups both exhibited significant symptom improvement, but the laser group scores showed greater improvement. There were significantly more recurrences in the laser group, and significantly longer hospital stay and time to oral intake in the stapler group.
2. Bergeron JL, Long JL, Chhetri DK. Dysphagia characteristics in Zenker's diverticulum. Otolaryngol Head Neck Surg. 2013;148:223–8. Preoperative assessment using fiberoptic endoscopic evaluation of swallowing demonstrated that post-swallow hypopharyngeal reflux was predictive of a diverticulum larger than 1 cm and may be useful in surgical planning.
3. Bloom JD, Bleier BS, Mirza N, Chalian AA, Thaler ER. Factors predicting endoscopic exposure of Zenker's diverticulum. Ann Otol Rhinol Laryngol. 2010;119:736–41. Factors that significantly correlated with endoscopic exposure failure included a short neck, short hyomental distance and high BMI.
4. Bonavina L, Bona D, Abraham M, Saino G, Abate E. Long-term results of endosurgical and open surgical approach for Zenker diverticulum. World J Gastroenterol. 2007;13:2586–9. Both endoscopic stapler and open stapled diverticulectomy groups reported good short and long-term outcomes. The authors advocate performing a longer myotomy in order to prevent recurrence. They also recommend small diverticula as a formal contraindication to endoscopic stapling.
5. Chang YC, Payyapilli RJ, Scher RL. Endoscopic staple diverticulostomy for Zenker's diverticulum: review of literature and experience in 159 consecutive cases. Laryngoscope. 2003;113:957–65. Compared to open techniques, endoscopic stapler produced shorter operative times, quicker time to PO, and lower complication and mortality rates. Compared to endoscopic laser, endoscopic stapler led to comparable operative times and mortality rates but fewer complications and more rapid convalescent times.
6. Ferreira LE, Simmons DT, Baron TH. Zenker's diverticula: pathophysiology, clinical presentation, and flexible endoscopic management. Dis Esophagus. 2008;22(21):1–8. Good description of the different cutting techniques of flexible endoscopic treatment, as well as the variety of accessories that improve exposure and optimize safety.
7. Gutschow CA, Hamoir M, Rombaux P, Otte JB, Goncette L, Collard JM. Management of pharyngoesophageal (Zenker's) diverticulum: which technique? Ann Thorac Surg. 2002;74:1677–83. This study demonstrated better symptomatic relief with open techniques compared to endoscopic, especially in smaller diverticula. Diverticula resection without CP myotomy predisposed to development of fistula and recurrence.

8. Koch M, Mantsopoulos K, Velegrakis S, et al. Endoscopic laser-assisted diverticulotomy versus open surgical approach in treatment of Zenker's diverticulum. Laryngoscope. 2011;121:2090–4. Although the operative time, hospital stay and complication rate were significantly lower in the endoscopic laser group, the recurrence rate was significantly lower in the open group.
9. Mantsopoulos K, Psychogios G, Kunzel J, Zenk J, Iro H, Koch M. Evaluation of the different transcervical approaches for Zenker diverticulum. Otolaryngol Head Neck Surg. 2012;146:725–9. Hospitalization times were significantly shorter in the inversion group compared to open diverticulectomy. There was no difference in operative time, recurrence rate or follow-up satisfaction with the surgery.
10. Pomerri F, Costantini M, Dal Bosco C, Battaglia G, Bottin R, Zanatta L, Ancona E, Muzzio PC. Comparison of preoperative and surgical measurements of Zenker's diverticulum. Surg Endosc. 2012;26:2010–5. This study confirms that preoperative barium radiography accurately evaluates diverticulum size compared to surgical measurements and is essential in surgical planning.
11. Siddiq MA, Sood S, Strachan D. Pharyngeal pouch (Zenker's diverticulum). Postgrad Med J. 2001;77:508–11. Succinct review of epidemiology, etiology, clinical presentation and treatment options of Zenker's diverticulum.
12. Simic A, Radovanovic N, Stojakov D, Bjelovic M, Kotarac M, Sabljak P, Skrobic O, Pesko P. Surgical experience of the national institution in the treatment of Zenker's diverticula. Acta Chir Iugosl. 2009;56:25–33. Compares three open approaches that were used based on diverticula size. Although hospital stay and time to oral intake were significantly longer in the resection group, good outcomes were achieved in all groups.
13. Veenker EA, Andersen PE, Cohen JI. Cricopharyngeal spasm and Zenker's diverticulum. Head Neck. 2003;25:681–94. Critical evaluation of histopathologic, manometric, fluoroscopic and retrospective clinical studies of cricopharyngeal spasm and its role in Zenker's diverticulum.
14. Whited C, Lee WT, Scher R. Evaluation of endoscopic harmonic diverticulostomy. Laryngoscope. 2012;122:1297–300. The largest study comparing endoscopic harmonic scalpel and stapler demonstrated a significantly higher complication rate for the harmonic scalpel.
15. Yuan Y, Zhao YF, Hu Y, Chen LQ. Surgical treatment of Zenker's diverticulum. Dig Surg. 2013;30:207–18. This systematic review provides cumulative data on morbidity, mortality and complications of all open and endoscopic techniques, as well as outcomes details from selected studies.
16. Zaninotto G, Narne S, Costantini M, Molena D, Cutrone C, Portale G, Costantino M, Rizzetto C, Basili U, Ancona E. Tailored approach to Zenker's diverticula. Surg Endosc. 2003;17:129–33. Both open and endoscopic groups demonstrated an UES pressure reduction, improved UES relaxation and lower intrabolus pressure on manometry, but persistent dysphagia was higher in the endoscopic group.

Chapter 10
Achalasia: Pathophysiology and Diagnostic Evaluation

Benedetto Mungo and Daniela Molena

Abstract Achalasia is a chronic, progressive disease characterized by a manometric pattern showing loss of peristalsis of the distal esophagus, failure of the lower esophageal sphincter (LES) to completely relax with deglutition, and elevated baseline intraluminal esophageal pressure. Even though achalasia is a relatively rare disease, it represents the most common primary esophageal motility disorder and the second functional esophageal disorder most likely to necessitate surgical intervention after gastroesophageal reflux disease (GERD). Esophageal achalasia is an idiopathic disease resulting in damage of the Auerbach myenteric plexus. Over the last decade, the use of high resolution manometry, has allowed for a deeper understanding of this disease.

Keywords Achalasia • Dysphagia • Barium Swallow • Endoscopy • Esophageal manometry • Ambulatory pH monitoring

Introduction

Achalasia is a chronic, progressive disease characterized by a manometric pattern showing loss of peristalsis of the distal esophagus, failure of the lower esophageal sphincter (LES) to completely relax with deglutition, and elevated baseline intraluminal esophageal pressure. Sir Thomas Willis first described this disease in 1672, and the word achalasia can be literarily translated from the Greek as "absence of relaxation," in referral to the impaired function of the LES. Achalasia is a rare

B. Mungo, MD • D. Molena, MD (✉)
Division of Thoracic Surgery, Department of Surgery, John Hopkins Medical School,
600 North Wolfe Street, Blalock 240, Baltimore, MD 21827, USA
e-mail: bmungo1@jhmi.edu; dmolena2@jhmi.edu

P.M. Fisichella et al. (eds.), *Esophageal Diseases*,
DOI 10.1007/978-3-319-04337-1_10,

disease with an incidence of 0.5–1.63 per 100,000 people per year in the United States and a prevalence of 10.82 cases per 100,000 individuals. It has an equal distribution across genders and can occur at any time in the lifespan, although it usually develops between 20 and 40 years of age. Despite its low prevalence, achalasia represents the most common primary esophageal motility disorder and the second functional esophageal disorder most likely to necessitate surgical intervention after gastroesophageal reflux disease (GERD).

Despite the improvements in quality of life and prognosis achieved through the development of effective therapeutic protocols, this condition remains incurable. The treatment of achalasia is substantially palliative and aims to improve passive esophageal transit of food from the esophagus into the stomach.

Pathophysiology

The timing of esophageal peristaltic contractions and LES relaxation has been demonstrated to be dependent on the activity of a subpopulation of enteric inhibitory neurons located in the Auerbach myenteric plexus of the esophagus. The pathophysiology of the impaired peristalsis in achalasia is thought to be the result of the progressive degeneration and destruction of these neuronal ganglion cells, containing NO (nitric oxide) and VIP (vasoactive intestinal polypeptide). Physiologically, inhibitory ganglionic neurons facilitate LES relaxation and sequence the peristaltic contraction in the distal esophagus. Their damage therefore results in failed relaxation of the LES with bolus swallowing and in loss of coordinated peristaltic propulsion, due to the imbalance between excitatory and inhibitory innervation. The histological features of this process have been observed in esophagomyotomy specimens from patients with early achalasia. The initial pathological changes consist of myenteric inflammation with injury to ganglion cells, leading to their progressive loss, and damage to myenteric nerves, resulting in fibrosis. This process leads to inflammatory degeneration of the nitric oxide producing inhibitory neurons of the esophagus, while the cholinergic neurons involved in the smooth muscle contraction, which contribute to LES tone, are relatively spared. Moreover, in an experimental setting, no relaxations can be evocated on surgical specimens of LES muscle from achalasia patients. Conversely, normal LES muscle strips mounted in organ baths and electrically stimulated show frequency-dependent relaxations mediated by NO.

While the process leading to impaired motility has been defined, its underlying cause remains unknown. In a small group of patients affected by Allgrove syndrome (triple A syndrome: alacrima, achalasia, adrenocorticotropic hormone deficiency), a mutation on chromosome 12 is implicated in the development of achalasia and in Central and South America, esophageal infection with a protozoan parasite (*Trypanosoma cruzi*) has been shown to cause neuron destruction in Chagas disease. Nevertheless, for the vast majority of patients, no clear etiology has been established. Achalasia is associated with an inflammatory response including CD3-/CD8-positive lymphocytic infiltrates in the myenteric ganglia, IgM antibodies, and evidence of complement activation, all factors that suggest the implication of an autoimmune, viral, or chronic degenerative process. In particular, there are reports in the literature supporting the evidence that the neural cells responsible for achalasia might be the targets for an autoimmune response, and anti-myenteric neuronal circulating antibodies have been demonstrated in some patients. The development of this immune reaction is postulated to take place preferentially in genetically susceptible hosts; the hypothesis of a genetic basis is supported by studies in twins and siblings, as well as by the association of achalasia with genetic diseases such as Allgrove syndrome, Down's syndrome, and Parkinson disease. The development of achalasia has also been reported to be associated with HLA-DR and -DQ alleles, hence showing a behavior consistent with an autoimmune disease, linked to MHC complex genes. In addition, autoimmune conditions such as type 1 diabetes, hypothyroidism, and Sjogren's syndrome have been reported to be more prevalent in patients with achalasia than in the general population, further supporting the association between achalasia and autoimmune disorders. The event rousing the cellular damage is yet to be determined; however, there are studies suggesting a triggering role of viral infections, such as herpes simplex virus-1 and measles, in initiating an immune response that subsequently becomes aberrant.

The above-described events lead to long-lasting contraction of the LES, resulting in stasis of food within the esophageal lumen. Moreover, damage to the inhibitory ganglion cells disrupts the coordination that physiologically delays the swallow-initiated peristaltic contraction, such that it occurs only after several seconds of LES relaxation. As a result, a pattern of premature distal esophageal contractions occurs, impairing the esophageal emptying and contributing to trap the bolus above the LES. In a later phase of the disease, the esophageal body's peristaltic disorder progresses to total aperistalsis, probably due to either degeneration of the excitatory cholinergic esophageal neurons or to progressive esophageal dilatation caused by chronic obstruction. This functional obstacle to food progression persists until the rising intraesophageal pressure overcomes the cardial spasm and the bolus slowly transits into the stomach. However, long food stasis inevitably causes over time increasing esophageal dilation. If the condition is left untreated, it will lead eventually to sigmoid megaesophagus (end-stage disease) (Fig. 10.1).

Three stages (Table 10.1), corresponding to progressive dilation, elongation, and tortuosity of the esophagus, have been individuated within the natural history of the disease.

Clinical Presentation

Patients with achalasia usually present with a history of dysphagia for both solids and liquids. Of note, dysphagia for liquids represents a key clue for esophageal motility disorder as this symptom is uncommon in mechanical causes of esophageal

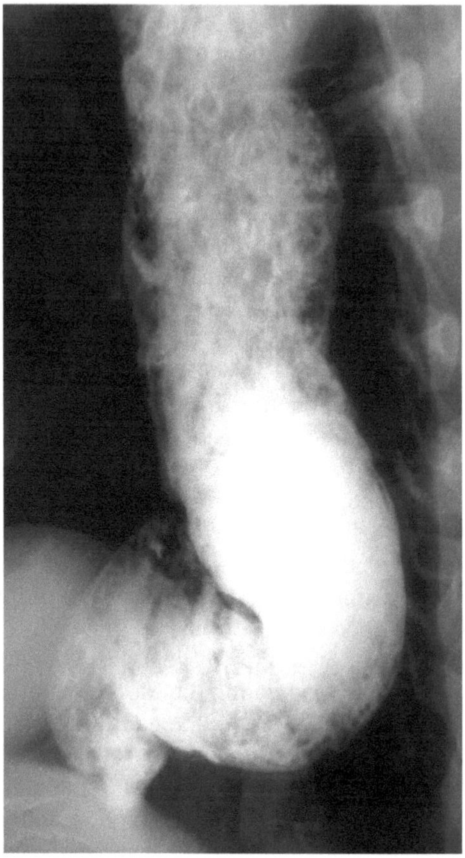

Fig. 10.1 End-stage achalasia on a barium swallow: the esophagus is massively dilated, elongated, tortuous, and sigmoid shaped above the diaphragmatic hiatus

Table 10.1 Stages of achalasia

Stage	Time frame	Description
1	*Onset* Presentation	The patient suddenly complains pain, dysphagia, and regurgitation never experienced before
2	*Silent period* Follows undiagnosed onset	Worsening of the symptoms due to esophageal dilatation and food retention in the absence of esophageal distention
3	*Final stage* More than two decades after initial diagnosis	Severe weight loss, malnutrition, and respiratory infection. Esophageal dilation and tortuosity

obstruction, exception made for extremely advanced disease. Dysphagia is present in >90 % of patients with achalasia. Other common symptoms (present in 70–90 % of patients) include regurgitation of indigested food and saliva occurring minutes to hours after the meal. Heartburn and chest pain during or after eating, that some patients relieve with the regurgitation of undigested food, may be present as well in 20–50 % of cases. Respiratory symptoms usually consist of nocturnal cough and aspiration; these complaints as well as weight loss are common in the more advanced

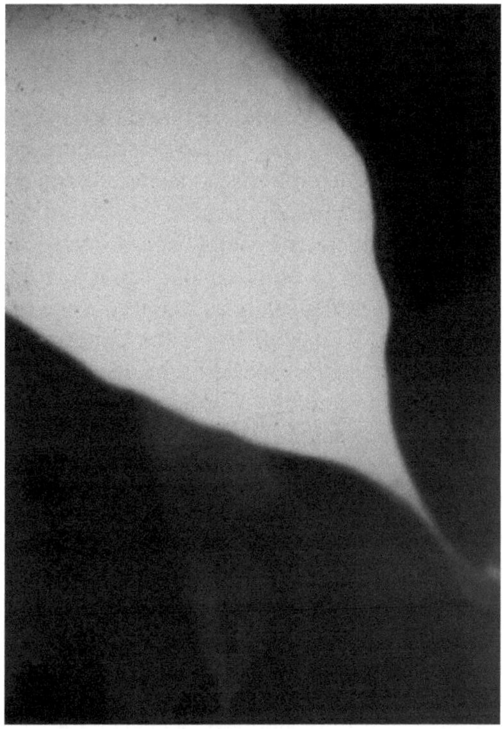

Fig. 10.2 The classic "bird's beak" appearance at the esophagogastric junction on a barium swallow

stages. Patients with achalasia typically describe themselves as "slow eaters" and avoid certain solid foods that are difficult to swallow. Malnutrition and recurrent aspiration pneumonia usually occur in the final stage of the disease and are therefore uncommon at the time of the first diagnosis. Of note, it is not uncommon to formulate the diagnosis of achalasia only at the late stages of the disease, due to a blurry initial presentation with nonspecific long-lasting symptoms and the rarity of the condition.

Diagnosis

In order to establish a diagnosis of achalasia, it is paramount to obtain evidence of defective LES relaxation and impaired peristalsis; at the same time, other causes of obstruction that could potentially mimic achalasia must be ruled out. These goals can be achieved using a combination of imaging studies and functional tests.

Barium swallow has the potential to show the loss of esophageal peristalsis along with distal esophageal tapering in almost every affected patient. The radiological aspect of narrowing of the esophagus delineated by the contrast in the esophagogram is known as the "bird's beak" appearance at the esophagogastric junction (EGJ) (Fig. 10.2). Moreover, barium swallow can demonstrate dilation of the distal esophagus, food retention above the cardiac, and esophageal tortuosity if the disease has already progressed. Finally, if performed as timed barium esophagogram protocol, it can also quantify the efficacy of esophageal emptying. With a sensitivity of 60 %, esophagogram alone is however not a sufficient diagnostic tool for achalasia.

Endoscopy should be performed in every patient who complains of dysphagia for the following reasons: (1) it is important to rule out cancer. If the endoscopy raises the suspicion of pseudoachalasia (manometric picture of achalasia due to an underlying cancer), endoscopic ultrasound or CT scan should be performed. (2) In advanced stages, endoscopy may directly visualize some features suggestive of achalasia, such as esophageal dilation and food or fluid retention. Esophagitis can also be observed, usually as a consequence of prolonged food stasis.

Esophageal manometry is the confirmatory test and should be performed in every patient with suspected achalasia.

Diagnostic findings on conventional manometry are the absence of esophageal peristalsis and failure of the LES to relax in response to swallowing. Elevated resting tone of the LES is present in about 50 % of patients. Conventional esophageal manometry requires, after the placement of the manometry catheter beyond the gastroesophageal junction, a slow retrograde pull through, in order to determine the position of the LES (pressure inversion point and high-pressure zone). LES relaxation is subsequently determined through pressure evaluation during water swallows. The recorded pressures are plotted on a graph as a linear manometry tracing. In the last decade, however, high-resolution manometry (HRM) and esophageal pressure topography (EPT) have revolutionized the performance of functional esophageal testing and have deepened the knowledge of functional impairments in patients with achalasia. This technique, now regarded as the gold standard for diagnosis of achalasia provides several advantages over conventional manometry. More than 30 closely spaced sensors allow for a more homogeneous and precise pressure recording throughout the whole esophagus. In addition, there is no need for catheter pull through and repositioning, and all the needed variables can be recorded with a single series of wet water swallows. Finally, the recorded data are plotted as color coded, spatiotemporal representations of pressure in the esophagus, delivering a more detailed, comprehensive, and intuitive reading.

The increased precision in defining the contractile characteristics of the esophagus and its sphincters prompted the development of a new classification for esophageal motility disorders, which parallels conventional manometric classifications enriched with the knowledge offered by the new technology (The Chicago Classification). A diagnostic algorithm, consisting of three major steps (assessment of the EGJ, characterization of esophageal contractility, and pressurization pattern) has been developed to help the clinician progressively identify the esophageal physiological dysfunction. The application of this technology to the assessment of patients with esophageal achalasia led to the identification of three clinically relevant groups based on the contractility pattern in the esophagus and the esophageal pressurization associated with LES dysfunction (Fig. 10.3a–c):

- *Type I*: absent peristalsis. In this subtype, also defined as classic achalasia, there is impaired LES relaxation, but no significant pressurization within the esophageal body.

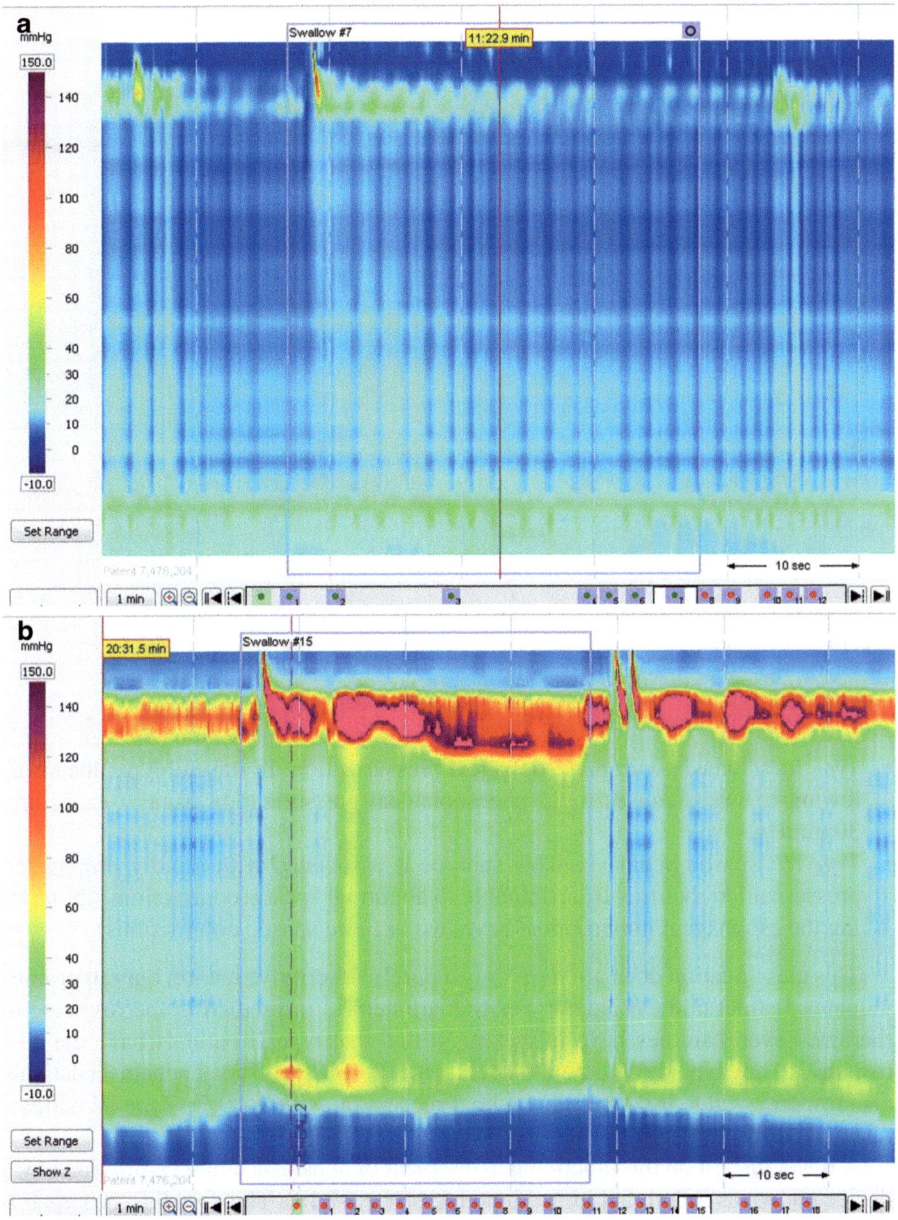

Fig. 10.3 (**a**–**c**) Classification of esophageal achalasia into three subtypes based on HRM and EPT. (**a**) Type I achalasia. (**b**) Type II achalasia. (**c**) Type III achalasia

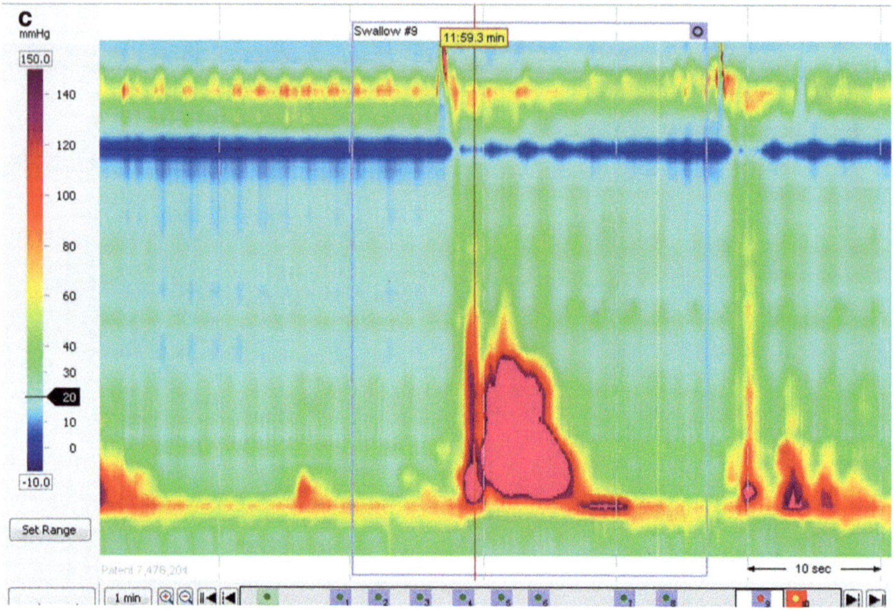

Fig. 10.3 (continued)

- *Type II*: achalasia with panesophageal pressurization. In this subtype, the swallowing of water causes rapid panesophageal pressurization usually exceeding 30 mmHg.
- *Type III*: spastic achalasia. This subtype is associated with rapidly propagated pressurization, but this is attributable to abnormal spastic contractions obliterating the esophageal lumen (must have two or more spastic contractions).

This classification does not have only a purely descriptive nature, but rather individuates distinct clinical phenotypes that are helpful in predicting the response to therapy. Several studies have in fact suggested that type II patients have the best response to any type of treatment (success rate 90–100 %). Type I achalasia patients also respond well to treatment, but with a success rate of 60–80 %. Type III patients respond poorly (about 30 % success rate).

A novel insight on the functional assessment of achalasia could be provided by a device known as functional lumen imaging probe (FLIP). This tool has the capability of measuring EGJ compliance during volume-controlled distension, thus complementing information yield by esophagogram and HRM. Results from a recent study showed a correlation between FLIP-measured EGJ distensibility in achalasia patients and symptom severity, thus suggesting a potentially relevant application of FLIP in the clinical practice.

Summary

- Achalasia is a chronic, benign, progressive esophageal disease.
- Achalasia is the most common primary esophageal motility disorder.
- Key features include absent esophageal peristalsis and failure of the lower esophageal sphincter (LES) to completely relax in response to swallowing.
- The presentation of the disease may be confusing, and diagnosis is often delayed.
- The pathophysiology of achalasia is thought to be the result of the progressive degeneration and destruction of inhibitory neuronal ganglion cells in the esophageal Auerbach plexus.
- The cause of this disease is unknown; a genetic and an autoimmune component are thought to play an important role
- Dysphagia is the most common symptom; regurgitation, heartburn, chest pain, respiratory symptoms, and weight loss may also be present
- Esophageal manometry (or HRM) is the most reliable test; it is pathognomonic for achalasia if it demonstrates absence of esophageal peristaltic contractions and failure of the LES to relax in response to swallowing.
- HRM delivers more detailed, comprehensive, and intuitive information than traditional manometry and allows achalasia classification in three different subtypes.
- Endoscopy and barium swallow should be performed to rule out different causes of dysphagia such as cancer. Both tests, if performed alone, will be diagnostic only in about half of patients with achalasia.

Selected Reading

1. Boeckxstaens GE, Zaninotto G, Richter JE. Achalasia. Lancet. 2014;383:83–93. *Comprehensive detailed and updated review on achalasia from renowned experts in the field.*
2. Carlson DA, Pandolfino JE. High-resolution manometry and esophageal pressure topography: filling the gaps of convention manometry. Gastroenterol Clin North Am. 2013;42:1–15. *A comprehensive work on features and innovation in HRM from renowned experts.*
3. Ellis FG. The natural history of achalasia of the cardia. Proc R Soc Med. 1960;53:663–6. *An historical perspective on the disease and classification based on natural history.*
4. Facco M, Brun P, Baesso I, Costantini M, Rizzetto C, Berto A, Baldan N, Palù G, Semenzato G, Castagliuolo I, Zaninotto G. T cells in the myenteric plexus of achalasia patients show a skewed TCR repertoire and react to HSV-1 antigens. Am J Gastroenterol. 2008;103:1598–609. *This study showed an aberrant response to a viral infection or to self-antigens triggered by the infection leading to an immune response against esophageal enteric neurons..*
5. Fisichella PM, Raz D, Palazzo F, Niponmick I, Patti MG. Clinical, radiological, and manometric profile in 145 patients with untreated achalasia. World J Surg. 2008;32:1974–9. *Detailing of features of untreated disease with commonly used diagnostic tests.*
6. Goldblum JR, Rice TW, Richter JE. Histopathologic features in esophagomyotomy specimens from patients with achalasia. Gastroenterology. 1996;111:648–54. *Analysis of histopathologic features of achalasia, important to yield better understanding of pathophysiology of the disease.*

7. Kahrilas PJ, Ghosh SK, Pandolfino JE. Esophageal motility disorders in terms of pressure topography: the Chicago Classification. J Clin Gastroenterol. 2008;42:627–35. *New classification for esophageal motility disorders using HRM and pressure topography plots..*
8. Pandolfino JE, de Ruigh A, Nicodeme F, Xiao Y, Boris L, Kahrilas PJ. Distensibility of the esophagogastric junction assessed with the functional lumen imaging probe (FLIP) in achalasia patients. Neurogastroenterol Motil. 2013;25:496–501. *Description of a novel tool with interesting potential in the study of achalasia patients.*
9. Pandolfino JE, Kahrilas PJ. Presentation, diagnosis, and management of achalasia. Clin Gastroenterol Hepatol. 2013;11:887–97. *Comprehensive detailed and updated review on achalasia from renowned experts in the field.*
10. Pandolfino JE, Kwiatek MA, Nealis T, Bulsiewicz W, Post J, Kahrilas PJ. Achalasia: a new clinically relevant classification by high-resolution manometry. Gastroenterology. 2008;135:1526. *Identification of 3 subtypes of achalasia with clinical and prognostic relevance.*
11. Park W, Vaezi MF. Etiology and pathogenesis of achalasia: the current understanding. Am J Gastroenterol. 2005;100:1404–14. *An interesting insight in hypothesis on pathophysiology and etiogenesis of achalasia.*
12. Sadowski DC, Ackah F, Jiang B, Svenson LW. Achalasia: incidence, prevalence and survival. A population-based study. Neurogastroenterol Motil. 2010;22:256–61. *The first North American population-based study of achalasia epidemiology using a governmental administrative database.*
13. Sandler RS, Nyren O, Ekbom A, Eisen GM, Yuen J, Josefsson S. The risk of esophageal cancer in patients with achalasia. A population-based study. JAMA. 1995;274:1359–62. *Large population study on risk of cancer in achalasia patients compared to general population.*
14. Triadafilopoulos G, Boeckxstaens GE, Gullo R, Patti MG, Pandolfino JE, Kahrilas PJ, et al. The Kagoshima consensus on esophageal achalasia. Dis Esophagus. 2012;25:337–48. *A summary of the state of the art of knowledge on achalasia from international experts in this field.*
15. Vaezi MF, Pandolfino JE, Vela MF. ACG clinical guideline: diagnosis and management of achalasia. Am J Gastroenterol. 2013;108:1238–49. *Detailed and updated review of key steps in diagnosis and treatment of achalasia.*
16. Verne GN, Hahn AB, Pineau BC, Hoffman BJ, Wojciechowski BW, Wu WC. Association of HLA-DR and -DQ alleles with idiopathic achalasia. Gastroenterology. 1999;117:26–31. *Experimental study showing an association between idiopathic achalasia and HLA alleles in a race-specific manner.*
17. Verne GN, Sallustio JE, Eaker EY. Anti-myenteric neuronal antibodies in patients with achalasia. A prospective study. Dig Dis Sci. 1997;42:307–13. *Study showing the presence of circulating neural antibodies in patients with achalasia..*

Chapter 11
Achalasia: Treatment

Marco E. Allaix, Fabrizio Rebecchi, Claudio Giaccone, and Mario Morino

Abstract The last 20 years have witnessed a shift in the treatment algorithm of esophageal achalasia. Laparoscopic Heller myotomy with partial fundoplication is considered in most centers the primary treatment modality, while endoscopic treatment such as pneumatic dilatation and endoscopic botulinum toxin injection is mainly reserved for the management of patients unfit for surgery or in case of surgical failure. Recently, a new approach to achalasia has been proposed: the peroral endoscopic myotomy (POEM).

Keywords Achalasia • Botulinum toxin injection • Endoscopic dilatation • Peroral endoscopic myotomy • Laparoscopic myotomy • Partial anterior fundoplication • Partial posterior fundoplication

---

Conflict of Interest
The authors have no conflicts of interest to declare.

M.E. Allaix, MD (✉) • F. Rebecchi, MD • C. Giaccone, MD • M. Morino, MD
Department of Surgical Sciences, University of Torino,
Corso A.M. Dogliotti 14, 10126 Torino, Italy
e-mail: meallaix@gmail.com

P.M. Fisichella et al. (eds.), *Esophageal Diseases*,
DOI 10.1007/978-3-319-04337-1_11, © Springer International Publishing Switzerland 2014

Introduction

Esophageal achalasia is a primary motility disorder characterized by the absence of esophageal peristalsis and by impaired lower esophageal sphincter (LES) relaxation in response to swallowing. These findings lead to abnormal emptying of food from the esophagus into the stomach with consequent stasis.

Because the pathogenesis of achalasia is unknown, treatment is palliative and aims to improve esophageal emptying by decreasing the functional obstruction at the level of the gastroesophageal junction. Treatment modalities include:

1. Endoscopic botulinum toxin injection;
2. Pneumatic dilatation;
3. Laparoscopic Heller myotomy;
4. Peroral endoscopic myotomy

This chapter will discuss the outcomes of the different treatment options for esophageal achalasia.

Endoscopic Botulinum Toxin Injection

The toxin is injected with a fine needle through the endoscope at the level of the gastroesophageal junction. It decreases the LES pressure by inhibiting the release of acetylcholine from the presynaptic cholinergic nerve endings. It is a safe procedure, with a negligible risk of complications. Symptom relief or improvement is achieved in approximately 80–85 % of patients at 1 month, but its effects progressively decrease over time (only 30–40 % of patients are symptom free at 12 months). Repeated toxin injections are needed in most patients, the effect is not long lasting and fibrosis can occur at the level of the gastroesophageal junction, making a further operation more difficult and the results less predictable. The most important prognostic factors for a poor response to further botulinum toxin injection include a lack of an initial symptomatic response and residual LES pressure of 18 mmHg or greater

Pneumatic Dilatation

Pneumatic dilatation of the LES has been standardized with the introduction of Rigiflex balloons (Boston Scientific Corporation, MA, USA). A balloon is inflated at the level of the gastroesophageal junction to rupture the muscle fibers leaving the mucosa intact.

In the 1980s, thanks to the introduction of low-compliance nonexpandable balloons of increasing diameters associated with a lower risk of perforation, pneumatic dilatation was considered the main treatment modality for patients with achalasia, and surgery had a secondary role in case of dilatation failure. In the last 20 years, the introduction of minimally invasive surgery has led to a gradual shift in the treatment algorithm of achalasia, and today endoscopic dilatation is mostly used for treating recurrent dysphagia after Heller myotomy.

Botulinum Toxin Injection Versus Pneumatic Dilatation

Compared to pneumatic dilatation, botulinum toxin injection is associated with significantly lower remission rates (36 % vs. 66 %) and higher relapse rates (50 % vs. 17 %) over a 12-month follow-up period. A randomized controlled trial showed at 2-year follow-up that about 66 % of patients undergoing botulinum toxin injection had symptom recurrence compared to 13.5 % of patients who had undergone laparoscopic Heller myotomy.

Therefore, in 2014, botulinum toxin injection should be reserved for patients not fit for more effective treatment modalities, such as pneumatic dilatation and laparoscopic Heller myotomy.

Surgical Treatment

In the last two decades, the wide acceptance gained by minimally invasive surgery has led to a gradual shift in the treatment algorithm of achalasia.

In 1991, the first minimally invasive esophageal myotomy was performed in the United States through a left thoracoscopic approach, followed a few months later by laparoscopic myotomy. Laparoscopy progressively became the approach of choice in most centers due to better results in terms of reduced postoperative discomfort, shorter hospital stay, quicker return to the daily activities, and relief of dysphagia compared to the open approach. The technical reasons for this switch included the better exposure of the gastroesophageal junction and the possibility to perform a fundoplication, therefore reducing the risk of postoperative gastroesophageal reflux which was about 60 % after the thoracoscopic approach.

Laparoscopic Heller Myotomy and Dor Fundoplication: Our Technique

- Five trocars are used (Fig. 11.1).
- The operation is started by dividing the gastro-hepatic ligament close to the apex of the right pillar of the crus.

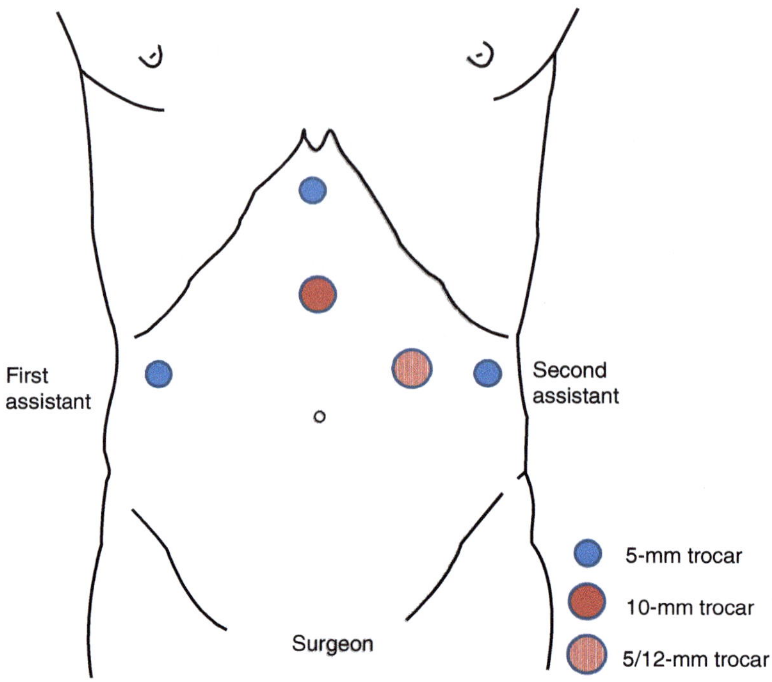

Fig. 11.1 Placement of the trocars

- The right and left pillars of the crus are separated by blunt dissection from the anterior wall of the esophagus after division of the phreno-esophageal ligament. The dissection is then continued in the posterior mediastinum, lateral and anterior to the esophagus, in order to expose 8–10 cm of the esophagus. During this part of the dissection, it is important to identify and preserve the anterior vagus nerve. No posterior dissection is necessary if a Dor fundoplication is planned. In patients with a sigmoid esophagus, it is important to extend the dissection more proximally in the posterior mediastinum to straighten of the esophageal axis.
- The gastric fundus is dissected and the gastrophrenic ligament is divided. The short gastric vessels are not routinely divided.
- Traction is then applied by a grasper to expose the right side of the esophageal wall. The myotomy is performed using the hook cautery in the 11 o'clock position. After reaching the submucosal plane in one point, about 2–3 cm above the gastroesophageal junction, the myotomy is then extended for about 6 cm upward and 2–2.5 cm onto the gastric wall.

At the end of the myotomy, an upper endoscopy is routinely performed to verify the complete section of the muscular fibers and the absence of mucosal injuries.

Because the main goal of the LHM is the relief of dysphagia while preventing reflux, the type of fundoplication is crucial. An LHM alone is associated with postoperative reflux in about 50–60 % of patients. If a Nissen fundoplication is performed, the risk of persistent or recurrent dysphagia is increased. A partial fundoplication added to the myotomy achieves better functional results when compared to a total fundoplication because it takes into account the lack of peristalsis. A recent multicenter, randomized controlled trial did not find significant differences in control of reflux after partial anterior and partial posterior fundoplication. A Dor fundoplication is often preferred because it is simpler to perform, covers the exposed esophageal mucosa, and keeps separated the edges of the myotomy.

- The Dor fundoplication is constructed by using two rows of sutures.
- The first row of sutures is on the left and consists of three stitches that incorporate the esophageal and the gastric wall only.
- The stomach is then folded over the exposed mucosa so that the greater curvature lies next to the right pillar of the crus.
- The right row of sutures also has three stitches. The uppermost stitch includes the gastric fundus, the right side of the esophageal wall and the right pillar of the crus. The second and the third stitches are placed between the greater curvature of the stomach and the right pillar of the crus.

LHM is associated with minimal postoperative pain, short hospital stay (2–3 days), and fast recovery to daily activities (2–3 weeks). Symptoms are improved in 90–95 % of patients at 5 years and in about 90 % at 10 years. Symptoms recurrence mainly occurs during the first 2–3 years of follow-up and may be secondary to fibrosis at the level of the distal edge of the myotomy. Most cases can be successfully treated with pneumatic dilatation.

Increased age and esophageal diameter are not predictors of poor outcomes. Therefore, LHM should be also performed in elderly patients and in those with a dilated and sigmoid esophagus, while esophagectomy should be considered only in case of LHM failure.

Postoperative gastroesophageal reflux is demonstrated by 24-h ambulatory pH monitoring in less than 15 % of patients when a partial fundoplication is performed, and it is usually well controlled by proton pump inhibitors.

Pneumatic Dilatation Versus LHM

Compared to pneumatic dilatation, LHM obtains better results in terms of dysphagia improvement and postoperative gastroesophageal reflux rates, with a significantly lower risk of re-intervention. While the results are similar at a short-term follow-up, long-term follow-up shows that most patients after LHM are asymptomatic, compared to only 50 % of patients even after multiple pneumatic dilatations. In addition, previous endoscopic treatment, such as botulinum toxin injection or pneumatic dilatation, may compromise the clinical outcome of LHM. Higher intraoperative complication rates and poorer long-term outcomes after LHM have been reported in several series of patients previously treated with endoscopic treatments. These findings may be related to scar tissue at the level of the gastroesophageal junction that makes surgical dissection of the anatomic planes more difficult.

In 2011, Boeckxstaens et al. reported the results of a multicenter, randomized trial comparing pneumatic dilatation to LHM with Dor fundoplication for untreated esophageal achalasia. The perforation rate during pneumatic dilatation and LHM was 4 and 12 %, respectively. Therapeutic success was defined as a drop in Eckardt score below 3. The study showed similar success rates after LHM (90 %) and pneumatic dilatation (86 %) over a 2-year follow-up period. However, the 2-year follow-up of this trial is short. Several studies have demonstrated that the success rate of pneumatic dilatation at 10–15 years is 40–50 % only, even after several endoscopic sessions.

In conclusion, while in the pre-laparoscopic era, pneumatic dilatation was the main treatment modality for achalasia, in 2014, laparoscopic surgery represents the treatment of choice, while endoscopic dilatation plays a major role in patients who are poor candidates for surgery or in case of recurrent dysphagia after LHM.

New Surgical Approaches to Heller Myotomy for Achalasia

A few studies have reported recently the results of single-port laparoscopic Heller myotomy as an alternative to the conventional laparoscopic approach. The relief of dysphagia seems similar, but the short follow-up period and the absence of objective data regarding the postoperative reflux do not allow drawing any conclusions.

Some authors have found that robotic Heller myotomy is superior to the conventional laparoscopic approach in terms of reduced intraoperative esophageal perforation rates, suggesting a key role of the three-dimensional visualization and increased surgeon dexterity. However, these conclusions are limited by the poor quality of the studies. In addition, the high cost of robotic instrumentation and the increased operative times do not seem to warrant a wide diffusion of the robotic instead of the LHM.

Peroral Endoscopic Esophageal Myotomy (POEM)

POEM has been recently introduced as a novel approach to achalasia. This endoscopic procedure is performed under general anesthesia with endotracheal intubation. A submucosal injection of about 10 ml saline with 0.3 % indigo carmine is performed in the mid esophagus, approximately 13 cm proximal to the gastroesophageal junction at the 2 o'clock position. A 2 cm longitudinal mucosal incision is made on the mucosal surface to create a mucosal entry to the submucosal space. Then, an anterior submucosal tunnel is created downwards, passing the gastroesophageal junction and about 3 cm into the proximal stomach. Additional indigo carmine solution is sequentially injected to mark progression of the tunnel, as well as to aid in hydrodissection and hemostasis. Once the submucosal tunnel is completed, section of the circular muscle fibers begins 2–3 cm distal to the mucosal entry, approximately 7 cm above the gastroesophageal junction. The myotomy is continued step by step distally until the gastric submucosa is reached, extending approximately 2–3 cm distal to the gastroesophageal junction. After identification and section of the circular muscle fibers of the lower esophagus and proximal stomach, the mucosal entry site is closed with hemostatic clips.

Several potential advantages of this technique have been proposed. First, the endoscopic approach should theoretically minimize postoperative pain. Second, a longer myotomy can be performed, extending to the medium third of the esophagus, just below the aortic arch. Finally, a concomitant antireflux surgery may not be required because of the selective section of the circular muscle fibers without any dissection at the level of the gastroesophageal junction.

Today, only few data are available regarding clinical outcomes in small series of patients over very short follow-up periods.

Inoue et al. published in 2010 their initial experience of POEM performed in 17 consecutive patients with achalasia. Mean operative time was 126 min, ranging from 100 to 180 min. The average length of the myotomy was 8.1 cm, being about 6 cm in the esophagus and 2 cm in the stomach. Pneumoperitoneum occurred in one patient, causing temporary elevation of intraperitoneal pressure; puncture of the abdominal wall using a needle allowed quick recovery without sequelae. None of the 17 patients had postoperative clinically evident subcutaneous emphysema. In all cases POEM significantly reduced the resting LES pressure (from mean 52.4 to 19.9 mmHg; $P=0.0001$). During a mean follow-up of 5 months, no patient developed recurrent symptoms of dysphagia, while reflux esophagitis (grade B according to Los Angeles classification) was diagnosed in one patient who was successfully treated with medical therapy. No patients required any further endoscopic or surgical treatment.

Swanstrom et al. published in 2012 6-month physiological and symptomatic outcomes in 18 patients undergoing POEM for achalasia. Median myotomy length was 9 (range, 7–12) cm, and the median operating time was 135 (range, 90–260) min. Three intraoperative complications (2 gastric mucosotomies and 1 full-thickness esophagotomy) were reported. All complications were repaired endoscopically with no sequelae. The median hospital stay was 1 day and median return to normal activity was 3 (range, 3–9) days. All patients had relief of dysphagia at a mean follow-up of 11.4 months. Postoperative manometry and barium swallows showed significant improvements in LES relaxation and esophageal emptying, respectively. Gastroesophageal reflux was objectively diagnosed by 24-h pH monitoring in 46 % of patients at 6 months after POEM.

In 2013, von Renteln et al. reported the outcomes of 70 achalasia patients treated with POEM in a prospective, international, multicenter trial of POEM conducted in Europe and North America. At 3 months after POEM, 97 % of patients were in symptom remission, and LES pressures were reduced from 28 to 9 mmHg ($P<0.001$). The percentage of patients in symptom remission at 6 and 12 months was 89 and 82 %, respectively. Symptoms of reflux were reported by 37 % of patients at 12 months after the procedure.

Only a few nonrandomized studies have compared retrospectively POEM and LHM. Hungness et al. compared 18 patients undergoing POEM to 55 patients treated by LHM. No differences were observed in terms of length of the myotomy, complication rate, and length of hospital stay. Veress needle decompression of the pneumoperitoneum was required intraoperatively in seven (39 %) patients undergoing POEM. Treatment success (Eckardt score ≤ 3) after POEM was achieved in 16 (89 %) patients at median 6-month follow-up. Six weeks after POEM, routine follow-up manometry and timed esophagram showed normalization of esophagogastric junction pressures and contrast column heights.

Bhayani et al. have recently published the results of a comparative study including 64 patients treated with LHM (42 % Toupet and 58 % Dor fundoplications) and 37 with POEM. Median operative time (149 vs 120 min, $P<0.001$) and mean hospitalization (2.2 vs 1.1 days, $P<0.0001$) were significantly higher for HM patients. No differences were observed in postoperative morbidity. POEM patients had a significantly better Eckardt scores at 1 month follow-up (1.8 vs. 0.8, $P<0.0001$), while no differences were observed at 6 months. LES resting pressures were higher after POEM than after HM (16 vs 7.1 mmHg, $P=0.006$). Postoperatively, 39 % of POEM patients and 32 % of HM patients had abnormal esophageal acid exposure.

Based on the limited evidence available, POEM seems to be a promising new procedure. However, there are some concerns about this new technique:

1. Endoscopic myotomy is a very demanding procedure, requiring major skills, with a steep learning curve.
2. Even though several studies have reported significant reduction of LES pressure as demonstrated by manometry, the LES pressure was often between 15 and 20 mmHg. As we know, a predictor of long-term success is a LES pressure around 10 mmHg;
3. Gastroesophageal reflux is reported in up to 50 % of patients after POEM, replicating the results obtained when a myotomy alone was performed without an antireflux operation.
4. Surgical revision in patients with recurrent dysphagia after POEM might be challenging. The presence of adhesion between the submucosal and the longitudinal muscular layer after POEM might make the dissection at this level very difficult.

Therefore, in 2014, POEM should be limited to patients included in prospective trials.

Summary

- Treatment modalities include endoscopic botulinum toxin injection, pneumatic dilation, laparoscopic Heller myotomy, and peroral endoscopic myotomy.
- Repeated toxin injections are needed in most patients, the effect is not long lasting, and fibrosis can occur at the level of the gastroesophageal junction, making a further operation more difficult and the results less predictable.

- Endoscopic dilatation is mostly used for treating recurrent dysphagia after Heller myotomy.
- Laparoscopic Heller myotomy is currently the approach of choice in most centers.
- Increased age and esophageal diameter are not predictors of poor outcomes.
- A partial fundoplication added to the myotomy achieves better functional results compared to a total fundoplication because it takes into account the lack of peristalsis.
- There are no significant differences in control of reflux after partial anterior (Dor) and partial posterior (Toupet) fundoplication.
- POEM is a novel promising approach to achalasia. Long-term results are needed to validate this procedure in the treatment of achalasia.

Selected Reading

1. Allescher HD, Storr M, Seige M, Gonzales-Donoso R, Ott R, Born P, et al. Treatment of achalasia: botulinum toxin injection vs. pneumatic balloon dilation. A prospective study with long-term follow-up. Endoscopy. 2001;33:1007–17.
2. Barry L, Ross S, Dahal S, Morton C, Okpaleke C, Rosas M, Rosemurgy AS. Laparoendoscopic single-site Heller myotomy with anterior fundoplication for achalasia. Surg Endosc. 2011;25:1766–74.
3. Bhayani NH, Kurian AA, Dunst CM, Sharata AM, Rieder E, Swanstrom LL. A comparative study on comprehensive, objective outcomes of laparoscopic Heller myotomy with Per-Oral Endoscopic Myotomy (POEM) for achalasia. Ann Surg. 2013 [Epub ahead of print].
4. Boeckxstaens GE, Annese V, des Varannes SB, Chaussade S, Costantini M, Cuttitta A, Elizalde JI, Fumagalli U, Gaudric M, Rohof WO, Smout AJ, Tack J, Zwinderman AH, Zaninotto G, Busch OR, European Achalasia Trial Investigators. Pneumatic dilation versus laparoscopic Heller's myotomy for idiopathic achalasia. N Engl J Med. 2011;364:1807–16.
5. Burpee SE, Mamazza J, Schlachta CM, Bendavid Y, Klein L, Moloo H, Poulin EC. Objective analysis of gastroesophageal reflux after laparoscopic Heller myotomy: an anti-reflux procedure is required. Surg Endosc. 2005;19:9–14.
6. Eckardt VF, Gockel I, Bernhard G. Pneumatic dilation for achalasia: late results of a prospective follow-up investigation. Gut. 2004;53:629–33.
7. Falkenback D, Johansson J, Oberg S, Kjellin A, Wenner J, Zilling T, Johnsson F, Von Holstein CS, Walther B. Heller's esophagomyotomy with or without a 360 degrees floppy Nissen fundoplication for achalasia. Long-term results from a prospective randomized study. Dis Esophagus. 2003;16:284–90.
8. Fisichella PM, Raz D, Palazzo F, Niponmick I, Patti MG. Clinical, radiological, and manometric profile in 145 patients with untreated achalasia. World J Surg. 2008;32:1974–9.
9. Inoue H, Minami H, Kobayashi Y, Sato Y, Kaga M, Suzuki M, Satodate H, Odaka N, Itoh H, Kudo S. Peroral endoscopic myotomy (POEM) for esophageal achalasia. Endoscopy. 2010;42:265–71.
10. Oelschlager BK, Chang L, Pellegrini CA. Improved outcome after extended gastric myotomy for achalasia. Arch Surg. 2003;138:490–7.
11. Patti MG, Arcerito M, De Pinto M, Feo CV, Tong J, Gantert W, Way LW. Comparison of thoracoscopic and laparoscopic Heller myotomy for achalasia. J Gastrointest Surg. 1998;2:561–6.
12. Patti MG, Feo CV, Arcerito M, De Pinto M, Tamburini A, Diener U, et al. Effects of previous treatment on results of laparoscopic Heller myotomy for achalasia. Dig Dis Sci. 1999;11:2270–6.

13. Patti MG, Fisichella PM, Perretta S, Galvani C, Gorodner MV, Robinson T, Way LW. Impact of minimally invasive surgery on the treatment of esophageal achalasia: a decade of change. J Am Coll Surg. 2003;196:698–705.
14. Patti MG, Pellegrini CA, Horgan S, Arcerito M, Omelanczuk P, Tamburini A, Diener U, Eubanks TR, Way LW. Minimally invasive surgery for achalasia. An 8-year experience with 168 patients. Ann Surg. 1999;230:587–93.
15. Pellegrini CA, Wetter LA, Patti MG, Leichter R, Mussan G, Mori T, Bernstein G, Way L. Thoracoscopic esophagomyotomy. Initial experience with a new approach for the treatment of achalasia. Ann Surg. 1992;216:291–6.
16. Rawlings A, Soper NJ, Oelschlager B, Swanstrom L, Matthews BD, Pellegrini C, Pierce RA, Pryor A, Martin V, Frisella MM, Cassera M, Brunt LM. Laparoscopic Dor versus Toupet fundoplication following Heller myotomy for achalasia: results of a multicenter, prospective, randomized-controlled trial. Surg Endosc. 2012;26:18–26.
17. Rebecchi F, Giaccone C, Farinella E, Campaci R, Morino M. Randomized controlled trial of laparoscopic Heller myotomy plus Dor fundoplication versus Nissen fundoplication for achalasia. Ann Surg. 2008;248:1023–30.
18. Richards WO, Torquati A, Holzman MD, Khaitan L, Byrne D, Lutfi R, Sharp KW. Heller myotomy versus Heller myotomy with Dor fundoplication. A prospective randomized double-blind clinical trial. Ann Surg. 2004;240:405–15.
19. Shaligram A, Unnirevi J, Simorov A, Kothari VM, Oleynikov D. How does the robot affect outcomes? A retrospective review of open, laparoscopic, and robotic Heller myotomy for achalasia. Surg Endosc. 2012;26:1047–50.
20. Smith CD, Stival A, Howell DL, Swafford V. Endoscopic therapy for achalasia before Heller myotomy results in worse outcomes than Heller myotomy alone. Ann Surg. 2006;243: 579–86.
21. Stefanidis D, Richardson W, Farrell TM, Kohn GP, Augenstein V, Fanelli RD, Society of American Gastrointestinal and Endoscopic Surgeons. SAGES guidelines for the surgical treatment of esophageal achalasia. Surg Endosc. 2012;26:296–311.
22. Sweet MP, Nipomnick I, Gasper WJ, Bagatelos K, Ostroff JW, Fisichella PM, Way LW, Patti MG. The outcome of laparoscopic Heller myotomy for achalasia is not influenced by the degree of esophageal dilatation. J Gastrointest Surg. 2008;12:159–65.
23. Vaezi MF, Richter JE, Wilcox CM, Schroeder PL, Birgisson S, Slaughter RL, et al. Botulinum toxin versus pneumatic dilatation in the treatment of achalasia: a randomised trial. Gut. 1999;44:231–9.
24. Von Renteln D, Fuchs KH, Fockens P, Bauerfeind P, Vassiliou MC, Werner YB, Fried G, Breithaupt W, Heinrich H, Bredenoord AJ, Kersten JF, Verlaan T, Trevisonno M, Rösch T. Peroral endoscopic myotomy for the treatment of achalasia: an international prospective multicenter study. Gastroenterology. 2013;145:309–11.
25. West RL, Hirsch DP, Bartelsman JFWM, de Borst J, Ferwerda G, Tytgat GNJ, et al. Long term results of pneumatic dilation in achalasia followed for more than 5 years. Am J Gastroenterol. 2002;97:1346–51.
26. Zaninotto G, Annese V, Costantini M, Del Genio A, Costantino M, Epifani M, et al. Randomized controlled trial of botulinum toxin versus laparoscopic Heller myotomy for esophageal achalasia. Ann Surg. 2004;239:364–70.

Chapter 12
Benign Esophageal Tumors: Evaluation and Treatment

Anahita Jalilvand and P. Marco Fisichella

Abstract The goal of this chapter is to describe the different varieties of benign esophageal tumors, their clinical presentation, and indications for treatment and provide an overview of the surgical management of patients with this rare benign esophageal pathology.

Keywords Benign esophageal tumors • Laparoscopic resection • Thoracoscopic resection • Esophageal leiomyoma • Duplication cysts

Benign tumors of the esophagus are rare and usually asymptomatic. Some of them can give rise to problems and warrant resection, which is accomplished by endoscopic means in most small intraluminal lesions and by minimally techniques for other larger intramural tumors, such as leiomyomas.

A. Jalilvand, MD
Department of Surgery, Loyola University Medical Center and Loyola Stritch School of Medicine, 2160 South 1st Ave, Maywood, IL 60153, USA

P.M. Fisichella, MD, MBA, FACS (✉)
Department of Surgery, Boston Veteran Administration Healthcare System, 1400 VFW Parkway, West Roxbury, MA 02132, USA

Department of Surgery, Brigham and Women's Hospital, Harvard Medical School, Boston, MA USA
e-mail: piero.fisichella@va.gov

P.M. Fisichella et al. (eds.), *Esophageal Diseases*,
DOI 10.1007/978-3-319-04337-1_12,

Classification

Benign esophageal tumors represent a broad category of lesions, which include esophageal leiomyomas, fibrovascular polyps, granular cell tumors, lipomas, esophageal hemangioma, and cysts and duplications. Of these pathologies, leiomyomas are the most common benign esophageal mass. Benign esophageal tumors can be classified in numerous ways, but most commonly they are categorized either by cell origin, location within the esophageal wall, or their appearance on imaging or endoscopy.

Epidemiology

Benign esophageal tumors are very rare and account for only 1–2 % of all resected esophageal masses. These masses are found incidentally in 0.5 % of the population on autopsy evaluation. The prevalence of benign esophageal tumors is equally distributed between men and women, although specific pathologies, such as esophageal granular cell tumors, are more common in men than in women.

Clinical Presentation

Since benign esophageal masses are usually found incidentally, patients are usually asymptomatic at diagnosis. If they are symptomatic, most often the presenting symptoms are correlated to the location of the lesions. For example, intraluminal lesions, such as cysts and fibrovascular polyps, are more likely to cause dysphagia than intramural lesions. Cervical esophageal tumors, particularly pedunculated lesions, can cause aspiration pneumonia. On the other hand, intramural lesions, such as leiomyomas and granular cell tumors, can become symptomatic if they are large enough to cause intraluminal obstruction. Additional symptoms can include cough, substernal pain, and weight loss. Esophageal hemangiomas can present with sometimes devastating and fatal hemorrhage.

Diagnostic Testing

Workup includes computed tomography of the chest, barium swallow, upper endoscopy, and endoscopic ultrasound.

Computed tomography is useful in determining the location of the tumor within the esophageal wall as well as determining anatomic relationships for large intraluminal or intramural tumors.

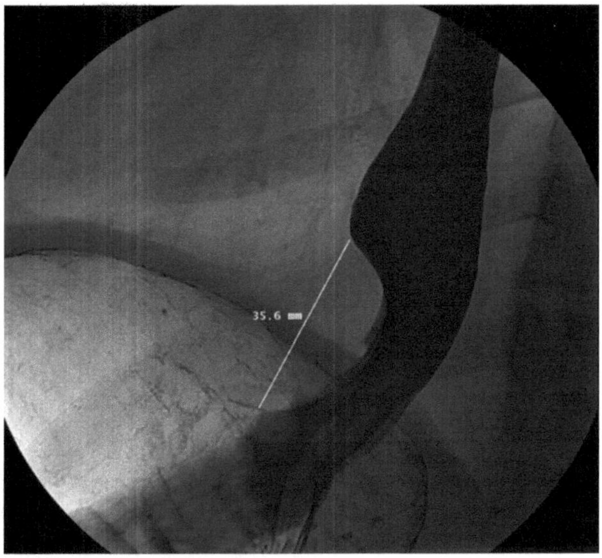

Fig. 12.1 Barium swallow showing an esophageal leiomyoma

A barium swallow can identify other pathologies, such as hiatal hernias or esophageal diverticula. In addition, it can highlight areas of filling defects within the esophagus and assess the laterality of the lesion for surgical planning during thoracoscopy (Figs. 12.1 and 12.2).

Upper endoscopy allows for direct visualization and biopsy of suspicious lesions. Therapeutic procedures can also be accomplished through endoscopy, such as endoscopic resection. Intraoperatively, upper endoscopy can help in locating the lesion when enucleation is planned using minimally invasive techniques.

Endoscopic ultrasound is frequently utilized during the upper endoscopy to rule out evidence of malignancy; findings consistent with malignancy include tumor size greater than 4 cm, heterogeneous echo patterns, and regional lymphadenopathy. Endoscopic ultrasound can also add further detail as to the location and appearance of a tumor within the layers of the esophagus and guide fine-needle aspiration, when needed.

Indications for Surgery

Since these lesions are benign, most patients who are asymptomatic can be managed with routine observation and periodic imaging. When patients become symptomatic, then surgical treatment is indicated. Specifically, small intraluminal or mucosal lesions can be resected endoscopically, whereas those suspicious for malignancy, tumors which are very large and symptomatic, or masses which are causing complications such as mucosal ulceration or hemorrhage should be resected in the operating room.

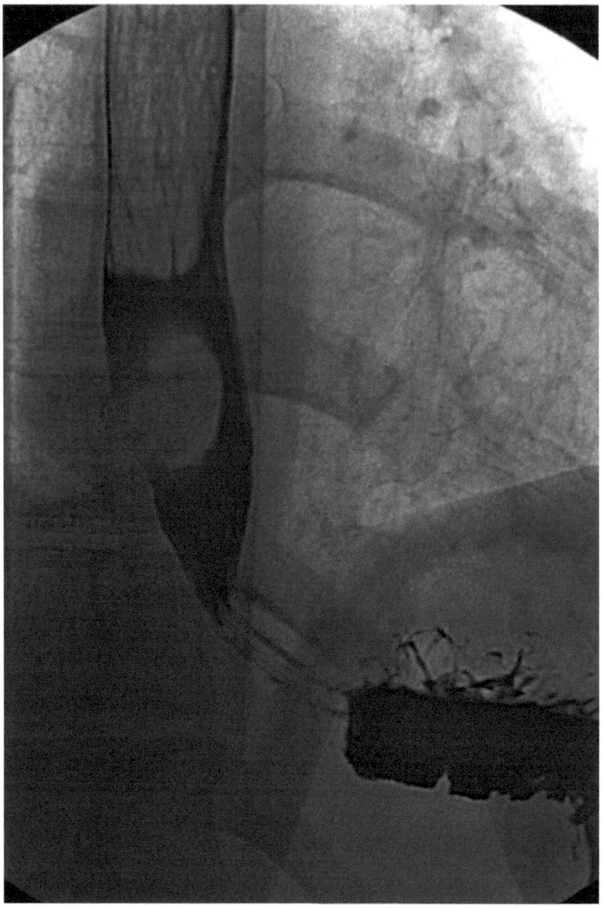

Fig. 12.2 Barium swallow showing an esophageal duplication cyst

Minimally invasive techniques have shown to have very good results in resection of benign esophageal tumors with low mortality and complication rates. Such techniques include using thoracoscopy and laparoscopy for tumor enucleation. Enucleation consists of incising and splitting the muscle fibers over the mass and then dissecting the mass from the muscle fibers and submucosa without violating it. When the enucleation is performed close to the gastroesophageal junction, a fundoplication should be performed to prevent reflux after the continence mechanisms of the distal esophagus are disrupted. A careful preoperative workup must be performed to determine the location of the tumor from the hiatus, which will influence the surgical approaches used: laparoscopic or thoracoscopic. Endoscopic resection is usually reserved for lesions that are intraluminal, polypoid, less than 2 cm in diameter, or intramural and originating no deeper than the muscularis mucosae. Snare polypectomy, endoscopic mucosal resection (EMR), and endoscopic submucosal dissection (ESD) are the most common endoscopic techniques today available.

Leiomyoma

Over 50 % of benign esophageal tumors are leiomyomas, making them the most common benign esophageal pathology. These are mesenchymal spindle-shaped tumors, which on histology demonstrate interlacing bundles of muscle cells. They are typically found intramurally and usually originate in the lower 2/3 of the esophagus from the muscularis propria or muscularis mucosa. A small percentage of these masses have been found intraluminally, although this occurs less than 10 % of the time. They are more commonly identified in men between the ages of 20 and 60. However when they are congenital lesions, they are most commonly seen in females. Leiomyomatosis, which is a very rare familial disorder, presents with numerous esophageal and gastric leiomyomas and is most commonly seen in females in conjunction with genital hypertrophy. Most resected leiomyomas are between 2 and 6 cm, averaging 4–5 cm in diameter. As these are commonly intramural masses, patients are often asymptomatic, although it has been reported that approximately 50 % of patients present with symptoms. The most commonly reported symptom, if they do become symptomatic, is dysphagia, followed by reflux symptoms, weight loss, and odynophagia. On imaging, a barium swallow will depict a round, sharply delineated defect (Fig. 12.1). A well-circumscribed, hypoechoic, and homogeneous mass is characteristically found on endoscopic ultrasound and can be very helpful in distinguishing it from other malignant pathologies. Fine-needle aspiration and cold forceps biopsy have not been shown to be helpful in the diagnosis and may cause complications such as bleeding and infection. Computed tomography of the chest is not useful in diagnosing the pathology, although it can be used to assess the extent of the tumor and its relationship with the surrounding anatomical structures. Distinguishing between GIST tumors and leiomyomas is necessary for determining process management options, and this usually requires histologic evaluation. Staining for desmin or actin can rule out GIST tumors, while CD34 and CD117 are present on GIST tumors.

Resection of a leiomyoma is reserved for symptomatic patients. Since malignant degeneration of esophageal leiomyoma is very rare, accounting only for 0.2 % of cases, this potential is not considered an indication for resection, although if features suggestive of such degeneration, including mucosal ulceration, tumor size greater than 5 cm, or interval growth, are present, resection should be considered. If resection is deemed necessary, it is traditionally approached through thoracoscopic and laparoscopic techniques, which involve enucleation. If the tumor is large or is presenting with malignant features, then segmental resection of the esophagus is appropriate.

Granular Cell Tumor

In contrast to leiomyomas, granular cell tumors are rare and are not commonly found in the gastrointestinal tract. Rather, these are submucosal tumors that are typically found in the tongue, skin, breast, and muscle. The first esophageal granular cell tumor was described by Abrikossoff in 1931. These tumors can be found in any part of the esophagus, although over 50 % of them are found in the distal esophagus. They are reported to be twice as common in women and are more prevalent in African Americans. On histopathologic evaluation, they appear to be derived from neural tissue, sharing similar characteristics with Schwann cells. Not unlike leiomyomas, granular cell tumors are submucosal and therefore do not usually present with significant symptomology, with over 90 % of patients not presenting with any symptoms at all. If the tumor is large enough, usually over 10 mm in diameter, dysphagia is usually the most common presenting symptom. Endoscopy is the diagnostic modality of choice, as it allows for both visualization and biopsy, and it will classically reveal a submucosal, yellow, polyploid lesion, typically found in the distal esophagus. Diagnosis is typically confirmed with multiple biopsies. In contrast to the hypoechoic leiomyomas, these lesions are hyperechoic on endoscopic ultrasound. It is important to note that these lesions have a 1–3 % risk of malignant conversion, although there has been no documented malignant conversion of granular cell tumors if the original pathology lacks malignant features.

Indication for removal of a granular cell tumor is reserved for symptomatic patients or if the tumor is larger than 1 cm. Resection can be accomplished endoscopically if the lesion is restricted to the submucosa. Minimally invasive techniques with both thoracoscopy and laparoscopy can also be used for enucleation.

Hemangioma

Hemangiomas are benign vascular tumors. They are extremely rare lesions and account for approximately 4.8 % of benign esophageal tumors. They are submucosal, and they can be found throughout the esophagus, although most commonly they are found in the upper half of the esophagus. Patients who have a history of Osler-Weber-Rendu disease may be at an increased risk of developing esophageal hemangiomas. Most reported cases have been in men and are diagnosed between the ages of 40 and 70. Most patients are asymptomatic, although hemangiomas can present with dysphagia and a significant risk of bleeding, which can be catastrophic and fatal. Endoscopy and endoscopic ultrasound, along with MRI and CT, can be used for diagnosis. A barium swallow will show a well-circumscribed mass, which may appear lobulated, making it difficult to distinguish it from other benign pathologies. Endoscopic evaluation will reveal a blue polypoid or sessile mass with sharp borders. Most lesions have been shown to measure between 5 mm and 20 cm in length. Under microscopic evaluation, these tumors are highly vascularized lesions, which can appear as blood clots. Diagnosis is therefore established using radiographic findings along with endoscopy and any reported symptomology. Biopsy is contraindicated, as this can lead to potentially fatal hemorrhage. Because of this risk of bleeding, intervention is typically always indicated. Traditionally, these lesions were managed with endoscopic resection. Currently, treatment modalities for hemangiomas include similar strategies used to manage esophageal varices, such as sclerotherapy and laser fulguration. Other options include EMR and minimally invasive techniques with laparoscopy and thoracoscopy for enucleation.

Lipoma

A lipoma is a benign proliferation of adipose tissue. Gastrointestinal lipomas account for a very small percentage of GI tumors, and most of these lipomas are found in the small intestine. Of all alimentary tract lipomas, only 2 % are found in the esophagus. Furthermore, only 2 % of all benign esophageal tumors are esophageal lipomas. Although gastrointestinal lipomas are more common in women than men overall, esophageal lipomas are more frequently found in men. The etiology of lipomas has not been clearly elucidated, although some have theorized that trauma can be an inciting factor for lipomatous growth. Esophageal lipomas can be found in the cervical and thoracic esophagus; in the cervical esophagus, lipomas are typically pedunculated intraluminal masses, while in the thoracic esophagus they are intramural lesions. There is some discussion as to whether pedunculated lipomas should be classified as fibrovascular polyps, as the latter can be described in terms of the composition of lipomatous, vascular, and fibrous tissue. The symptomology of a lipoma depends on its location. For example, cervical lipomas can present with symptoms such as regurgitation of undigested food, aspiration pneumonia, and dysphagia if they are large enough. Asphyxiation by a cervical lipoma has also been described in the literature. Cervical esophageal lipomas can be detected on imaging as an intraluminal filling defect. On endoscopy, they are yellow, soft, submucosal masses. "Tenting," which is described as the ability to retract normal mucosa over the suspected lesion, and the "cushion" sign, which is a "spongelike" characteristic of the lipomatous tissue, have both been identified as potential diagnostic findings on endoscopy. While tenting is seen in most cases, some have been reported with ulcerated mucosa, thought to be secondary to distal inflammation from acid reflux. Endoscopic ultrasound will reveal hyperechoic, well-circumscribed, homogeneous submucosal masses. Treatment of lipomas is almost always surgical, since lipomas have been shown to grow over time and because of the potential for very severe complications. Other possible indications include symptomatic patients, especially those with large lipomas of the cervical esophagus, given the risk for aspiration pneumonia. For pedunculated lesions, endoscopic ligation has been shown to be a useful treatment strategy.

Fibrovascular Polyps

Despite being the most common intraluminal benign esophageal neoplasm, fibrovascular polyps are very rare. They are most commonly found in Killian's triangle, which is bounded inferiorly by the cricopharyngeus and laterally and superiorly by the oblique lines of the thyropharyngeus on either side. Fibrovascular polyps arise from the submucosa and are propelled into the lumen over time through the action of repetitive peristaltic waves. These lesions can grow over time, some becoming large enough to extend into the cardia of the stomach. The largest fibrovascular polyp described was 25 cm in length. Despite this growth, they remain attached to the cervical esophagus by a discrete pedicle or stalk, which is an important feature when considering proper resection of the tumor. On histologic review, these lesions are composed of fibrous, lipomatous, and vascular tissue with an overlying squamous mucosa, although the composition of each tissue differs in each polyp. There has been no documented case of malignant conversion.

As they are mostly found in the cervical esophagus, presenting symptoms are similar to those of a Zenker's diverticulum or cervical esophageal lipoma and include dysphagia, regurgitation of undigested food, airway obstruction, and aspiration pneumonia. In some studies, over 50 % of patients with cervical fibrovascular polyps presented with regurgitation of the polyp into the oral cavity. If the polyp is very large, superficial ulceration can occur and cause bleeding and anemia. As with cervical lipomas, asphyxiation is also a risk.

The diagnosis of fibrovascular polyps can be easily made if the polyp is visualized in the oral cavity. A barium swallow will depict a "smooth, elongated" filling defect. A CT and MRI can also be used to diagnose the pathology; however, it is important to note that they may appear with varying densities on imaging, as each polyp may have different compositions of fibrous, vascular, and adipose tissue. Endoscopy is used to identify the site of origin of the polyp. If the lesion is large, this may be obvious on imaging, but if the polyp is small, it may be missed even on endoscopy as the lesion is characteristically covered with normal-appearing mucosa. The use of endoscopic ultrasound is particularly useful for determining the vascularity of the polyp, as this is important to consider during resection. Large polyps may have large feeding vessels, which may increase the risk of significant bleeding after a resection.

For larger polyps, given their location in the cervical esophagus, the risk of airway obstruction or aspiration pneumonia is significant, and for that reason, all large fibrovascular polyps typically require resection even if these complications have not emerged in the patient. Emergent tracheotomy has been documented in patients who have had large polyps causing airway obstruction.

Resection of all polyps involves removal of the base of the polyp, which requires adequate visualization of the pedicle. This not only allows for compete removal of the polyp but also decreases the risk of recurrence. For some polyps, this can be achieved through endoscopy, thus allowing for snare polypectomy and endoscopic mucosal resection. Large polyps may have to be removed through a cervical esophagectomy. For smaller polyps, endoscopic mucosal resection or snare polypectomy can be sufficient.

Duplication Cysts

Esophageal duplication cysts are congenital malformations that usually occur in the fourth week of embryologic development, during which the primitive foregut separates into an anterior diverticulum, which becomes the upper airway, and a posterior division, which eventually develops into the gastrointestinal tract. While no specific pathogenesis has been established for these lesions, some have hypothesized that aberrant persistence of an embryonic diverticula is the causative link, while others have proposed these cysts are caused by endodermal traction from the notochord during development. This group of esophageal tumors includes esophageal duplication cysts, bronchogenic cysts, gastric cysts, inclusion cysts, neuroenteric cysts, and acquired esophageal cysts. Esophageal duplication cysts must meet three criteria in order to be classified as such: they must be intramural lesions; they must be covered by at least two muscle layers; and the lining of the cyst must be from an esophageal embryologic origin (such as pseudostratified, columnar, cuboid, or ciliated mucosa) or squamous cell mucosa. The prevalence of esophageal duplication cysts is rare, and because so few cases have been described, the incidence is unknown. Since these are congenital lesions, they are most commonly identified in childhood.

For the most part, patients with esophageal duplication cysts are asymptomatic. Symptomatic cysts are usually the result of compression of nearby structures. When this occurs, the most common reported symptoms are of respiratory nature and include wheezing, coughing, and shortness of breath, if the cyst is located high in the esophagus. Cysts located behind the heart have been known to cause cardiac arrhythmias. Other symptoms include infection, erosion, and hemorrhage of the cyst, which can lead to fistulization and perforation. Cysts can very rarely undergo malignant transformation, with documented cases of adenocarcinoma and rhabdosarcoma.

While diagnosing this pathology may prove difficult, as with other benign esophageal pathologies, diagnosis should be accomplished using a combination of barium swallow, computed tomography of the chest, upper endoscopy, and endoscopic ultrasound. Barium swallow and endoscopy may reveal a small indentation at the site of the lesion, which is not useful in distinguishing this pathology from other benign esophageal masses (Fig. 12.2). Cold knife biopsy of the lesion can complicate future resection attempts and is therefore not recommended for definitive diagnosis. Biopsy of the lesion is also discouraged, as this can cause adhesions around the lesion and render future resection attempts more difficult. Endoscopic ultrasound can be useful in determining the location of the cyst within the esophageal wall and is also useful for distinguishing this pathology from esophageal leiomyomas. A CT/MRI can be used to determine the extent of the lesion and whether there are any anatomic relationships to consider before removing the cyst.

Because of the potential for infection, erosion, fistulization, as well as the small risk of malignant conversion, all cysts should be removed, even if patients are asymptomatic. Cyst resection involves enucleation and resection. A posterolateral thoracotomy was commonly used to accomplish this. Care should be made to resect the entire cyst along with its wall, as recurrence of cysts has been reported. However, in some cases where there are inflammation and dense adhesions, partial cyst removal may be the only appropriate solution. With the advent of minimally invasive procedures, both thoracoscopy and laparoscopy have become well-established modalities that have largely replaced open approaches.

Summary

- Benign tumors of the esophagus are rare and usually asymptomatic.
- Some of them can give rise to problems and warrant resection.
- Resection is accomplished by endoscopic means in most small intraluminal lesions and by minimally techniques for other larger intramural tumors, such as leiomyomas.
- Diagnosis should be accomplished using a combination of barium swallow, computed tomography of the chest, upper endoscopy, and endoscopic ultrasound.
- Leiomyomas are submucosal and intramural lesions and are the most common benign esophageal tumor. Resection is reserved for symptomatic tumors or those suspicious for malignancy.
- Granular cell tumors are submucosal lesions derived from neural tissue. Upper endoscopy is used to diagnose the lesion, and resection is reserved for tumors greater than 1 cm. There is a 1–3 % risk of malignant conversion.
- Hemangiomas are submucosal vascular tumors; because these lesions can present with significant bleeding, needle biopsy is contraindicated, and treatment with sclerotherapy, laser fulguration, or other resection techniques is indicated.
- Lipomas may either be pedunculated in the cervical esophagus or intramural lesions in the thoracic esophagus. Cervical lipomas may cause aspiration pneumonia and should be resected if they are large enough.
- Fibrovascular polyps are the most common intraluminal lesions. Resection is reserved for cervical polyps, which may obstruct the patient's airway. This can be accomplished using EMR, snare polypectomy, or cervical esophagectomy if the lesion is very large.
- Duplication cysts are congenital malformations, which are typically resected given the risk of infection, mucosal erosion, and fistulization.

Selected Reading

1. Azzie G, Beasley S. Diagnosis and treatment of foregut duplications. Semin Pediatr Surg. 2003;12(1):46–54.
2. Bardini R, Segalin A, Asolati M, Bonavina L, Pavanello M. Thoracoscopic removal of benign tumours of the oesophagus. Endosc Surg Allied Technol. 1993;1(5–6):277–9.
3. Choong CK, Meyers BF. Benign esophageal tumors: introduction, incidence, classification, and clinical features. Semin Thorac Cardiovasc Surg. 2003;15(1):3–8.
4. Espeso A, Verma S, Jani P, Sudhoff H. Mediastinal foregut duplication cyst presenting as a rare cause of breathing difficulties in an adult. Eur Arch Otorhinolaryngol. 2007;264(11): 1357–60.
5. Geller A, Wang KK, DiMagno EP. Diagnosis of foregut duplication cysts by endoscopic ultrasonography. Gastroenterology. 1995;109(3):838–42.
6. Herbella FA, Tedesco P, Muthusamy R, Patti MG. Thoracoscopic resection of esophageal duplication cysts. Dis Esophagus. 2006;19(2):132–4.
7. Hirose S, Clifton MS, Bratton B, Harrison MR, Farmer DL, Nobuhara KK, et al. Thoracoscopic resection of foregut duplication cysts. J Laparoendosc Adv Surg Tech A. 2006;16(5):526–9.

8. Kang CU, Cho DG, Cho KD, Jo MS. Thoracoscopic stapled resection of multiple esophageal duplication cysts with different pathological findings. Eur J Cardiothorac Surg. 2008;34(1):216–8.
9. Kent M, d'Amato T, Nordman C, Schuchert M, Landreneau R, Alvelo-Rivera M, et al. Minimally invasive resection of benign esophageal tumors. J Thorac Cardiovasc Surg. 2007;134(1):176–81.
10. Kim TS, Song SY, Han J, Shim YM, Jeong HS. Giant fibrovascular polyp of the esophagus: CT findings. Abdom Imaging. 2005;30(6):653–5.
11. Kinney T, Waxman I. Treatment of benign esophageal tumors by endoscopic techniques. Semin Thorac Cardiovasc Surg. 2003;15(1):27–34.
12. Lee LS, Singhal S, Brinster CJ, Marshall B, Kochman ML, Kaiser LR, et al. Current management of esophageal leiomyoma. J Am Coll Surg. 2004;198(1):136–46.
13. Mutrie CJ, Donahue DM, Wain JC, Wright CD, Gaissert HA, Grillo HC, et al. Esophageal leiomyoma: a 40-year experience. Ann Thorac Surg. 2005;79(4):1122–5.
14. Ordonez NG, Mackay B. Granular cell tumor: a review of the pathology and histogenesis. Ultrastruct Pathol. 1999;23(4):207–22.
15. Rice TW. Benign esophageal tumors: esophagoscopy and endoscopic esophageal ultrasound. Semin Thorac Cardiovasc Surg. 2003;15(1):20–6.
16. Seremetis MG, Lyons WS, de Guzman VC, Peabody Jr JW. Leiomyomata of the esophagus. An analysis of 838 cases. Cancer. 1976;38(5):2166–77.
17. Sogabe M, Taniki T, Fukui Y, Yoshida T, Okamoto K, Okita Y, et al. A patient with esophageal hemangioma treated by endoscopic mucosal resection: a case report and review of the literature. J Med Invest. 2006;53(1–2):177–82.
18. Solerio D, Gasparri G, Ruffini E, Camandona M, De Angelis C, Raggio E, et al. Giant fibrovascular polyp of the esophagus. Dis Esophagus. 2005;18(6):410–2.
19. von Rahden BH, Stein HJ, Feussner H, Siewert JR. Enucleation of submucosal tumors of the esophagus: minimally invasive versus open approach. Surg Endosc. 2004;18(6):924–30.
20. Weigel TL, Schwartz DC, Gould JC, Pfau PR. Transgastric laparoscopic resection of a giant esophageal lipoma. Surg Laparosc Endosc Percutan Tech. 2005;15(3):160–2.
21. Zaninotto G, Portale G, Costantini M, Rizzetto C, Salvador R, Rampado S, et al. Minimally invasive enucleation of esophageal leiomyoma. Surg Endosc. 2006;20(12):1904–8.

Chapter 13
Gastroesophageal Reflux Disease: From Heartburn to Cancer

Marco E. Allaix, Bernardo A. Borraez, and Marco G. Patti

Abstract The pathophysiology of gastroesophageal reflux disease (GERD) is multifactorial. Barrett's esophagus is the result of continuous injury to the esophageal mucosa exposed to gastric refluxate. This condition can progress to low-grade and high-grade dysplasia (HGD) and eventually to adenocarcinoma. HGD and intramucosal carcinoma have traditionally been treated by esophagectomy. Today, however, most patients with HGD and intramucosal carcinoma are treated with endoscopic modalities, while esophagectomy is reserved for selected cases.

Keywords Gastroesophageal reflux disease • Heartburn • Barrett's esophagus • Dysplasia • Adenocarcinoma • Fundoplication • Endoscopic mucosal resection • Radiofrequency ablation • Esophagectomy

---

Conflict of Interest
The authors have no conflicts of interest to declare.

M.E. Allaix, MD
Department of Surgical Sciences, University of Torino,
Corso A.M. Dogliotti 14, 10126 Torino, Italy

B.A. Borraez, MD • M.G. Patti, MD, FACS (✉)
Department of Surgery, Center for Esophageal Diseases,
University of Chicago Pritzker School of Medicine,
5841 S. Maryland Ave, MC 5095, Room G-207, Chicago, IL 60637, USA
e-mail: mpatti@surgery.bsd.uchicago.edu

P.M. Fisichella et al. (eds.), *Esophageal Diseases*,
DOI 10.1007/978-3-319-04337-1_13, © Springer International Publishing Switzerland 2014

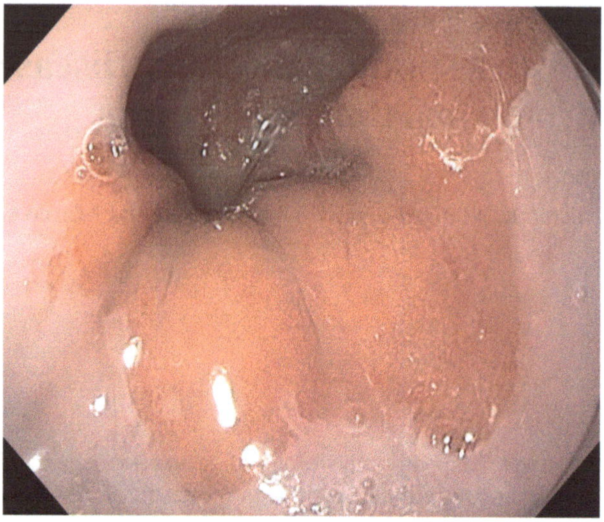

Fig. 13.1 Endoscopic view of Barrett's esophagus

Introduction

Gastroesophageal reflux disease GERD is the most common upper gastrointestinal condition diagnosed in Western countries, and it accounts for about 75 % of esophageal disorders. As a consequence of continuous injury to the esophageal mucosa secondary to gastric refluxate, about 10–15 % of patients with GERD develop columnar esophageal metaplasia containing goblet cells (Barrett's esophagus) (Fig. 13.1). Subsequently, Barrett's esophagus might progress to low-grade dysplasia (LGD) and high-grade dysplasia (HGD) and eventually to adenocarcinoma (Fig. 13.2). Barrett's esophagus with HGD is considered a precursor of invasive adenocarcinoma. Thus, adenocarcinoma represents the final step of a sequence of events in which a benign disease (GERD) evolves into a preneoplastic disease and eventually into cancer.

The adenocarcinoma of the esophagus, which occurs in most cases as a consequence of chronic gastroesophageal reflux, is currently the malignancy with the fastest increase of incidence in the United States, and has become the most prevalent histopathologic type of esophageal cancer.

This chapter focuses on the sequence of pathophysiologic events that lead from GERD to a preneoplastic disease, and eventually to cancer, and on the treatment options currently available.

Pathophysiology of GERD

The pathophysiology of GERD is multifactorial, since the physiologic control of gastric refluxate is based on several different components, including esophageal clearance, competence of the gastroesophageal junction, and gastric emptying.

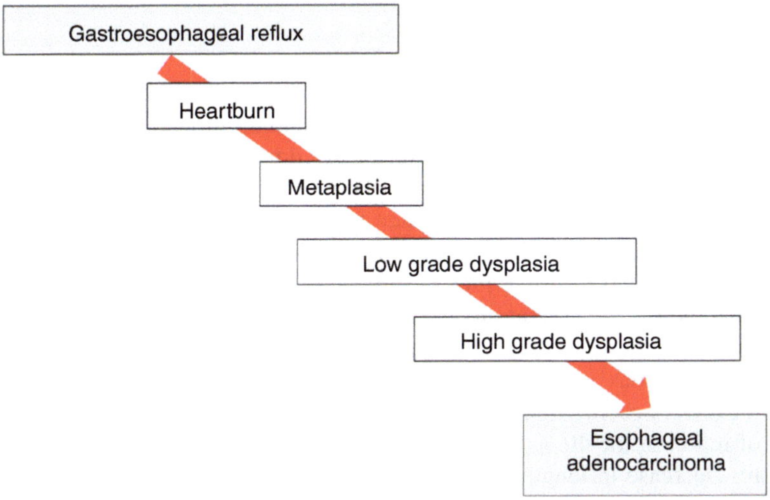

Fig. 13.2 Progression fron GERD to esophageal cancer

Esophageal clearance is promoted by esophageal peristalsis and saliva production, while competence of the gastroesophageal junction is governed by the lower esophageal sphincter (LES), the diaphragm, the angle of His, and the phrenoesophageal membrane.

Esophageal Peristalsis

Esophageal peristalsis plays a fundamental role in the antireflux mechanism because it governs esophageal clearance of the gastric contents. As a consequence, defective peristalsis is associated with symptoms and mucosal injury secondary to gastroesophageal reflux. Two indirect measurements of esophageal clearance are included in the DeMeester score: (1) number of reflux episodes longer than 5 min and (2) length of the longest episode. In addition, the average esophageal clearance time can be calculated by dividing the total time spent with pH below 4 by the number of reflux episodes. Therefore, severe symptoms and a higher degree of esophagitis (including Barrett's esophagus) are reported more likely in GERD patients with abnormal peristalsis and in systemic diseases that impair esophageal peristalsis, such as connective tissue disorders.

Abnormal peristalsis is present in 40–50 % of patients with GERD, and in about 20 % of them, it is particularly severe with very low amplitude and/or abnormal propagation of the peristaltic waves (ineffective esophageal motility).

There are no medications that improve esophageal peristalsis, while an effective fundoplication has been shown to ameliorate the impaired peristalsis in most patients.

Lower Esophageal Sphincter

The LES consists of tonically contracted smooth muscle that determines a 3–4 cm long high pressure zone between the esophagus and the stomach that prevents gastroesophageal reflux. The resting pressure of a competent LES ranges between 15 and 35 mmHg. At the time of swallowing, the LES relaxes for 5–10 s to allow the food bolus to enter the stomach and then regains its resting tone. The LES has a tendency to relax periodically independently from swallowing. These periodic relaxations are called *transient lower esophageal sphincter relaxations* (TLESR) to distinguish them from relaxations triggered by swallows. TLESRs account for the physiologic gastroesophageal reflux present in any individual. The cause of these transient relaxations is not known, but gastric distention probably plays a role. When TLESRs become more prolonged and frequent, they are the most common cause of reflux in the 40 % of patients with GERD who have normal resting LES pressure. Decrease in length and/or pressure of the LES is responsible for pathologic reflux in the remaining patients with GERD.

While TLESR is thought to be the most common mechanism of reflux in patients with either absent or mild mucosal injury, the prevalence of a mechanically defective LES increases in patients with severe esophagitis and when Barrett's esophagus is present.

At this moment, there are no medications that act on the LES, underlining that an incompetent LES represents a defect of the gastroesophageal barrier that can only be surgically corrected by a fundoplication.

Diaphragm

The left and right pillars of the crus have a synergistic action with the LES. This pinchcock action of the diaphragm is particularly important because it protects against reflux caused by sudden increases of intra-abdominal pressure, such as with coughing or bending. This synergistic action of the diaphragm is lost when a hiatal hernia is present, as the gastroesophageal junction is displaced above the diaphragm. The size of the hiatal hernia is associated with a more incompetent LES, impaired peristalsis, and increased acid exposure. Not surprisingly, a hiatal hernia is common in patients with Barrett's esophagus.

Increase of Thoracoabdominal Pressure Gradient and Obesity

Increased thoracoabdominal pressure gradient can contribute to GERD. Morbid obesity is a well-known cause of increased thoracoabdominal pressure gradient secondary to the increased abdominal pressure and intragastric pressure. Several studies have evaluated the relationship between increasing body mass index (BMI) and prevalence of GERD and its complications. BMI is independently associated with the severity of GERD in obese patients. Notably, a low prevalence of defective LES and higher peristaltic waves amplitude have been reported among obese patients with GERD, suggesting a physiologic compensatory mechanism to the increased thoracoabdominal pressure gradient.

It has been speculated that the increased negative intrathoracic pressure that occurs in some patients with lung disease may induce GERD. Thus, even with a manometrically normal LES, reflux can occur as a consequence of stressors that lead to a thoracoabdominal pressure gradient that exceeds the resting LES pressure.

Finally, abnormal gastric emptying might contribute to GERD by increasing intragastric pressure. If delayed gastric emptying is diagnosed, appropriate therapy should be considered, including medication such as metoclopramide and total fundoplication that are shown to increase gastric emptying.

Type of Refluxate

The gastroesophageal refluxate contains agents of gastric origin, such as hydrochloric acid and pepsin, and duodenal origin, including bile salts and pancreatic enzymes that are both noxious to the esophageal mucosa. It is well known that bile reflux causes symptoms and may be associated with the development of Barrett's esophagus and esophageal adenocarcinoma. Both symptom perception and mucosal injury are linked to a high proximal exposure and large amount of reflux.

Treatment of Barrett's Esophagus

Metaplasia

The treatment options are similar to those of patients with GERD without metaplasia: medical therapy (PPIs) and laparoscopic antireflux surgery.

A surgical approach might offer an advantage over medical therapy for the following reasons:

1. Successful elimination of reflux symptoms with PPIs does not guarantee control of acid reflux. When pH monitoring is performed in asymptomatic Barrett patients treated with these medications, up to 80 % of them still have abnormal acid reflux.
2. PPIs do not eliminate the reflux of bile, a major contributor to the pathogenesis of Barrett's esophagus. In contrast, an antireflux operation prevents any form of reflux by restoring the competence of the gastroesophageal junction.

The effect of both medical and surgical therapy on regression of the columnar epithelium is under evaluation. The current evidence supports the concept that antireflux surgery can promote regression only in short-segment Barrett's esophagus, but not in long-segment Barrett's esophagus. There is today no conclusive evidence that either medications or antireflux surgery can prevent development of cancer in patients with GERD and metaplasia.

Radiofrequency ablation (*RFA*) is based on the application of direct thermal energy to the esophageal mucosa using electrodes embedded in circumferential balloon or focal device. Potential complications of RFA include noncardiac chest pain, esophageal lacerations, and stenosis.

However, because the risk of progression of non-dysplastic Barrett's esophagus to adenocarcinoma is estimated by recent studies at 0.12–0.27 % per year and complications with RFA are present even though minimal, RFA is not currently recommended for patients with non-dysplastic Barrett's esophagus or LGD, until further risk stratification for this subgroup of patients will be available.

Low-Grade Dysplasia

Patients diagnosed with LGD should be treated for about 2 months with high doses of PPI (3–4 pills per day), and subsequently the endoscopy should be repeated with multiple biopsies. The rationale is to decrease the mucosal inflammation by blocking acid secretion, allowing the pathologist a more accurate reading. If the repeated biopsies show metaplasia or HGD, the patient will be treated accordingly. If LGD is confirmed, the same treatment as in case of metaplasia, i.e., laparoscopic fundoplication, should be proposed along with RFA. Nevertheless, endoscopic surveillance, aiming to detect recurrence and subsquamous glands, should be performed every 6 months because these patients have a risk of developing esophageal cancer greater than patients with non-dysplastic Barrett's esophagus.

High-Grade Dysplasia

Patients with HGD are at a higher risk for adenocarcinoma than patients with Barrett's esophagus without dysplasia or with LGD.

Esophagectomy has been the treatment of choice for HGD in the setting of Barrett's esophagus for many years, due to the high prevalence of occult esophageal cancer in patients undergoing esophagectomy for HGD reported to be as high as 40 %.

A recent review of studies that provided adequate differentiation between intramucosal (IMC, T1a) and submucosal invasion (T1b or beyond) has suggested that the prevalence of T1b cancer in the setting of HGD is about 13 %. The risk of lymph node metastases is 0 % for HGD and about 1–3 % for T1a cancer, while it is between 20 and 30 % for T1b cancer. These findings along with the development of new endoscopic techniques, including endoscopic mucosal resection (EMR) and endoscopic ultrasound (EUS), have determined a shift in the approach to most patients with HGD and IMC from esophagectomy to local endoscopic treatment, while esophagectomy is still the treatment of choice in T1b cancer patients.

Endoscopic eradication can be achieved through resection techniques (tissue-acquiring modalities) or through ablative therapies (non-tissue-acquiring modalities). Endoscopic tissue-acquiring techniques include focal EMR, complete Barrett's EMR, and endoscopic submucosal dissection. Ablative therapies include radiofrequency ablation and cryotherapy.

The main stem of the endoscopic evaluation of patients with Barrett's esophagus is a detailed white light examination with high-resolution endoscopy. Long-segment ($\geq$3 cm) Barrett's esophagus and visible lesions in the setting of HGD are at higher risk of cancer. In particular, the risk of submucosal invasion is higher for protruding or depressed lesions than those slightly raised or flat.

The standard protocol to detect early cancer in patients with Barrett's esophagus and HGD is to biopsy visible lesions and then perform 4 quadrant jumbo biopsies at 1 cm intervals throughout length of Barrett's esophagus.

Once a neoplastic lesion in the setting of HGD has been identified, EUS should be performed to rule out the presence of lymph node involvement, which identifies patients not eligible for endoscopic therapy. Regarding the T staging, however, EUS is not as reliable for differentiation between T1a and T1b cancer as EMR.

The major advantage of EMR is the ability to provide intact resection samples of appropriate size and depth for an accurate histopathologic diagnosis. Multifocal HGD and moderately to poorly differentiated cancers are risk factors for submucosal invasion, while lymphovascular invasion, neural invasion, and moderately to poorly differentiated cancers are risk factors for lymph node metastases.

In addition, this *en bloc* resection technique allows lateral and deep resection margins to be assessed for the need of further treatments. In case of positive lateral margins, further endoscopic treatment is necessary, while the detection of positive deep margins is an indication for esophagectomy.

EMR for treatment of macroscopically visible lesions suspicious for malignancy arising in Barrett's esophagus is associated with complete regression rates about 97 % at 5 years. These patients, however, need to be enrolled in a very strict endoscopic follow-up program to detect possible early recurrence.

The major drawback of using focal EMR as the only treatment for Barrett's neoplasia is the possible development of recurrent lesions, arising in the residual Barrett's epithelium (14–47 %). Complete Barrett's esophagus eradication EMR, also known as wide area EMR or stepwise radical endoscopic resection, aims to resect the entire Barrett's esophagus segment along with the visible lesions. However, stricture rates as high as 88 % have been reported.

Ablative therapies include RFA and cryotherapy. *RFA* of HGD in Barrett's esophagus can be achieved locally or circumferentially. A recent multicenter, sham-controlled trail randomly assigned 127 patients with dysplastic Barrett's esophagus to RFA alone or a sham procedure. In the subgroup of patients with HGD, complete eradication was reported in 81 % of patients undergoing RFA compared to 19 % of the control group ($p<0.001$). Globally, the rate of esophageal stricture reported in patients treated with RFA was 6 %, significantly lower than that reported with EMR.

In order to reduce the risk of stenosis after EMR, a combination of EMR and RFA of the remaining Barrett's esophagus has been recently proposed, with complete remission in 96–98 % of patients and stenosis in 14 % of cases. To date, no study evaluating the role of RFA alone in the treatment of intramucosal carcinoma has been published.

Cryotherapy is a relatively new ablation modality. This therapy is based on application of sprayed liquid nitrogen or carbon dioxide that produces freeze-thaw cycles with tissue destruction. Recently, initial success with complete HGD eradication rates of 94–97 % has been reported. Stenosis (about 8 %) and chest pain are the most common complications.

While EMR is effective in most patients with either HGD or a superficial cancer (T1a), esophagectomy remains the treatment of choice when:

- Positive tumor margins or T1b are detected on the EMR specimen.
- Endoscopic expertise is not available.
- Preoperative EUS staging is greater than a T1aN0.
- Lymph node involvement is shown.
- Young patients.
- Patients who cannot have a rigid follow-up.
- Multifocal dysplasia is present in a long segment.
- Complete eradication is not possible

Patients with invasive esophageal cancer (T1b and T2) are considered candidates for esophagectomy if the following criteria are met: (1) no evidence of distant metastases and (2) good functional status.

The best treatment for patients with locally advanced cancer (T3-4-N0-3, T2-N1-3) includes a preoperative combination of radiotherapy and chemotherapy used in order to improve local (radiotherapy) and distant control of the disease (chemotherapy), followed by surgery. Overall, it seems that the combination of neoadjuvant therapy followed by surgery offers the best survival benefit. This is particularly true in the subgroup of patients (about 20 %) who have a "complete pathologic response" (no tumor found in the specimen).

Summary

- Severe symptoms and a higher degree of esophagitis (including Barrett's esophagus) are reported more likely in GERD patients with abnormal peristalsis and in systemic diseases that impair esophageal peristalsis, such as connective tissue disorders.
- The prevalence of a mechanically defective LES increases in patients with severe esophagitis and when Barrett's esophagus is present.

- A hiatal hernia is common in patients with Barrett's esophagus.
- Bile reflux causes symptoms and may be associated with the development of Barrett's esophagus and esophageal adenocarcinoma.
- Antireflux surgery can promote regression of the columnar epithelium only in short-segment Barrett's esophagus, but not in long-segment Barrett's esophagus.
- EMR is the treatment modality of choice in case of HGD and T1aN0 esophageal cancer.
- Esophagectomy is the procedure of choice for more invasive adenocarcinoma of the esophagus.

Selected Reading

1. Abraham NS. Proton pump inhibitors: potential adverse effects. Curr Opin Gastroenterol. 2012;28:615–20.
2. American Gastroenterological Association, Spechler SJ, Sharma P, Souza RF, Inadomi JM, Shaheen NJ. American Gastroenterological Association medical position statement on the management of Barrett's esophagus. Gastroenterology. 2011;140:1084–91.
3. Ancona E, Rampado S, Cassaro M, Battaglia G, Ruol A, Castoro C, Portale G, Cavallin F, Rugge M. Prediction of lymph node status in superficial esophageal carcinoma. Ann Surg Oncol. 2008;15:3278–88.
4. Ayazi S, DeMeester SR, Hsieh CC, Zehetner J, Sharma G, Grant KS, Oh DS, Lipham JC, Hagen JA, DeMeester TR. Thoraco-abdominal pressure gradients during the phases of respiration contribute to gastroesophageal reflux disease. Dig Dis Sci. 2011;56:1718–22.
5. Ayazi S, Hagen JA, Chan LS, DeMeester SR, Lin MW, Ayazi A, Leers JM, Oezcelik A, Banki F, Lipham JC, DeMeester TR, Crookes PF. Obesity and gastroesophageal reflux: quantifying the association between body mass index, esophageal acid exposure, and lower esophageal sphincter status in a large series of patients with reflux symptoms. J Gastrointest Surg. 2009;13:1440–7.
6. Blonski W, Vela MF, Castell DO. Comparison of reflux frequency during prolonged multichannel intraluminal impedance and pH monitoring on and off acid suppression therapy. J Clin Gastroenterol. 2009;43:816–20.
7. Boshier PR, Anderson O, Hanna GB. Transthoracic versus transhiatal esophagectomy for the treatment of esophagogastric cancer: a meta-analysis. Ann Surg. 2011;254:894–906.
8. Brandt MG, Darling GE, Miller L. Symptoms, acid exposure and motility in patients with Barrett's esophagus. Can J Surg. 2004;47:47–51.
9. Bredenoord AJ, Tutuian R, Smout AJ, Castell DO. Technology review: esophageal impedance monitoring. Am J Gastroenterol. 2007;102:187–94.
10. Buttar NS, Wang KK, Sebo TJ, Riehle DM, Krishnadath KK, Lutzke LS, Anderson MA, Petterson TM, Burgart LJ. Extent of high-grade dysplasia in Barrett's esophagus correlates with risk of adenocarcinoma. Gastroenterology. 2001;120:1630–9.
11. Cameron AJ. Barrett's esophagus: prevalence and size of hiatal hernia. Am J Gastroenterol. 1999;94:2054–9.
12. Casanova C, Baudet JS, del Valle VM, Martin JM, Aguirre-Jaime A, de Torres JP, Celli BR. Increased gastro-oesophageal reflux disease in patients with severe COPD. Eur Respir J. 2004;23:841–5.
13. Connor MJ, Sharma P. Chromoendoscopy and magnification endoscopy for diagnosing esophageal cancer and dysplasia. Thorac Surg Clin. 2004;14:87–94.
14. Courrech Staal EF, Aleman BM, Boot H, van Velthuysen ML, van Tinteren H, van Sandick JW. Systematic review of the benefits and risks of neoadjuvant chemoradiation for oesophageal cancer. Br J Surg. 2010;97:1482–96.

15. Dent J, El Serag HB, Wallander MA, Johansson S. Epidemiology of gastro-oesophageal reflux disease: a systematic review. Gut. 2005;54:710–7.
16. Diener U, Patti MG, Molena D, Fisichella PM, Way LW. Esophageal dysmotility and gastroesophageal reflux disease. J Gastrointest Surg. 2001;5:260–5.
17. Ell C, May A, Gossner L, Pech O, Günter E, Mayer G, Henrich R, Vieth M, Müller H, Seitz G, Stolte M. Endoscopic mucosal resection of early cancer and high-grade dysplasia in Barrett's esophagus. Gastroenterology. 2000;118:670–7.
18. Feo CV, Villaflor VM, Patti MG. Should esophageal resections for cancer be performed in high-volume centers only? Updates Surg. 2011;63:147–50.
19. Fisichella PM, Patti MG. Gastroesophageal reflux disease and morbid obesity: is there a relation? World J Surg. 2009;33:2034–8.
20. Fleisher DE, Overholt BF, Sharma VK, Reymunde A, Kimmey MB, Chuttani R, Chang KJ, Muthasamy R, Lightdale CJ, Santiago N, Pleskow DK, Dean PJ, Wang KK. Endoscopic radiofrequency ablation for Barrett's esophagus: 5-year outcomes from a prospective multicenter trial. Endoscopy. 2010;42:781–9.
21. Gurski RR, Peters JH, Hagen JA, DeMeester SR, Bremner CG, Chandrasoma PT, DeMeester TR. Barrett's esophagus can and does regress after antireflux surgery: a study of prevalence and predictive features. J Am Coll Surg. 2003;196:706–12.
22. Herbella FA, Sweet MP, Tedesco P, Nipomnick I, Patti MG. Gastroesophageal reflux disease and obesity. Pathophysiology and implications for treatment. J Gastrointest Surg. 2007;11:286–90.
23. Hvid-Jensen F, Pedersen L, Drewes AM, Sørensen HT, Funch-Jensen P. Incidence of adenocarcinoma among patients with Barrett's esophagus. N Engl J Med. 2011;365:1375–83.
24. Kahrilas PJ. Anatomy and physiology of the gastroesophageal junction. Gastroenterol Clin North Am. 1997;26:467–86.
25. Katz D, Rothstein R, Schned A, Dunn J, Seaver K, Antonioli D. The development of dysplasia and adenocarcinoma during endoscopic surveillance of Barrett's esophagus. Am J Gastroenterol. 1998;93:536–41.
26. Katzka DA, Castell DO. Successful elimination of reflux symptoms does not insure adequate control of acid reflux in patients with Barrett's esophagus. Am J Gastroenterol. 1994;89:989–91.
27. Kauer WK, Peters JH, DeMeester TR, Ireland AP, Bremner CG, Hagen JA. Mized reflux of gastric and duodenal juices is more harmful to the esophagus than gastric juice alone. The need for surgical therapy re-emphasized. Ann Surg. 1995;222:525–31.
28. Kim RH, Takabe K. Methods of esophagogastric anastomoses following esophagectomy for cancer: a systematic review. J Surg Oncol. 2010;101:527–33.
29. Konda VJ, Ross AS, Ferguson MK, Hart JA, Lin S, Naylor K, Noffsinger A, Posner MC, Dye C, Cislo B, Stearns L, Waxman I. Is the risk of concomitant invasive esophageal cancer in high-grade dysplasia in Barrett's esophagus overestimated? Clin Gastroenterol Hepatol. 2008;6:159–64.
30. Konda VJ, Waxman I. Endotherapy for Barrett's esophagus. Am J Gastroenterol. 2012;107:827–33.
31. Lindeboom MY, Ringers J, van Rijn PJ, Neijenhuis P, Stokkel MP, Masclee AA. Gastric emptying and vagus nerve function after laparoscopic partial fundoplication. Ann Surg. 2004;240:785–90.
32. Lord RV, DeMeester SR, Peters JH, Hagen JA, Elyssnia D, Sheth CT, DeMeester TR. Hiatal hernia, lower esophageal sphincter incompetence, and effectiveness of Nissen fundoplication in the spectrum of gastroesophageal reflux disease. J Gastrointest Surg. 2009;13:602–10.
33. Luketich JD, Pennathur A, Awais O, Levy RM, Keeley S, Shende M, Christie NA, Weksler B, Landreneau RJ, Abbas G, Schuchert MJ, Nason KS. Outcomes after minimally invasive esophagectomy: review of over 1000 patients. Ann Surg. 2012;256:95–103.
34. McCallum R, Polepalle S, Davenport K, Frierson H, Boyd S. Role of anti-reflux surgery against dysplasia in Barrett's esophagus. Gastroenterology. 1991;100:A121.
35. Meneghetti AT, Tedesco P, Damani T, Patti MG. Esophageal mucosal damage may promote dysmotility and worsen esophageal acid exposure. J Gastrointest Surg. 2005;9:1313–7.

36. Nelsen EM, Hawes RH, Iyer PG. Diagnosis and management of Barrett's esophagus. Surg Clin North Am. 2012;92:1135–54.
37. Nigro JJ, Hagen JA, DeMeester TR, DeMeester SR, Theisen J, Peters JH, Kiyabu M. Occult esophageal adenocarcinoma: extent of disease and implications for effective therapy. Ann Surg. 1999;230:433–8.
38. Oelschlager BK, Barreca M, Chang L, Oleynikov D, Pellegrini CA. Clinical and pathologic response of Barrett's esophagus to laparoscopic antireflux surgery. Ann Surg. 2003;238:458–64.
39. Oh DS, DeMeester SR. Pathophysiology and treatment of Barrett's esophagus. World J Gastroenterol. 2010;16:3762–72.
40. Parrilla P, Martinez de Haro LF, Ortiz A, Minutiz V, Molina J, Bermejo J, Canteras M. Long-term results of a randomized prospective study comparing medical and surgical treatment of Barrett's esophagus. Ann Surg. 2003;237:291–8.
41. Patti MG, Arcerito M, Feo CV, Worth S, DePinto M, Gibbs VC, Gantert W, Tyrrell D, Ferrell LF, Way LW. Barrett's esophagus: a surgical disease. J Gastrointest Surg. 1999;3:397–403.
42. Patti MG, Goldberg HI, Arcerito M, Bortolasi L, Tong J, Way LW. Hiatal hernia size affects lower esophageal sphincter function, esophageal acid exposure, and the degree of mucosal injury. Am J Surg. 1996;171:182–6.
43. Patti MG, Perretta S. Gastro-oesophageal reflux disease: a decade of changes. Asian J Surg. 2003;26:4–6.
44. Pech O, Behrens A, May A, Nachbar L, Gossner L, Rabenstein T, Manner H, Guenter E, Huijsmans J, Vieth M, Stolte M, Ell C. Long-term results and risk factor analysis for recurrence after curative endoscopic therapy in 349 patients with high-grade intraepithelial neoplasia and mucosal adenocarcinoma in Barrett's esophagus. Gut. 2008;57:1200–6.
45. Pech O, Günther E, Ell C. Endosonography of high-grade intra-epithelial neoplasia/early cancer. Best Pract Res Clin Gastroenterol. 2009;23:639–47.
46. Peters JH, Avisar N. The molecular pathogenesis of Barrett's esophagus: common signaling pathways in embryogenesis metaplasia and neoplasia. J Gastrointest Surg. 2010;14 Suppl 1:S81–7.
47. Peters FP, Brakenhoff KP, Curvers WL, Rosmolen WD, Fockens P, ten Kate FJ, Krishnadath KK, Bergman JJ. Histologic evaluation of resection specimens obtained at 293 endoscopic resections in Barrett's esophagus. Gastrointest Endosc. 2008;67:604–9.
48. Pouw RE, Gondrie JJ, Sondermeijer CM, ten Kate FJ, van Gulik TM, Krishnadath KK, Fockens P, Weusten BL, Bergman JJ. Eradication of Barrett esophagus with early neoplasia by radiofrequency ablation, with or without endoscopic resection. J Gastrointest Surg. 2008;12:1627–36.
49. Raz DJ, Tedesco P, Herbella FA, Nipomnick I, Way LW, Patti MG. Side-to-side stapled intrathoracic esophagogastric anastomosis reduces the incidence of leaks and stenosis. Dis Esophagus. 2008;21:69–72.
50. Shaheen NJ, Greenwald BD, Peery AF, Dumot JA, Nishioka NS, Wolfsen HC, Burdick JS, Abrams JA, Wang KK, Mallat D, Johnston MH, Zfass AM, Smith JO, Barthel JS, Lightdale CJ. Safety and efficacy of endoscopic spray cryotherapy for Barrett's esophagus with high-grade dysplasia. Gastrointest Endosc. 2010;71:680–5.
51. Shaheen NJ, Sharma P, Overholt BF, Wolfsen HC, Sampliner RE, Wang KK, Galanko JA, Bronner MP, Goldblum JR, Bennett AE, Jobe BA, Eisen GM, Fennerty MB, Hunter JG, Fleischer DE, Sharma VK, Hawes RH, Hoffman BJ, Rothstein RI, Gordon SR, Mashimo H, Chang KJ, Muthusamy VR, Edmundowicz SA, Spechler SJ, Siddiqui AA, Souza RF, Infantolino A, Falk GW, Kimmey MB, Madanick RD, Chak A, Lightdale CJ. Radiofrequency ablation in Barrett's esophagus with dysplasia. N Engl J Med. 2009;360:2277–88.
52. Stein E, Katz PO. Reflux monitoring. Rev Gastroenterol Disord. 2009;9:E54–62.
53. Sweet MP, Patti MG, Hoopes C, Hays SR, Golden JA. Gastro-oesophageal reflux, aspiration in patients with advanced lung disease. Thorax. 2009;64:167–73.
54. Tack J, Koek G, Demedts I, Sifrim D, Janssens J. Gastroesophageal reflux disease poorly responsive to single-dose proton pump inhibitors in patients without Barrett's esophagus: acid reflux, bile reflux, or both? Am J Gastroenterol. 2004;99:981–8.

55. Tamhankar AP, Peters JH, Portale G, Hsieh CC, Hagen JA, Bremner CG, DeMeester TR. Omeprazole does not reduce gastroesophageal reflux: new insights using multichannel intraluminal impedance technology. J Gastrointest Surg. 2004;8:890–7; discussion 897–98.
56. Tharavej C, Hagen JA, Peters JH, Portale G, Lipham J, DeMeester SR, Bremner CG, DeMeester TR. Predictive factors of coexisting cancer in Barrett's high-grade dysplasia. Surg Endosc. 2006;20:439–43.
57. Theisen J, Peters JH, Fein M, Hughes M, Hagen JA, Demeester SR, Demeester TR, Laird PW. The mutagenic potential of duodenoesophageal reflux. Ann Surg. 2005;241:63–8.
58. Van Vilsteren FG, Pouw RE, Seewald S, Alvarez Herrero L, Sondermeijer CM, Visser M, Ten Kate FJ, Yu Kim Teng KC, Soehendra N, Rösch T, Weusten BL, Bergman JJ. Stepwise radical endoscopic resection versus radiofrequency ablation for Barrett's oesophagus with high-grade dysplasia or early cancer: a multicenter randomized trial. Gut. 2011;60:765–73.
59. Wang KK, Sampliner RE. Updated guidelines 2008 for the diagnosis, surveillance and therapy of Barrett's esophagus. Am J Gastroenterol. 2008;103:788–97.
60. Wani S, Falk G, Hall M, Gaddam S, Wang A, Gupta N, Singh M, Singh V, Chuang KY, Boolchand V, Gavini H, Kuczynski J, Sud P, Reddymasu S, Bansal A, Rastogi A, Mathur SC, Young P, Cash B, Lieberman DA, Sampliner RE, Sharma P. Patients with nondysplastic Barrett's esophagus have low risks for developing dysplasia or esophageal adenocarcinoma. Clin Gastroenterol Hepatol. 2011;9:220–7.
61. Wernly JA, DeMeester TR, Bryant GH, Wang CI, Skinner DB. Intra-abdominal pressure as a cause of gastroesophageal reflux: a study in man. Surg Forum. 1978;29:434–7.
62. Wetscher GJ, Gadenstaetter M, Klingler PJ, Weiss H, Obrist P, Wykypiel H, Klaus A, Profanter C. Efficacy of medical therapy and antireflux surgery to prevent Barrett's metaplasia in patients with gastroesophageal reflux disease. Ann Surg. 2001;234:627–32.
63. Zaninotto G, DeMeester TR, Schwizer W, Johansson KE, Cheng SC. The lower esophageal sphincter in health and disease. Am J Surg. 1988;155:104–11.

Chapter 14
Barrett's Esophagus: Treatment Options

Ajaypal Singh and Irving Waxman

Abstract Barrett's esophagus (BE) is an asymptomatic condition, but it is the most significant known risk factor for the development of esophageal adenocarcinoma (EAC). More than half of short segment BE patients do not have any reflux symptoms. Cancer develops in BE through a sequence of genetic and epigenetic changes that activate oncogenes and silence tumor suppressor genes and cause progression from metaplasia through dysplasia to esophageal adenocarcinoma. Treatment approaches to BE mainly focus on eradication of high-grade dysplasia and neoplasia as well as prevention of progression of metaplasia to neoplasia. The treatment options for BE have undergone a significant change over the last few years due to improvement in our understanding of pathogenesis and progression of Barrett's esophagus as well as availability of endoscopic treatment modalities.

Keywords *Gastroesophageal reflux disease* • Barrett's esophagus • Metaplasia • Low-grade dysplasia • High-grade dysplasia • Radiofrequency ablation • Endoscopic mucosal resection • Cryotherapy • Esophagectomy

Barrett's esophagus (BE) is an asymptomatic condition, but it is the most significant known risk factor for the development of esophageal adenocarcinoma (EAC). More than half of short segment BE patients do not have any reflux symptoms. Cancer develops in BE through a sequence of genetic and epigenetic changes that activate oncogenes and silence tumor suppressor genes and cause progression from metaplasia through dysplasia to esophageal adenocarcinoma.

A. Singh, MD • I. Waxman, MD, FASGE (✉)
Department of Medicine, Center for Esophageal Diseases, University of Chicago Pritzker School of Medicine, 5700 S. Maryland Avenue, MC 8043, Chicago, IL 60637, USA
e-mail: iwaxman@medicine.bsd.uchicago.edu

P.M. Fisichella et al. (eds.), *Esophageal Diseases*,
DOI 10.1007/978-3-319-04337-1_14, © Springer International Publishing Switzerland 2014

Treatment approaches to BE mainly focus on eradication of high-grade dysplasia and neoplasia as well as prevention of progression of metaplasia to neoplasia. The treatment options for BE have undergone a significant change over the last few years due to improvement in our understanding of pathogenesis and progression of Barrett's esophagus as well as availability of endoscopic treatment modalities.

Medical Treatment

Acid Suppression Therapy: All patients with BE and symptoms of GERD or reflux esophagitis seen on endoscopy should be treated with high-dose proton-pump inhibitor (PPI) therapy, unless there are contraindications for the use of PPIs in which case H2 receptor blockers should be used. The use of PPI therapy in patients with BE but no symptoms of reflux or endoscopic evidence of reflux esophagitis is not clear. The main argument for the use of PPIs in this group will be only to reduce the risk of progression of dysplasia or development of cancer. There are a few observational and retrospective studies that have shown that the use of PPIs is associated with lower risk of developing high-grade dysplasia (HGD) and adenocarcinoma and even partial regression of intestinal metaplasia, but no randomized controlled trials are available to support these findings. The American Gastroenterology Association (AGA) recommends discussion of risks and potential benefits of long-term acid suppression therapy with BE patients in the context of their overall health status and medication use. Currently we recommend acid suppression therapy for all patients with BE unless there are specific contraindications. The assessment of reflux symptoms in patients on high-dose acid suppression therapy has not shown to be a reliable indicator of acid suppression, and up to 40 % of these patients can have persistent acid reflux as judged by 24-h pH studies despite resolution of reflux symptoms. Even though pH monitoring might be needed to titrate doses of acid suppression, routine pH monitoring to confirm efficacy of acid suppression therapy is not currently recommended.

Aspirin and Nonsteroidal Anti-inflammatory Drugs: Multiple published studies have shown that aspirin (ASA) and nonsteroidal anti-inflammatory drugs (NSAIDS) might have potential chemopreventative effects in patients with BE. Both ASA and NSAIDs have been shown to reduce the risk of developing esophageal adenocarcinoma by as much as 33 %. Currently no prospective, randomized control trials to support this chemopreventative effect are available, but a large clinical trial is currently underway, the results of which are eagerly awaited. Most of the patients with BE are elderly males with obesity or other cardiovascular risk factors, so use of low-dose aspirin should be considered in patients with cardiovascular risk factors and BE. The biggest concern for the use of ASA is risk of bleeding, but the patients with BE should also be on a PPI, which should minimize the gastrointestinal toxicity associated with aspirin use.

Endoscopic Treatment

Who to Treat and Who to Watch?

The patients at highest risk for the development of invasive cancer are candidates for eradication of Barrett's epithelium. Currently the best available marker for predicting development of cancer in BE is dysplasia. The incidence of adenocarcinoma in high-grade dysplasia (HGD) is around 6 % per year with one study showing incidence of 19 % in 1 year. Thus, endoscopic eradication is recommended in all patients with HGD. Intense endoscopic surveillance every 3 months is an option for patients who decline eradication therapy or those who are not candidates for Barrett's eradication. The incidence of lymph node metastases is only 1–2 % in adenocarcinomas confined to the mucosa but increases to around 15 % with submucosal involvement. Thus, endoscopic therapy is also currently recommended in all patients with intramucosal carcinoma (IMC). This underlines the importance of accurate T-staging of the esophageal adenocarcinoma. Endoscopic ultrasound has been shown to have an accuracy of only 50–60 % in identifying the T-stage of early esophageal cancers. However, preoperative EMR specimens have excellent agreement with histology from esophagectomy specimens in patients with BE and neoplasia. Hence, in addition to being a therapeutic procedure, endoscopic mucosal resection is a very important staging tool. The incidence of adenocarcinoma is very low (0.1 % per year) in low-grade dysplasia (LGD) and there is no international consensus regarding eradication therapy, but most societies do not recommend eradication therapy in this patient population. One of the issues with managing low-grade dysplasia in BE is the interobserver variability among pathologists regarding the diagnosis, with studies reporting only 15 % cases of low-grade dysplasia that were confirmed by expert pathologists. A recent cost-effectiveness study concluded that radiofrequency ablation of low-grade dysplasia might be cost-effective if the diagnosis is accurate and it is assumed that risk of progression to cancer for low-grade dysplasia is at least 50 % more than that for non-dysplastic BE. In its latest medical position statement, the American Gastroenterological Association (AGA) "strongly supports the concept of shared decision-making where the physician and patient together consider whether endoscopic surveillance or eradication therapy is the preferred management option."

Surveillance for Barrett's Esophagus

The main aim of surveillance is to detect progression of dysplasia as well as early esophageal cancer. Even though there are no randomized, prospective trials showing direct benefits of regular surveillance, there are multiple retrospective studies that have shown improved survival if esophageal cancer is detected endoscopically rather than when it is symptomatic. Esophageal cancers detected during surveillance have a lower staging and improved survival. All patients with new diagnosis of BE should have two endoscopies within the first year and if no dysplasia is noted on either, they can be followed by serial endoscopy every 3–5 years. Due to high variability in reporting of low-grade dysplasia, if LGD is noted on biopsies, this diagnosis must be confirmed by an expert GI pathologist. Once low-grade dysplasia is confirmed, a repeat endoscopy is recommended within 6 months to make sure there is no high-grade dysplasia. All patients with low-grade dysplasia should undergo annual surveillance endoscopy until non-dysplastic BE is noted on two consecutive occasions after which surveillance can be done as for non-dysplastic BE (every 3–5 years). As mentioned above, all high-grade dysplasia patients should undergo eradication therapy unless they are not candidates for this or they decline treatment, in which case, surveillance endoscopy should be done every 3 months.

During surveillance endoscopy, current guidelines recommend 4-quadrant biopsies every 1–2 cm of the Barrett's segment (Seattle protocol). All areas of nodularity or mucosal irregularity should be sampled separately. Strict adherence to Seattle protocol is important since only around 40 % of high-grade dysplasia and esophageal adenocarcinomas were identified as endoscopically suspicious locations during high-definition white light endoscopy in one study. But due to multiple number of biopsies needed, adherence to the Seattle protocol in community practice has been low, with some studies reporting an adherence of only 30 % with BE of more than 10 cm (notably, this population is at higher risk of esophageal cancer). The time spent during inspection of Barrett's epithelium has been shown to be directly proportional to the number of suspicious lesions as well as HGD/EAC lesions identified, with 1 min per centimeter of Barrett's epithelium suggested as optimal Barrett's inspection time. Given the poor adherence to dysplasia surveillance by extensive biopsies, other markers of dysplasia as well as endoscopic imaging techniques are being studied. Currently the use of biomarkers for detection of dysplasia is only in the investigational stages and no professional gastroenterology society recommends their use for clinical decision-making. Various different modalities including chromoendoscopy, narrow band imaging with magnification, and confocal laser endomicroscopy are being study to identify high-risk lesions during visual inspection. The AGA currently recommends detailed examination under white light endoscopy and these additional imaging techniques are not currently recommended. The endoscopic surveillance should be performed using high-definition, high-resolution endoscopes and strict adherence to the biopsy protocol should be followed. We utilize these resources as adjuncts to our endoscopic examination to help us target the biopsies toward areas of interest.

How to Treat?

An international, multidisciplinary, systematic, evidence-based review of management strategies for BE in 2012 recommended that endoscopic treatment of BE with HGD or T1m esophageal adenocarcinoma is preferred over surveillance strategies or surgical treatment. It further went on to recommend that endoscopic treatment of HGD or T1m BE should be performed in tertiary referral centers after proper training of both endoscopists and pathologists involved. The goal of all endoscopic therapies is complete eradication of intestinal metaplasia leading to regeneration of squamous epithelium.

Endoscopic Treatment

Endoscopic treatment of BE includes endoscopic ablative therapies and endoscopic mucosal resection (EMR).

Ablative Therapies

The ablative therapies include thermal therapies (argon plasma coagulation, radiofrequency ablation, cryotherapy) and photodynamic therapy that utilizes photochemical energy. Even though the ablative methods are technically easier to adopt, they do not provide any tissue for histopathological analysis. Another major concern about ablative therapies is that they can leave behind foci of metaplastic Barrett's epithelium that is covered by squamous epithelium during regeneration and is thence not visible during routine endoscopic surveillance. These residual columnar foci, also known as buried glands, have neoplastic potential and can cause progression of BE despite complete Barrett's eradication visually.

Radiofrequency Ablation (RFA)

Radiofrequency ablation (RFA) involves mucosal ablation via superficial thermal injury generated by a high-frequency electromagnetic field from electrodes placed in an ablation catheter. Commercially available RFA catheters as Barrx ablation system, it includes an RFA energy generator and RFA delivery catheters. There are three kinds of ablation catheters: a balloon catheter (Barrx 360) for circumferential ablation, over the scope catheters of various sizes (Barrx 90, Barrx 60, and Barrx Ultra Long Catheter) and a recently developed through the scope catheter (Barrx Channel RFA Catheter). RFA is currently the most commonly used mucosal ablation technique for BE given its efficacy, ease of use, and low risk of complications. After cleaning the esophageal mucosa with 1 % *N*-acetylcysteine, the RFA catheter is applied to the surface at a dose of 12 J/cm^2. A second round of ablation is done after cleaning the mucosa and removing the debris. Some endoscopists use 10 J/cm^2 for low-grade dysplasia. Usually multiple sessions of RFA are required till complete ablation of dysplastic mucosa is achieved. It is very important to note that RFA is indicated only for flat Barrett's mucosa and patients with nodular disease should undergo resection of visible nodular lesions for staging purposes before the remaining flat Barrett's mucosa is ablated.

In a multicenter, randomized, sham-controlled study from the United States, complete eradication of intestinal metaplasia at 12 months was achieved in 74 % patients with high-grade dysplasia and 81 % patients with low-grade dysplasia. Progression of high-grade dysplasia to esophageal cancer was reduced from 19 % in shams to 2.4 % in the ablation group, though the total number of cancers in the study population was low. The number of high-grade dysplasia patients needed to treat (NNT) to prevent one esophageal cancer in the study was 6. Major complication of RFA is esophageal stricture that is seen in 6–8 % of cases, while bleeding and mediastinitis have been reported but are uncommon. The major disadvantage of RFA is the lack of tissue for histopathology. Though there is no long-term data about the durability of RFA, a recent study showed 93 % complete remission of intestinal metaplasia and neoplasia at 5 years in patients treated with a combination of EMR and RFA. Further, buried glands were found only in the 0.08 % of neosquamous biopsies. The recurrence can be successfully treated with repeat RFA sessions with good results. Further follow-up data is still needed to confirm the long-term efficacy of eradication and the optimal interval for surveillance endoscopies in these patients.

Argon Plasma Coagulation

Argon plasma coagulation (APC) was the most common eradicative therapy before RFA became widely available. APC utilizes a monopolar high-frequency probe that causes surface coagulation of the epithelium through ionized argon plasma. In a single center from the United Kingdom, 86 % remission of Barrett's metaplasia was seen after a mean follow-up period of 37 months, while 14 % developed esophageal adenocarcinoma over a follow-up period of 90 patient-years. Other studies have also shown that buried glands are noted in up to 30 % of patients treated with APC therapy, which is much higher than that reported for radiofrequency ablation. Stricture formation is the most common adverse event, while the risk of perforation is very low. Currently APC is not widely used as a primary ablative therapy for HGD but has an important role as an adjunct to endoscopic mucosal resection where it is used to ablate the edges of the resection.

Photodynamic Therapy

Photodynamic therapy (PDT) was one of the earliest used modalities for Barrett's ablation. It involves systemic administration of a photosensitizer that is activated during endoscopy by using light waves of appropriate wavelength. The photosensitizer can be administered either orally or intravenously. Porfimer sodium is the most extensively studied photosensitizer for BE and has been approved by the U.S. Food and Drug Administration. It is administered intravenously at a dose of 2 mg/kg approximately 48 h before the procedure. The required wavelength is delivered to the esophagus under endoscopic visualization using a cylindrical balloon advanced over a wire. The desired dose for successful therapy is 130 J/cm that allows calculation of application time if the power density of the instrument is known. The mucosal injury is usually evaluated 2 days after PDT when an additional dose of 50 J/cm can be delivered to the skip areas. The side effects of PDT include chest pain (20 %), nausea (11 %), vomiting (32 %), hiccups (10 %), dysphagia (19 %), esophageal perforation (less than 1 %), pleural effusion (2 %), and photosensitivity reaction (7–18 %). The major complication of PDT is stricture formation occurring 3–4 weeks after PDT, with a reported incidence of up to 36 % in some studies. These are more commonly seen in areas of treatment overlap and in patients with long segment BE and are treated with serial dilations. Patients should also avoid sun and bright light for at least 30 days and sometimes up to 90 days due to risk of photosensitivity. Known history of porphyria and porphyria sensitivity is a contraindication for PDT. In an international, multicenter, partially blinded phase III trial of PDT in 208 patients with HGD, 77 % patients with PDT had complete ablation of HGD at 2 years compared to 39 % in the control arm ($p<0.0001$). The incidence of esophageal adenocarcinoma decreased from 28 % in the control arm to 13 % in the PDT group ($p=0.006$). A 5-year follow-up study of the same patient cohort was subsequently published and it confirmed the long-term efficacy for HGD ablation (77 % for PDT vs. 39 % for control group, $p<0.001$) and lower risk of progression to cancer after PDT (15 % vs. 29 %, $p=0.027$).

Due to systemic absorption of porfimer sodium and high incidence of photosensitivity after exposure to sunlight, various other photosensitizers have been studied. Aminolevulinic acid has been used as an oral photosensitizer administered on the day of photoradiation and has lesser systemic absorption along with shorter duration of skin photosensitivity (24–48 h). In one of the earlier studies using ALA, eradication of HGD and mucosal cancer was noted in 100 % (10/10) and 77 % (17/22) patients, respectively, after a mean follow-up of 9.9 months. In a subsequent study to evaluate the long-term efficacy of PDT with ALA, 66 patients with HGIN and early adenocarcinoma were treated with PDT using ALA and complete response was documented in 97 and 100 % patients, respectively, at 37 months. Currently ALA is not approved for use in the United States. Further randomized studies comparing PDT with other ablation modalities are required. Given its ease of application, better adverse effect profile, and good efficacy at Barrett's eradication, radiofrequency ablation has replaced photodynamic therapy as the most commonly used ablation technique.

Cryotherapy

It is a noncontact ablation technique that induces cell damage with minimal fibrosis by using alternating cycles of rapid freezing and slow thawing. It is a relatively newer technique and has the most limited experience of all the ablation techniques. Commonly used gases include liquid nitrogen and carbon dioxide. In a multicenter, retrospective cohort study, 98 patients with BE and HGD underwent 333 cryotherapy treatment sessions with 97 % complete eradication of HGD and

57 % complete eradication of all intestinal metaplasia after a mean of 3.4 treatments per patient. Two percent patients developed severe chest pain requiring narcotics and 3 % patients developed esophageal strictures treated with endoscopic dilation. There were no perforations in the study population. Cryotherapy has also been shown to provide complete luminal response in patients with intramucosal cancer who failed or refused conventional therapy. But long-term data on the efficacy is lacking and this modality is available only at select centers in the country.

Endoscopic Mucosal Resection

Endoscopic mucosal resection or EMR refers to endoscopic removal of neoplastic epithelium using the standard polypectomy technique usually after raising the area of interest by saline injection. EMR has been shown to be effective and safe along with the advantage of providing tissue of histological evaluation, making it both a therapeutic and a staging procedure as discussed above. All patients with any nodular disease and absence of submucosal disease should undergo EMR. Currently it is being widely used for treatment of mucosal adenocarcinoma in patients with BE. The role of EMR in diagnosis of dysplasia and early cancer as well as staging of BE is very important. Any area of mucosal irregularity noted on endoscopy for Barrett's surveillance should ideally be removed by EMR. Endoscopic biopsies of these areas have several limitations including small sample size, lesser depth, poor orientation, and crush artifact. The EMR has the advantage of providing larger and well-oriented specimens. Diagnosis and staging of dysplasia in BE is a difficult decision and has shown to be observer dependent. Analysis of EMR specimens has shown to improve the interobserver agreement for diagnosis of dysplasia when compared to endoscopic biopsies.

The most commonly used techniques for EMR are the cap-assisted technique and multiband ligation technique. The cap technique is the more commonly used of the two and it uses a transparent cap (flat or oblique) and a snare to resect the mucosa. The target area is first lifted by injection of a fluid in the submucosal layer (saline or diluted epinephrine). After that a snare is fitted into the inside of the cap, the injected mucosa is suctioned into the cap, captured by already placed snare, and resected using blended current electrocautery. In the band and ligate technique, which can be performed without submucosal injection, a banding device (modification of the traditional variceal bander) is used to band areas of interest creating pseudopolyps which are then resected using a snare and electrocoagulation. In a randomized trial comparing cap technique with submucosal injection and band ligation without submucosal injection for early esophageal cancers, no difference in efficacy or safety profiles were noted. Multiband technique has been shown to be more efficient for resection of larger mucosal specimens, but the final decision is usually based on the endoscopist's preference, level of comfort, and experience with a particular modality.

Most of the initial studies used EMR focally for the treatment of mucosal adenocarcinoma. Long-term success with complete response rates of around 95 % at 5 years had been reported for focal EMR done to treat intramucosal carcinoma (IMC). In one of the earlier studies of focal EMR for patients with IMC (only 3 patients in the study with HGD), local recurrence or metachronous carcinoma was noted in up to 17 % patients after a mean follow-up interval of 10 months. Other studies have shown recurrence rate as high as 47 % after focal EMR. Seewald et al. for the first time reported successful use of circumferential EMR (75 % of luminal circumference at one setting) in patients with HGD and IMC but no visible lesions. Complete eradication of BE was noted in all patients after a median follow-up of 9 months. This technique is also known as stepwise radical endoscopic resection or wide area EMR and involves resection of the entire Barrett's segment. Multiple studies have shown the effectiveness of complete Barrett's eradication using EMR only with reported success rate of 76–100 %. Esophageal strictures are very common after circumferential EMR with one study reporting an incidence of up to 88 %. These can be successfully treated using serial dilations.

Combination or Hybrid Therapy

Complete eradication of Barrett's using EMR should be performed only at high volume referral centers with adequate surgery backup (Fig. 14.1). A combination approach is used in a significant number of cases, where all visible lesions are treated with EMR while the remaining of Barrett's epithelium is treated with ablative therapies (RFA being the most common) (Fig. 14.2). This approach has been shown to have good outcomes with neoplasia and metaplasia eradication rates of 83–95 % and 79–88 %, respectively. This might be a safer alternative to long segment BE with segments longer than 10 cm where risks of esophageal strictures is very high after complete eradication using EMR.

Surgical Options

Fundoplication

Fundoplication is primarily performed in patients with refractory reflux symptoms not responding to medical therapy. Some surgeons have suggested that fundoplication might be more effective than acid suppression therapy in preventing cancer in BE patients, but published literature on this topic is limited. Nissen fundoplication has been associated with regression of low-grade dysplasia at 12–18 months in up to 93 % patients compared to 63 % in patients treated with medical therapy alone. In addition to promoting regression of Barrett's metaplasia, some studies have demonstrated lower risk of progression to adenocarcinoma after fundoplication in Barrett's patients. This has been proposed to be secondary to decreased exposure of the esophageal epithelium to bile acids, in addition to gastric secretions. Currently,

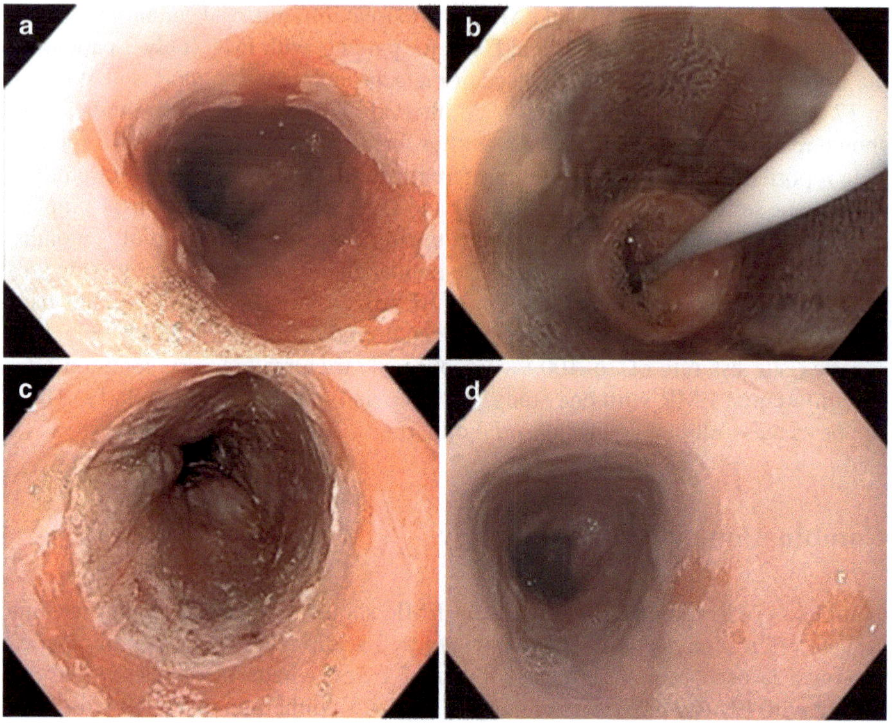

Fig. 14.1 (**a**) Patient with long-standing BE with focal high-grade dysplasia above the GE junction that was previously treated with focal EMR. (**b**) Barrett's ablation using 360° RFA balloon catheter. (**c**) Endoscopic view immediately after RFA. (**d**) Neosquamous epithelium with few islands of BE after 9 months and 3 RFA sessions. The Barrett's islands were treated with focal RFA

surgical attempts at reducing acid exposure solely for the purpose of reducing cancer risk in BE are not recommended.

Esophagectomy

Esophagectomy was the standard of care for patients with high-grade dysplasia and intramucosal carcinoma till the endoscopic eradication techniques became more available. Even though esophagectomy can be done using a laparoscopic and thoracoscopic approach now, it is still associated with significant morbidity and long hospital stays compared to endoscopic treatment that can be done as an outpatient. Patients who were treated with a combination of photodynamic therapy and endoscopic mucosal resection were shown to have similar 5-year mortality as those who underwent esophagectomy for high-grade dysplasia (9 % vs. 8.5 %). None of the deaths in either group was from esophageal adenocarcinoma. Intramucosal cancer (m1) has only 1–2 % incidence of lymph node metastasis, while submucosal

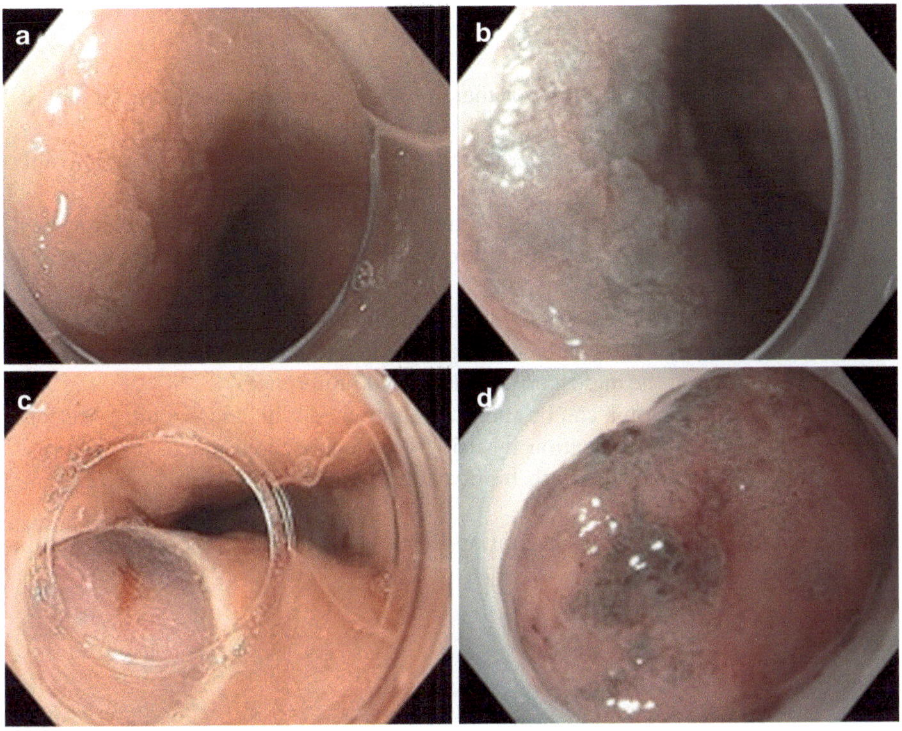

Fig. 14.2 (**a**) A flat area of nodularity (IIA) noted during surveillance endoscopy for BE (white light with magnification). (**b**) Same lesion seen under narrow band imaging and magnification. (**c**) Endoscopic mucosal resection (EMR) using saline injection followed by cap and snare was performed. (**d**) Mucosectomy specimen, pathology was consistent with high-grade dysplasia

involvement is associated with 15 % incidence of nodal involvement. When performed in appropriately selected patients, esophagectomy has a mortality of less than 5 % with good quality of life; it should be discussed with all patients who have high-grade dysplasia, especially for younger, otherwise healthy patients.

Follow-Up After Ablation

Close follow-up and surveillance of patients is needed after eradication therapy, but no guidelines have been established due to lack of data about recurrence of metaplasia and dysplasia after eradication. After eradication therapy, these patients should initially have surveillance according to the highest grade of dysplasia that was noted. Biopsies should be obtained from entire area of prior BE at appropriate intervals until complete ablation is documented on at least three consecutive endoscopies with reasonable certainty, following which the surveillance intervals can be increased.

Summary

- High-dose proton-pump inhibitor therapy for acid suppression is recommended for all patients with BE.
- Patients with HGD should undergo eradication therapy, either endoscopic ablation or endoscopic resection.
- All patients with non-dysplastic BE and LGD should undergo regular surveillance endoscopies with high-definition scopes and adequate Barrett's inspection time.
- All visible or nodular lesions should be treated with endoscopic mucosal resection and the residual BE can be eradicated with either ablation or mucosal resection depending on the endoscopists' skills and preference.
- Intramucosal carcinoma can be successfully treated with endoscopic resection.
- Complete Barrett's eradication by using only endoscopic mucosal resection is possible but is associated with high stricture rate, which can be easily treated endoscopically.
- All patients who undergo eradication therapy should have appropriate surveillance endoscopies.

Chapter 15
Esophageal Cancer: Evaluation

Henner M. Schmidt and Donald E. Low

Abstract In recent years esophageal adenocarcinoma incidence increased rapidly and esophageal cancer is now the seventh leading cause of all cancer-related deaths. Over the last decades treatment approaches for esophageal cancer have evolved, with esophagectomy remaining a central component in the curative treatment of resectable esophageal cancer. Esophagectomy is a demanding procedure and with the availability of a wide variety of treatment regimes, accurate staging and evaluation became even more important. The management of patients is determined by patients physiology as well as tumor histology, location and clinical stage. This chapter describes a complete evaluation of esophageal cancer patients, including physiologic work-up, clinical staging modalities and treatment decision making.

Keywords Esophageal cancer • Staging • Evaluation • Physiologic work-up • treatment decision

H.M. Schmidt, MD
Department for General, Thoracic and Vascular Surgery, Virginia Mason Medical Center, 1100 Ninth Ave, Seattle, WA 98101, USA
e-mail: henner.schmidt@vmmc.org, henner.schmidt@yahoo.de

D.E. Low, FACS, FRCS(c), FRCSI (Hon.) (✉)
Department for General, Thoracic and Vascular Surgery, Virginia Mason Medical Center, 1100 Ninth Ave, Seattle, WA 98101, USA

Department of Thoracic Surgery and Thoracic Oncology, Director Esophageal Center of Excellence, Scientific Director Ryan Hill Research Fellowship, Digestive Disease Institute, Seattle, WA, USA
e-mail: donald.low@vmmc.org

P.M. Fisichella et al. (eds.), *Esophageal Diseases*,
DOI 10.1007/978-3-319-04337-1_15,

Introduction

Epidemiology, Etiology, and Pathophysiology

The incidence of esophageal cancer remains relatively rare, accounting only for 1 % of all malignancies worldwide; however, it is the seventh leading cause of cancer-related deaths [1]. According to the Surveillance, Epidemiology, and End Results program (SEER), the annual incidence of esophageal carcinoma for 2012 in the United States is 4.7 cases per 100.000 [1]. Esophagectomy remains a central component of curative therapy, although treatment approaches became increasingly diversified, making an accurate evaluation even more important.

The two most common histological types of esophageal cancer are squamous cell carcinoma (SCC) and adenocarcinoma (AC) representing over 95 % of all esophageal cancers. Historically squamous cell carcinoma was the leading histology worldwide; however, currently in Western industrialized countries adenocarcinoma has become by far the most prevalent form of esophageal carcinoma. In the last decades, a 460 % increase in the incidence of esophageal adenocarcinoma has been documented making it the fastest growing cancer in the United States [2]. While AC rapidly increases the incidence of SCC has demonstrated a steady decline in the western world. Well-established etiologic factors for SCC include smoking, alcohol consumption, and low socioeconomic status [3]. While smoking is also a risk factor for the development of AC obesity, gastroesophageal reflux disease (GERD) and Barrett's esophagus are the most current common risk factors [4]. High-grade dysplasia in Barrett's esophagus is a well-described precancerous lesion with up to 30 % of patients with documented high-grade dysplasia developing esophageal AC within 5 years. There is some data suggesting that high intakes of fresh fruits, antioxidants, as well as aspirin and other nonsteroidal anti-inflammatory drugs may have a protective effect for the development of AC. As the prevalence for esophageal cancer is eightfold higher in males, the effect of estrogen on the occurrence of AC is currently being assessed [5].

As the location of esophageal carcinoma strongly influences its behavior and the treatment approach, the esophagus is divided into four distinct anatomic regions: the cervical, the upper thoracic, the mid thoracic, and the lower thoracic esophagus. AC is typically located in the mid and lower esophagus typically distal to the carina. SCC is found in up to 65 % of cases in the mid and upper esophagus. Second primary squamous cell malignancies in the pharyngeal and laryngeal location occur in up to 10 % in patients presenting with SCC of the esophagus. Tumors originating at the region of the gastroesophageal junction (EGJ) incorporating the very distal esophagus and the very proximal stomach can be classified according to the Siewert classification [6]. In this classification, type I is defined as tumors in which the center is located 1–5 cm above the esophagogastric junction (EGJ), type II as tumors invading the EGJ in which the center is located between 1 cm above and 2 cm below the EGJ, and type III as tumors invading the EGJ in which the center is located 2–5 cm below the EGJ (Fig. 15.1). The revised 7th edition of the AJCC staging systems classifies tumors whose midpoints are in the lower esophagus, EGJ, or within the proximal 5 cm of stomach that extends into the EGJ (Siewert type I and

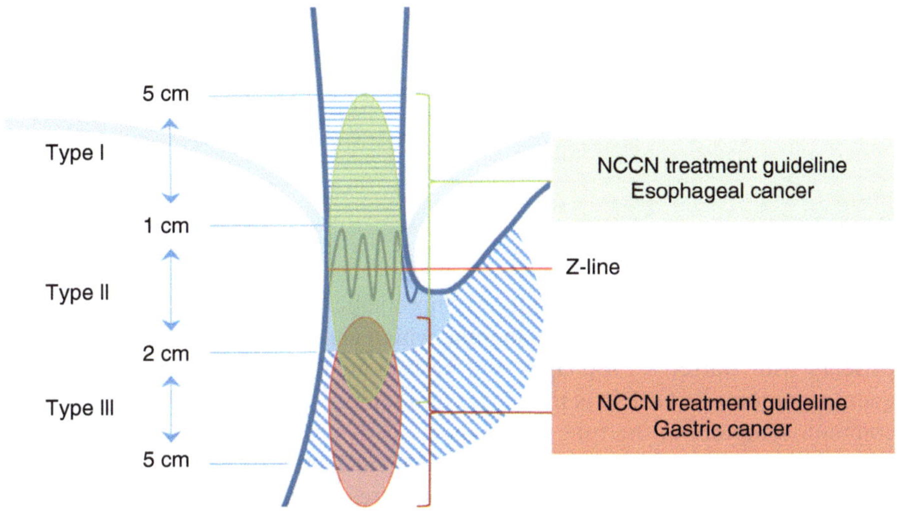

Fig. 15.1 Siewert classification type I–III for esophagogastric junction carcinomas and corresponding NCCN treatment guidelines for esophageal and gastric cancers

II) as esophageal tumors, whereas cancers with a midpoint within 5 cm of the EGJ (Siewert type III) but not extending into the EGJ are staged using the gastric cancer staging system. Although the Siewert classification is routinely used internationally, there is the need to apply a single classification in research and outcomes reporting, and, therefore, the AJCC system is recommended.

Esophageal resection remains an important component of the treatment for early and regional esophageal cancer. Despite significant advances in the diagnosis and treatment of esophageal cancer, overall survival remains poor with 5-year survival rates increasing from 5 % in the 1980s to 19 % in 2007 for all patients presenting with esophageal cancer [1]. Simultaneously over the last several decades, there has been an evolution of treatment approaches to esophageal cancer. These advances include the application of endoscopic techniques in the treatment of superficial cancer, the evolution of minimally invasive techniques, as well as the addition of neoadjuvant therapy to the treatment of regional esophageal cancer. With the availability of a diversified treatment approach, an accurate evaluation becomes even more important. The management of patients is determined by patient's physiology, location of the primary cancer, and clinical tumor stage at presentation.

Medical Evaluation

Esophagectomy is a major procedure requiring a preoperative evaluation to assess the patient's physiologic suitability for the operation. The assessment of cardiopulmonary health and nutritional status is an important issue to minimizing morbidity and mortality. Esophagectomy typically requires access to the abdominal and thoracic cavities; it remains one of the most demanding surgical procedures. Treatment decisions are best assigned after presentation at multidisciplinary tumor board where the patient's staging assessment and physiologic and psychologic health and nutritional status can be reviewed.

Symptoms

Early esophageal cancer is typically asymptomatic, although ulceration can lead to gastroesophageal bleedings or anemia, which can result in early detection. For patients with Barrett's esophagus and early adenocarcinoma, a history of frequent symptoms of GERD is the most common preexisting condition. The most common symptom at the time of diagnosis is dysphagia. This most commonly occurs when the cancer narrows the esophageal lumen to a third of its normal width. Persistent solid food dysphagia or progressive dysphagia associated with weight loss should always be investigated. Patients can also experience odynophagia and regurgitation as an expression of advanced regional disease and upper GI bleeding can be present at all stages. In addition hoarseness can be a sign of advanced cancers because of compression or involvement of the recurrent nerve. Similarly, frequent hiccups can be triggered by phrenic nerve or diaphragmatic involvement and a persistent postprandial cough may indicate the presence of a malignant esophagotracheal or bronchial fistula. At the time of diagnosis, most patients have locally advanced or metastatic disease. Only 22 % are diagnosed with early stage disease although this component is increasing due to Barrett's surveillance programs [1].

Past Medical History

In patients presenting with adenocarcinoma, a history of gastroesophageal reflux disease is common. Furthermore, a component of especially elderly patients will have undergone previous upper gastrointestinal surgical procedures which can affect the surgical approach. If previous gastric surgery is present, the complete extent of such surgery must be assessed, including obtaining previous operative reports, as prior surgery can necessitate reconstruction with colon or small bowel.

Age

Considering that life expectancy and the incidence of esophageal cancer are both increasing it is expected that more elderly patients will present with esophageal cancer. Advanced age is routinely associated with a higher prevalence of comorbidities with the associated risk of pulmonary and cardiac complications. However, many studies have shown improved outcomes in elderly patients when treated in specialized high-volume centers [7–9]. In addition definitive chemoradiotherapy showed increased morbidity and treatment-related mortality rates in elderly patients, and a substantial part of these patients will have difficulty receiving the entire course of therapy. Age itself is not a contraindication for surgery but physiological status and coexisting diseases are more likely to affect morbidity and mortality. However, a complete assessment of mental and physical comorbidities in these patients is critically important when considered for surgery [7].

Cardiopulmonary Status

Pulmonary complications are the most common cause for postoperative morbidity and mortality [10]. Preoperative pulmonary function test can be helpful to assess patient's baseline lung function prior to esophagectomy. In addition certain techniques of esophagectomy require one-sided lung ventilation and impaired pulmonary function test can increase the complexity of the operation. Forced vital capacity (FVC) of less than 70 % and forced expiratory volume in 1 s (FEV_1) of less than 60 % are associated with an increased incidence of prolonged mechanical ventilation and are at higher risk for pulmonary complications [11]. Smokers are at higher risk of developing pulmonary complications and smoking cessation at time of diagnosis is beneficial and should be recommended [12].

Supraventricular arrhythmias are the most common cardiac complication in patients undergoing esophagectomy reported in 20–30 % of all cases [13]. The causes remain unclear but arrhythmia is more prevalent in patients sustaining anastomotic leakage and mediastinitis. Current rates of perioperative infarction are 1–2 % [10]. A preoperative cardiac work-up is electively advisable in patients presenting with risk factors such as preexisting arrhythmia, documented coronary disease, previous myocardial infarction, positive family history, smoking, hypertension, and diabetes. High-risk patients for cardiac complications include those with congestive heart failure, preexisting arrhythmia, valvular disease, angina symptoms, and prior myocardial infarction. These patients are recommended for objective cardiac assessment according to the guidelines of American College of Cardiology (ACC) and the American Heart Association (AHA) [14]. Limited research focused on medical prevention of arrhythmia in patients undergoing esophagectomy. Dilitiazem and amiodarone have been effective in preventing arrhythmias, but because of side effects of these drugs (especially lung fibrosis for amiodarone), the overall benefit remains unclear [15, 16]. Beta blockers should be continued perioperatively if patients are taking these medications for other clinical indications [17]. According to the ACC/AHA guidelines, esophagectomy represents an intermediate risk for arrhythmia. The risk group that should be considered for the initiation of β blockers includes patients with diabetes, prior myocardial infarction, compensated heart failure, and untreated renal insufficiency. Patient with documented coronary disease on aspirin should be maintained on aspirin throughout the perioperative period. Other antiplatelet agents such as clopidogrel (SP) need to be discontinued prior to esophagectomy.

Nutrition

Dysphagia is the most common symptom of esophageal cancer and can result in a portion of patients presenting with significant weight loss and malnutrition. Malnutrition is most commonly assessed based on the extent of weight loss and albumin levels and has been shown to increase rates of postoperative morbidity and mortality, mainly due to postoperative infections [18]. Patients with greater than 10 % loss of body weight, presenting BMI of ≤18.5, albumin levels <3.25 mg/dl, or dysphagia to all solid food should be considered for enteric nutritional supplementation prior to neoadjuvant therapy and surgery. Jejunostomy tubes can be placed either with endoscopic, open, or laparoscopic techniques and can be done in conjunction with other necessary procedures such as Port-A-Cath placement or diagnostic laparoscopy. Percutaneous endoscopic or radiologic gastrostomy tubes have been utilized by some centers but have the hypothetical risk of affecting blood supply to the stomach which could impact the outcome of esophagectomy. More recently, the utilization of short-term placement of removable esophageal stents prior to neoadjuvant therapy has shown to provide a nonoperative possibility to improve oral nutrition. Stent placement can be performed during initial endoscopic staging but should be orchestrated to be done at the end of the staging process as stents can alter diagnostic findings on CT and PET/CT scans. These stents should be considered for elective removal 4–5 weeks following initiation of radiation/chemotherapy which seems to decrease the incidence of stent-related complications [19–21].

The incidence of obesity in patients presenting with adenocarcinoma is increasing. Although surgery in obese patients is technically more challenging and postoperative wound infections rates are higher, studies show that the overall operative risk is not increased [22].

Staging

With the availability of different treatment options such as endoscopic resection, esophagectomy, neoadjuvant chemotherapy, and/or radiation and definitive chemoradiotherapy, staging information in addition to physiologic status is crucial for determining the appropriate treatment approach. Esophageal cancers should be staged according to the 7th edition of the TNM classification system (see Table 15.1) published by the American Joint Committee on Cancer (AJCC) in 2010 [23]. The

Table 15.1 TNMG descriptors, AJCC 7th edition

Primary tumor T	
Tx	Primary tumor cannot be assessed
T0	No evidence of primary tumor
Tis	High-grade dysplasia
T1a	Tumor invades lamina propria or muscularis mucosae
T1b	Tumor invades submucosa
T2	Tumor invades muscularis propria
T3	Tumor invades adventitia
T4a	Resectable tumor invading pleura, pericardium, diaphragm
T4b	Unresectable tumor invading aorta, trachea, heart, vertebral body, etc.
Regional lymph nodes N	
Nx	Regional lymph nodes cannot be assessed
N0	No evidence of regional lymph nodes
N1	Metastasis in 1–2 regional lymph nodes
N2	Metastasis in 3–6 regional lymph nodes
N3	Metastasis in ≥7 regional lymph nodes
Distant metastasis M	
M0	No distant metastasis
M1	Distant metastasis
Histological grade G	
Gx	Grade cannot be assessed
G1	Well differentiated
G2	Moderately differentiated
G3	Poorly differentiated
G4	Undifferentiated

introduction of the 7th edition included major changes in the staging of esophageal cancer compared to the 6th edition. These changes are based on evidence for the increased importance of nodal burden rather than nodal location as contributors to outcome as well as differing prognoses of squamous cell carcinoma and adenocarcinoma (see Tables 15.2 and 15.3). In general changes affect the anatomic characteristics like TNM descriptors and tumor location as well as the nonanatomic cancer characteristics such as histologic type and grade.

Appropriate staging currently includes endoscopy (EGD) with biopsy, endoscopic ultrasound (EUS) ± EUS-guided fine needle aspiration of paraesophageal and perigastric nodes (EUS-FNA), contrast-enhanced computed tomography (CT), and fused computed tomography and FDG positron emission tomography (PET/CT). Upper endoscopy with biopsy is typically the initial diagnostic tool to establish the histologic type and grade of the tumor as well as providing information about the localization and length of the tumor. Specifically the relation of the tumor origin to the esophagogastric junction (EGJ) should be measured. Additionally satellite lesions, extent of underlying Barrett's or prior foregut surgery, can be identified and described. An upper gastrointestinal contrast study is no longer a routine part of pretreatment staging [23].

Table 15.2 Stage grouping – squamous cell carcinoma, AJCC 7th edition

Stage	T	N	M	G	Location
0	Tis	N0	M0	1, x	Any
IA	T1	N0	M0	1, x	Any
IB	T1	N0	M0	2–3	Any
	T2-3	N0	M0	1, x	Lower, x
IIA	T2-3	N0	M0	1, x	Upper, middle
	T2-3	N0	M0	2–3	Lower, x
IIB	T2-3	N0	M0	2–3	Upper, middle
	T1-2	N1	M0	Any	Any
IIIA	T1-2	N2	M0	Any	Any
	T3	N1	M0	Any	Any
	T4a	N0	M0	Any	Any
IIIB	T3	N2	M0	Any	Any
IIIC	T4a	N1-2	M0	Any	Any
	T4b	Any	M0	Any	Any
	Any	N3	M0	Any	Any
IV	Any	Any	M1	Any	Any

Table 15.3 Stage grouping – adenocarcinoma, AJCC 7th edition

Stage	T	N	M	G
0	Tis	N0	M0	1, x
IA	T1	N0	M0	1–2, x
IB	T1	N0	M0	3
	T2	N0	M0	1, x
IIA	T2	N0	M0	1–2, x
IIB	T3	N0	M0	3
	T1-2	N1	M0	Any
IIIA	T1-2	N2	M0	Any
	T3	N1	M0	Any
	T4a	N0	M0	Any
IIIB	T3	N2	M0	Any
IIIC	T4a	N1-2	M0	Any
	T4b	Any	M0	Any
	Any	N3	M0	Any
IV	Any	Any	M1	Any

T Category

This category corresponds to the extent of the local tumor invasion ranging from Tis (high-grade dysplasia) to T4b (not resectable tumor invades adjacent structures). Accurate information about depth of tumor invasion is important for treatment planning. The 7th edition introduced major changes in the T category when compared to the older version. With the new version Tis was redefined as high-grade dysplasia (HGD) including all noninvasive neoplastic epithelium that was previously called

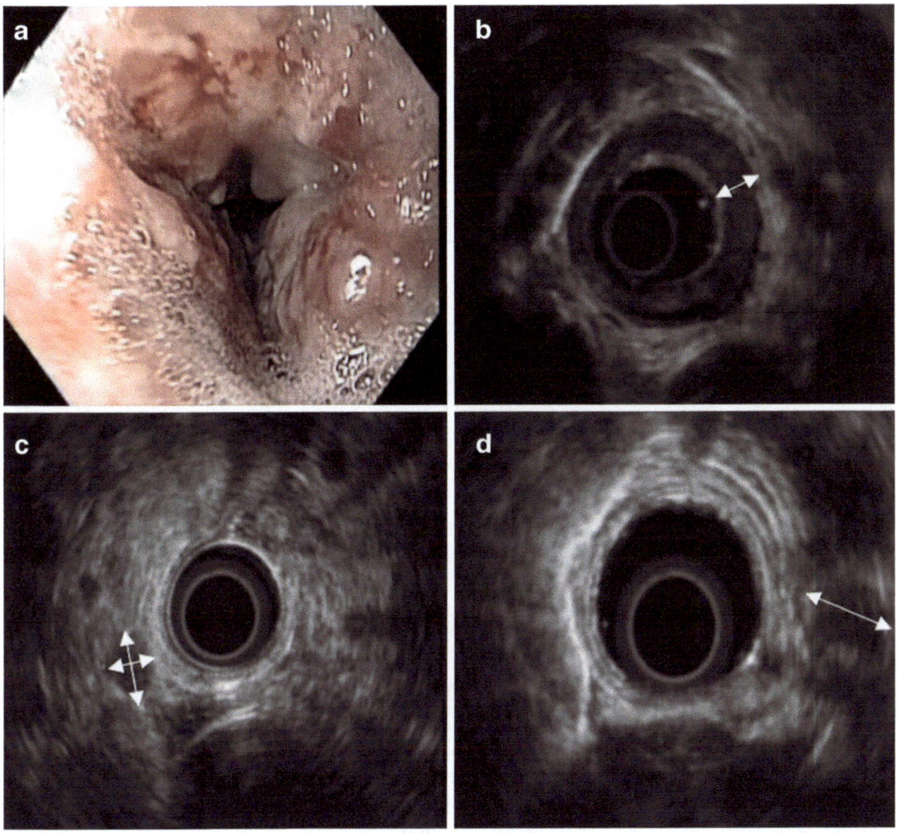

Fig. 15.2 (**a**) Gastroscopic view of distal esophagus, circumferential Barrett's segment with severe nodularity. (**b**) Endoscopic ultrasound showing thickening of esophageal wall (*arrow*) staged as uT2. (**c**, **d**) Endoscopic ultrasound showing paraesophageal lymph nodes (*arrows*)

carcinoma in situ. The T1 and the T4 categories are now subdivided into T1a (intramucosal cancer confined to the mucosa), T1b (submucosal invasion), T4a (invasive to surrounding structures but resectable cancer), and T4b (invasive non-resectable cancer) (see Table 15.1) [23].

Best assessment of depth of tumor invasion is achieved by endoscopic ultrasound (EUS) which can assess invasion of the different histological layers of the esophageal wall (Fig. 15.2). EUS accuracy regarding depth of tumor invasion ranges from 81 to 92 %, but accuracy in distinguishing between T1a and T1b cancers is less reliable [24, 25]. Best clinical information for differentiating T1a and T1b cancers is provided by diagnostic endoscopic mucosal resection (EMR) which is frequently applied in high-volume centers (Fig. 15.3). Histologic differentiation between HGD, T1a, and T1b cancer as well as additional information about lymphovascular invasion can be histologically confirmed. Perforation and bleeding rates are the most severe complications associated with EMR ranging between 1 and 2 % in experienced centers [26].

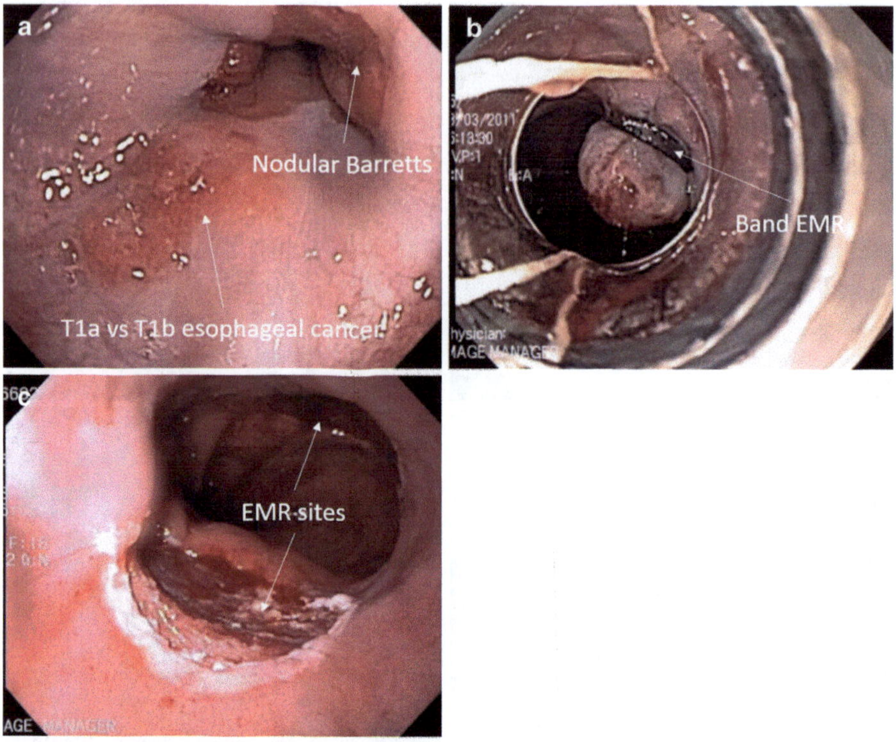

Fig. 15.3 (**a**) Endoscopic view of the distal esophagus, cancer lesion, and nodular Barrett's esophagus. (**b**) Endoscopic mucosal resection (EMR) with band technique of an area with nodular Barrett's esophagus. (**c**) After completion of 2 simultaneous EMRs, view of the muscularis propria layer at the EMR sites

Contrast-enhanced computed tomography (CT) can assess the tumor bulk but has limited sensitivity for accurately assessing depth of tumor invasion (Fig. 15.4). CT scans can provide valuable information in evaluating tumor extension into adjacent structures. Invasion may be suggested if the tumor contacts the aorta in over 90° of circumference or if the tumor bulges into the trachea [27]. In that case bronchoscopy for confirmation should be performed.

Most esophageal cancers are FDG avid and PET/CT can identify metastatic deposits not evident on CT (Fig. 15.5). However, invasion through the esophageal wall and adjacent structures cannot be assessed with any greater accuracy than CT [28].

N Category

The assessment of involvement of locoregional and distant lymph nodes is described in the N category. In general cervical and upper thoracic cancers typically drain to cervical lymph nodes, whereas lower thoracic and EGJ carcinomas tend to drain to

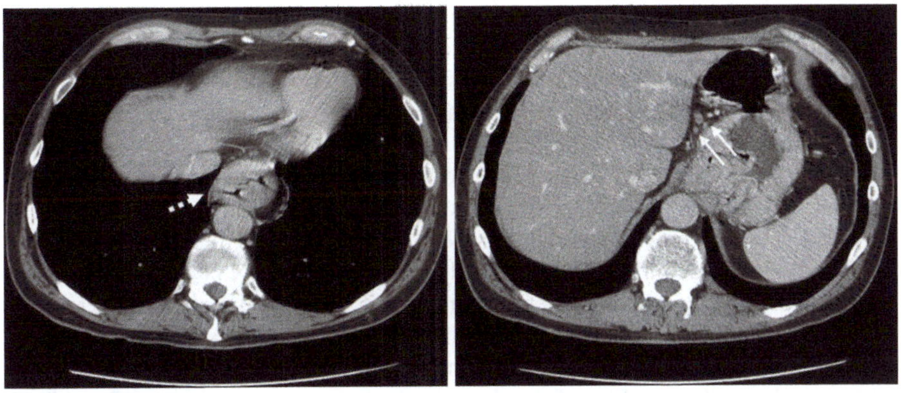

Fig. 15.4 Primary staging of distal esophageal tumor with IV contrast-enhanced CT: axial view of enlarged distal esophageal wall (*dashed arrow*) and enlarged perigastric lymph nodes (*arrows*)

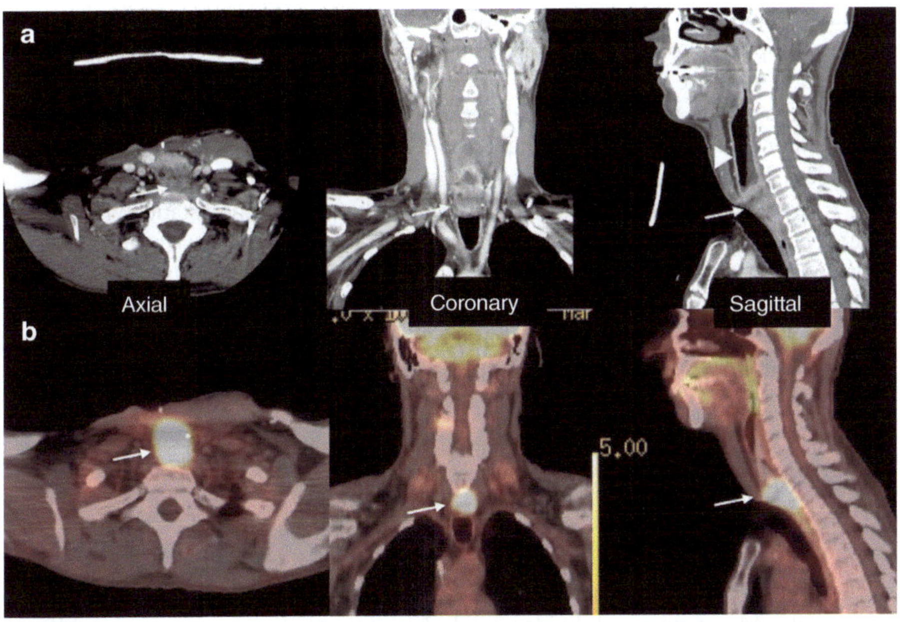

Fig. 15.5 Primary staging for cervical esophageal cancer: (**a**) IV contrast-enhanced CT showing bulky tumor in the cervical esophagus (*arrow*) with compression of posterior trachea and prestenotic dilation of cervical esophagus (*triangle*). (**b**) Corresponding fused PET/CT showing SUV uptake in bulky tumor (*arrow*) of cervical esophagus

the distal mediastinum and the celiac and perigastric nodes. Under the AJCC 7th edition, all paraesophageal and paragastric lymph nodes from the cervical to the celiac region are included under the term "locoregional" regardless of the location of the primary tumor [23]. These changes mostly contribute to two issues regarding lymphatic metastases. Firstly lymphatic metastatic disease occurs early in esophageal cancers as the lymphatic vessels are localized in the submucosal layer. The rate of lymph node metastases increases exponentially by T-stage with low incidences of lymphatic involvement less than 2 % in T1a cancers, whereas in T1b cancers the rate can be as high as 50 %. In T3 cancers lymphatic metastases are present in up to 80 % of cases [29]. Additionally tumor depth correlates to the number of involved nodes and the risk for metastatic disease. The number of involved nodes is now categorized as N0 (no lymph node metastasis), N1 (1–2 positive lymph nodes), N2 (3–6 positive lymph nodes), and N3 (≥7 positive lymph nodes). Clinical staging at most can distinguish if there are lymph node metastases or not, but at the present time cannot define the true extent of lymph node involvement. Regional lymph node involvement is best assessed with EUS (sensitivity 85 %, specificity 97 %) (Fig. 15.2) which has been proven superior to CT and PET/CT (sensitivity 50–60 %, specificity 80–85 %) [30]. Additionally EUS provides the opportunity for ultrasound-guided fine needle assessment (FNA) of suspicious lymph nodes [24]. EUS can only assess lymph nodes adjacent to the esophagus and stomach. Sampling lymph nodes directly adjacent to the tumor is not feasible because biopsies should not be done if the primary tumor needs to be traversed by the FNA. Therefore, EGD/EUS in combination with CT and CT/PET is the best method to evaluate the N status. However, a high SUV-uptake signal from the primary tumor can "spill over" to make the assessment of adjacent regional lymph nodes less accurate on CT/PET.

CT scans can provide information about regional and metastatic lymph node spread, but the evaluation depends predominantly on lymph node size (Fig. 15.3). A short axis of the lymph node greater than 1 cm is considered highly suspicious for malignancy. However, smaller lymph nodes may be involved and larger lymph nodes may simply reflect inflammation. PET/CT scans provide the best opportunity to identify nonregional positive nodes (Fig. 15.6a).

M Category

Seventy-five percent of patients presenting with esophageal cancer will have metastatic disease at initial presentation. In the 7th edition of the TNM classification system, the M category subdivides solely between no distant metastases (M0) or distant metastases (M1) [23]. M1 diseases typically reflect an incurable disease with a 3 % 5-year survival rate. Distant metastases include those lymph node stations outside of "regional" area involved in the N designation. Visceral metastases are most commonly seen in the liver followed by lung, bones, and adrenal glands [31].

Chest, abdominal, and pelvic CT scans are the most common initial diagnostic tests for the evaluation of metastatic diseases. Many metastases are readily detectable by CT (sensitivity 81 %). However, specificity especially for the evaluation of pulmonary metastases is impaired as differentiation between indeterminate pulmonary nodules and metastases cannot be readily made. It is currently estimated that 20 % hematogenous and peritoneal metastases will be occult on CT imaging [32].

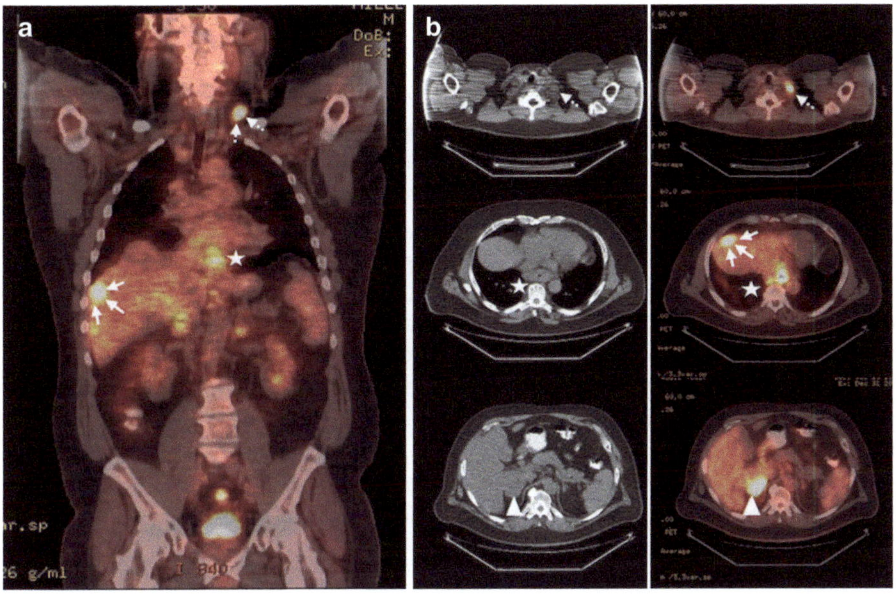

Fig. 15.6 Primary staging with fused PET/CT showing metastatic diseases in distal esophageal cancer. (**a**) Coronary view with SUV uptake in left cervical lymph node (*dashed arrow*), distal esophagus (*star*), and focal hepatic lesion (*solid arrows*). (**b**) Corresponding axial view with focal cervical, esophageal, and hepatic uptake, bottom pictures showing additional right adrenal SUV uptake (*triangle*)

Best results are achieved in a combination of CT and PET/CT, which has a sensitivity of 69–81 % and a specificity of 92 % (Fig. 15.6) [33]. It has been shown that PET/CT will detect up to 20 % of metastatic lesions not detected on other image modalities [34]. With the use of PET/CT, determination of resectability improves and ultimately will decrease the percentage of patients found unresectable at surgery. However, one must be aware of the limitations of PET/CT imaging. FDG avidity may not always represent malignant diseases as it can be seen at sites of infection, inflammation, and fracture as well as a reflection of physiological processes involving the bowel, skeletal muscle, liver, and kidney. Therefore, FDG avid lesions should be evaluated by histologic assessment depending on the location of the suspicious lesion either by EUS-FNA, EBUS-FNA, percutaneous CT- or US-guided FNA or excision biopsy. A lack of FDG uptake may occur in necrotic or mucinous tumors and small regional nodal or visceral metastases (<8 mm) may not be reliably detected as they may be masked by the normal SUV uptake of the surrounding tissue [35].

Patients who present with the epicenter of their cancer located in the stomach should be considered for diagnostic staging laparoscopy and peritoneal lavage. Laparoscopy following CT and EGD-US increases sensitivity and specificity for detecting distant lymph node and visceral metastases especially in patients with lower esophageal and EGJ cancers. Peritoneal metastases not detected on CT were seen in up to 20 % of the cases being additionally staged laparoscopically [36].

Treatment Decision

According to the NCCN treatment guidelines for esophageal cancer, treatment planning is optimally delivered in a multidisciplinary setting. There is increasing support for esophageal cancer staging and treatment planning being done in specialized high-volume centers with expertise in esophageal cancer treatment in all participating disciplines. Treatment options are most effectively reviewed in the setting of multidisciplinary tumor board. The disciplines that optimally should be participating include surgical oncology, medical and radiation oncology, gastroenterology, radiology, and pathology. The presence of nutritional services, nursing, palliative care team, social workers, and other supportive disciplines is desirable. A treatment decision should only be developed after complete staging and physiologic work-up. In patients receiving neoadjuvant treatment, it is potentially helpful to review the treatment response, restaging tests, and nutritional and physiologic status at tumor board.

The main factors that guide the treatment decision are tumor stage, location, and histology (Tables 15.2 and 15.3) as well as patient medical condition and preferences.

Limited Locoregional Disease (Stage I and IIA)

In patients staged with high-grade dysplasia or early intramucosal cancer without suspected lymph node involvement (Tis-T1a N0 M0), historically surgery has been the standard treatment. Today endoscopic mucosal resection is an accepted treatment option as specialized centers report similar cure rates when compared to surgery [38, 39]. Additionally any underlying Barrett's esophagus should be eradicated either by endoscopic mucosal resection alone or in combination with ablational therapies (such as radiofrequency ablation or cryotherapy). For tumor invasion into the submucosal layer but not into the muscularis propria (T1b), primary surgery is the standard treatment. Current data does not support endoscopic submucosal dissection in cancers with submucosal invasion only (T1b) as lymph node metastases may be present in 20–50 % of cases [40, 41].

Localized cancers clinically staged T2 N0 M0 are a matter of controversy as this particular group is staged accurately in only 13 % of cases and 37 % of cases are understaged. Primary surgery may be appropriate in 63 % of cases clinically staged with T2. However, one-third could benefit from undergoing neoadjuvant therapy. Understaged patients undergoing surgery can be considered for adjuvant therapy.

Locoregional Disease (Stage IIB–IIIC)

Only 30–40 % of patients presenting with esophageal cancer have resectable disease, and lymph node involvement is common. Neoadjuvant therapy with either chemotherapy alone or in combination with chemoradiation is indicated in locoregional cancers. Currently R0 resection rates over 85 % and complete pathologic response rates of 26 % have been documented following neoadjuvant chemoradiotherapy resulting in an overall survival benefit. In patients with squamous cell carcinoma, neoadjuvant chemoradiation showed higher complete tumor resection rates and improved overall survival rates when compared to neoadjuvant chemotherapy alone. Neoadjuvant therapy for adenocarcinoma in the United States most commonly involves chemotherapy in combination with radiation. The randomized control trial from the Netherlands including 366 patients (CROSS study), comparing outcomes between surgery alone and surgery following neoadjuvant chemoradiotherapy, showed a survival benefit for those patients undergoing neoadjuvant chemoradiation without increased perioperative morbidity or mortality [37]. While the location and treatment response of the primary tumor is a prognostic factor in patients with squamous cell carcinoma, the extent of lymph node involvement in patients with adenocarcinoma is more important for prognosis. Squamous cell carcinoma involving the cervical esophagus should be considered for definitive chemoradiotherapy.

Metastatic Disease (Stage IV) or Nonsurgical Patients

Patients unfit for esophagectomy or presenting with non-resectable or metastatic disease can be considered for different options of palliative treatment depending on their personal wishes and general and psychological health status. Definitive chemoradiotherapy in nonsurgical patients with regional squamous cell carcinoma is the most common treatment option. Chemotherapy is indicated in patients with metastatic esophageal carcinoma and a good performance status (Karnofsky performance score ≥60 %). The value of chemotherapy in patients with metastatic squamous cell carcinoma is less proven and response rates are inferior to those in patients with adenocarcinoma.

Best supportive care includes treatment for dysphagia and nutritional supplementation as well as pain control and antiemetic treatment. In patients experiencing severe dysphagia secondary to cancer-related esophageal obstruction, permanent endoscopic self-expandable metallic stent can provide significant relief in swallowing symptoms. Alternatively single-dose brachytherapy may be an option, even in patients who have received previous radiation. Enteric feeding tubes particularly endoscopic gastrostomy or jejunostomy tubes are potential alternatives for nutritional support in selected patients.

References

1. Siegel R, DeSantis C, Virgo K, Stein K, Mariotto A, Smith T, et al. Cancer treatment and survivorship statistics, 2012. CA Cancer J Clin. 2012;62(4):220–41.
2. Lagergren J. Adenocarcinoma of oesophagus: what exactly is the size of the problem and who is at risk? Gut. 2005;54 Suppl 1:i1–5.
3. Brown LM, Hoover R, Silverman D, Baris D, Hayes R, Swanson GM, et al. Excess incidence of squamous cell esophageal cancer among US Black men: role of social class and other risk factors. Am J Epidemiol. 2001;153(2):114–22.

4. Shaheen N, Ransohoff DF. Gastroesophageal reflux, Barrett esophagus, and esophageal cancer: clinical applications. JAMA. 2002;287(15):1982–6.
5. Pohl H, Wrobel K, Bojarski C, Voderholzer W, Sonnenberg A, Rosch T, et al. Risk factors in the development of esophageal adenocarcinoma. Am J Gastroenterol. 2013;108(2):200–7.
6. Siewert JR, Stein HJ. Classification of adenocarcinoma of the oesophagogastric junction. Br J Surg. 1998;85(11):1457–9.
7. Markar SR, Low DE. Physiology, not chronology, dictates outcomes after esophagectomy for esophageal cancer: outcomes in patients 80 years and older. Ann Surg Oncol. 2013;20(3):1020–6.
8. Moskovitz AH, Rizk NP, Venkatraman E, Bains MS, Flores RM, Park BJ, et al. Mortality increases for octogenarians undergoing esophagogastrectomy for esophageal cancer. Ann Thorac Surg. 2006;82(6):2031–6.
9. Cijs TM, Verhoef C, Steyerberg EW, Koppert LB, Tran TC, Wijnhoven BP, et al. Outcome of esophagectomy for cancer in elderly patients. Ann Thorac Surg. 2010;90(3):900–7.
10. Law S, Wong KH, Kwok KF, Chu KM, Wong J. Predictive factors for postoperative pulmonary complications and mortality after esophagectomy for cancer. Ann Surg. 2004;240(5):791–800.
11. Kuwano H, Sumiyoshi K, Sonoda K, Kitamura K, Tsutsui S, Toh Y, et al. Relationship between preoperative assessment of organ function and postoperative morbidity in patients with oesophageal cancer. Eur J Surg. 1998;164(8):581–6.
12. Zingg U, Smithers BM, Gotley DC, Smith G, Aly A, Clough A, et al. Factors associated with postoperative pulmonary morbidity after esophagectomy for cancer. Ann Surg Oncol. 2011;18(5):1460–8.
13. Murthy SC, Law S, Whooley BP, Alexandrou A, Chu KM, Wong J. Atrial fibrillation after esophagectomy is a marker for postoperative morbidity and mortality. J Thorac Cardiovasc Surg. 2003;126(4):1162–7.
14. Eagle KA, Berger PB, Calkins H, Chaitman BR, Ewy GA, Fleischmann KE, et al. ACC/AHA guideline update for perioperative cardiovascular evaluation for noncardiac surgery–executive summary: a report of the American College of Cardiology/American Heart Association Task Force on Practice Guidelines (Committee to Update the 1996 Guidelines on Perioperative Cardiovascular Evaluation for Noncardiac Surgery). J Am Coll Cardiol. 2002;39(3):542–53.
15. Tisdale JE, Wroblewski HA, Wall DS, Rieger KM, Hammoud ZT, Young JV, et al. A randomized, controlled study of amiodarone for prevention of atrial fibrillation after transthoracic esophagectomy. J Thorac Cardiovasc Surg. 2010;140(1):45–51.
16. Tisdale JE, Wroblewski HA, Kesler KA. Prophylaxis of atrial fibrillation after noncardiac thoracic surgery. Semin Thorac Cardiovasc Surg. 2010;22(4):310–20.
17. Fleisher LA, Beckman JA, Brown KA, Calkins H, Chaikof E, Fleischmann KE, et al. ACC/AHA 2006 guideline update on perioperative cardiovascular evaluation for noncardiac surgery: focused update on perioperative beta-blocker therapy: a report of the American College of Cardiology/American Heart Association Task Force on Practice Guidelines (Writing Committee to Update the 2002 Guidelines on Perioperative Cardiovascular Evaluation for Noncardiac Surgery) developed in collaboration with the American Society of Echocardiography, American Society of Nuclear Cardiology, Heart Rhythm Society, Society of Cardiovascular Anesthesiologists, Society for Cardiovascular Angiography and Interventions, and Society for Vascular Medicine and Biology. J Am Coll Cardiol. 2006;47(11):2343–55.
18. Bollschweiler E, Herbold T, Plum P, Holscher AH. Prognostic relevance of nutritional status in patients with advanced esophageal cancer. Expert Rev Anticancer Ther. 2013;13(3):275–8.
19. Lopes TL, Eloubeidi MA. A pilot study of fully covered self-expandable metal stents prior to neoadjuvant therapy for locally advanced esophageal cancer. Dis Esophagus. 2010;23(4):309–15.
20. Siddiqui AA, Sarkar A, Beltz S, Lewis J, Loren D, Kowalski T, et al. Placement of fully covered self-expandable metal stents in patients with locally advanced esophageal cancer before neoadjuvant therapy. Gastrointest Endosc. 2012;76(1):44–51.
21. von Rahden BH, Stein HJ. Staging and treatment of advanced esophageal cancer. Curr Opin Gastroenterol. 2005;21(4):472–7.

22. Morgan MA, Lewis WG, Hopper AN, Escofet X, Harvard TJ, Brewster AE, et al. Prognostic significance of body mass indices for patients undergoing esophagectomy for cancer. Dis Esophagus. 2007;20(1):29–35.
23. Edge SB, Compton CC. The American Joint Committee on Cancer: the 7th edition of the AJCC cancer staging manual and the future of TNM. Ann Surg Oncol. 2010;17(6):1471–4.
24. Puli SR, Reddy JB, Bechtold ML, Antillon D, Ibdah JA, Antillon MR. Staging accuracy of esophageal cancer by endoscopic ultrasound: a meta-analysis and systematic review. World J Gastroenterol. 2008;14(10):1479–90.
25. Young PE, Gentry AB, Acosta RD, Greenwald BD, Riddle M. Endoscopic ultrasound does not accurately stage early adenocarcinoma or high-grade dysplasia of the esophagus. Clin Gastroenterol Hepatol. 2010;8(12):1037–41.
26. Seerden TC, Larghi A. Staging of early adenocarcinoma in Barrett's esophagus. Gastrointest Endosc Clin N Am. 2011;21(1):53–66.
27. Rasanen JV, Sihvo EI, Knuuti MJ, Minn HR, Luostarinen ME, Laippala P, et al. Prospective analysis of accuracy of positron emission tomography, computed tomography, and endoscopic ultrasonography in staging of adenocarcinoma of the esophagus and the esophagogastric junction. Ann Surg Oncol. 2003;10(8):954–60.
28. Kato H, Nakajima M. The efficacy of FDG-PET for the management of esophageal cancer: review article. Ann Thorac Cardiovasc Surg. 2012;18(5):412–9.
29. Prenzel KL, Holscher AH, Drebber U, Agavonova M, Gutschow CA, Bollschweiler E. Prognostic impact of nodal micrometastasis in early esophageal cancer. Eur J Surg Oncol. 2012;38(4):314–8.
30. van Vliet EP, Heijenbrok-Kal MH, Hunink MG, Kuipers EJ, Siersema PD. Staging investigations for oesophageal cancer: a meta-analysis. Br J Cancer. 2008;98(3):547–57.
31. Quint LE, Hepburn LM, Francis IR, Whyte RI, Orringer MB. Incidence and distribution of distant metastases from newly diagnosed esophageal carcinoma. Cancer. 1995;76(7):1120–5.
32. Luketich JD, Friedman DM, Weigel TL, Meehan MA, Keenan RJ, Townsend DW, et al. Evaluation of distant metastases in esophageal cancer: 100 consecutive positron emission tomography scans. Ann Thorac Surg. 1999;68(4):1133–6.
33. van Westreenen HL, Westerterp M, Bossuyt PM, Pruim J, Sloof GW, van Lanschot JJ, et al. Systematic review of the staging performance of 18F-fluorodeoxyglucose positron emission tomography in esophageal cancer. J Clin Oncol. 2004;22(18):3805–12.
34. Weber WA, Ott K. Imaging of esophageal and gastric cancer. Semin Oncol. 2004;31(4):530–41.
35. van Westreenen HL, Plukker JT, Cobben DC, Verhoogt CJ, Groen H, Jager PL. Prognostic value of the standardized uptake value in esophageal cancer. AJR Am J Roentgenol. 2005;185(2):436–40.
36. Krasna MJ, Jiao X, Mao YS, Sonett J, Gamliel Z, Kwong K, et al. Thoracoscopy/laparoscopy in the staging of esophageal cancer: Maryland experience. Surg Laparosc Endosc Percutan Tech. 2002;12(4):213–8.
37. van Hagen P, Hulshof MC, van Lanschot JJ, Steyerberg EW, van Berge Henegouwen MI, Wijnhoven BP, et al. Preoperative chemoradiotherapy for esophageal or junctional cancer. N Engl J Med. 2012;366(22):2074–84.
38. Pech O, Bollschweiler E, Manner H, Leers J, Ell C, Holscher AH. Comparison between endoscopic and surgical resection of mucosal esophageal adenocarcinoma in Barrett's esophagus at two high-volume centers. Ann Surg 2011;254(1):67–72.
39. Pech O, May A, Manner H, Behrens A, Pohl J, Weferling M, et al. Long-term efficacy and safety of endoscopic resection for patients with mucosal adenocarcinoma of the esophagus. Gastroenterology 2014;146(3):652–60.
40. Leers JM, DeMeester SR, Oezcelik A, Klipfel N, Ayazi S, Abate E, et al. The prevalence of lymph node metastases in patients with T1 esophageal adenocarcinoma a retrospective review of esophagectomy specimens. Ann Surg 2011;253(2):271–8.
41. Bollschweiler E, Holscher AH. Early adenocarcinoma of the esophagus - clinical relevance of depth of infiltration into the submucosa. Clin Gastroenterol Hepatol 2011;9(3):277–8.

Chapter 16
Esophageal Cancer: Surgical Treatment

Henner M. Schmidt and Donald E. Low

Abstract Treatment approaches varies according to the stage of esophageal cancer and the majority of patients present with advanced disease. Despite being a challenging surgical procedure, historically associated with high morbidity and mortality, esophagectomy remains a central treatment component in patients with early-stage and loco regional esophageal cancer. This chapter describes the indications for esophagectomy, with an emphasis of the technical aspects of the surgical approaches available, common post-operative complications and outcomes following esophagectomy.

Keywords Esophageal cancer • Esophagectomy • Surgery • Indication • Complication

Introduction

Outcomes of treatment of esophageal cancer remain poor with an overall 5-year survival rate of 19 % [1]. As expected the treatment approach varies according to the stage of disease at presentation although the majority of patients present with advanced disease [2]. Esophageal resections in patients with esophageal cancer are

H.M. Schmidt
Department for General, Thoracic and Vascular Surgery, Virginia Mason Medical Center, 1100 Ninth Ave, Seattle, WA 98101, USA
e-mail: henner.schmidt@vmmc.org, henner.schmidt@yahoo.de

D.E. Low, FACS, FRCS(c), FRCSI (Hon.) (✉)
Department for General, Thoracic and Vascular Surgery, Virginia Mason Medical Center, 1100 Ninth Ave, Seattle, WA 98101, USA

Department of Thoracic Surgery and Thoracic Oncology, Scientific Director Ryan Hill Research Fellowship, Director Esophageal Center of Excellence, Digestive Disease Institute, Seattle, WA, USA
e-mail: donald.low@vmmc.org

P.M. Fisichella et al. (eds.), *Esophageal Diseases*,
DOI 10.1007/978-3-319-04337-1_16,

challenging procedures, rated as high risk procedures by the Leapfrog Group, and are historically associated with high morbidity and mortality rates and concerns that the operation can negatively impact quality of life [3]. However, surgery remains the best option for cure in certain patients with early-stage disease and provides superior local control and improved survival for regional cancers [4]. Additionally, mortality rates have steadily declined over the past decades due to the improvement in staging techniques, patient selection, and the application of enhanced recovery protocols and standardized clinical pathways. Surgical approaches have also continued to evolve especially with the introduction of minimally invasive techniques [5].

In a US nationwide study assessing 57,000 esophagectomies between 1998 and 2006, a decrease in mortality rates from 12 to 7 % has been reported [6]. Furthermore, several studies showed a strong relationship between operative mortality when procedures are performed in high volume centers [7, 8]. In specialized high volume centers for esophagcetomy, mortality rates of 0.3–5 % have been reported [9]. However, morbidity rates following esophagectomy continue to be appreciably higher when compared to other complex oncologic operations such as pancreatectomy, gastrectomy, or hepatectomy. Several studies have demonstrated that postoperative quality of life is negatively impacted by postoperative complications [10]. However, it has been shown that in the absence of major perioperative complications, a comparable normal baseline level of quality of life can typically be achieved 6 months after surgery [11, 12].

Indications for Esophagectomy

The current NCCN treatment guidelines for esophageal cancer recommend surgery for all physiological fit patients clinically staged with resectable cancers (T1b-T4a N0-3 M0) [4]. After accurate staging patients presenting with T1b N0 cancer are currently recommended to be treated with surgical resection, although certain specialized centers have advocated that selected "low risk" T1b N0 cancers can be treated endoscopically. These "low-risk" cancers are described as tumor infiltration only in the superficial submucosal layer (sm1), tumor differentiation grades 1 and 2, and no evidence of lymphovascular invasion [13]. However, the majority of high volume centers would recommend primary surgical resection due to the potential for inaccuracy in the assessment of depth of submucosal invasion and the risk of lymph node metastases. Clinically staged T3 and T4a cancers with or without suspected lymph node involvement are currently recommended for multimodality therapy which involves neoadjuvant therapy with either chemotherapy alone or in combination with radiation to improve local control and survival. The most appropriate treatment for patients clinically staged with T2 N0 cancers remains controversial with surgery alone or multimodality both identified as appropriate treatment [14]. However, up to 37 % of patients with clinically staged T2 N0 cancers will be found on final pathology to be understaged and would therefore potentially benefit from neoadjuvant treatment. If those patients are upstaged regarding the final surgical pathology, adjuvant chemotherapy can be considered.

Surgical Approach

Esophageal resection may be accomplished by a variety of different approaches, but no one technical approach will be appropriate for all patients. To understand the reasoning for selecting one approach over another, it is important to understand the fundamental aspects of various esophageal resection strategies. Factors involved in the choice of procedure include disease stage, tumor location and histology, patient-related factors such as comorbidities and previous surgeries, as well as personal preference and experience of the surgeon [2].

Transhiatal Esophagogastrectomy

The transhiatal esophagectomy is performed using a laparotomy and left cervical incision [15]. Mobilization of the stomach is performed with dissection of the celiac and left gastric nodes, division of the left gastric artery, and preservation of the right gastroepiploic and proximal right gastric arteries. The majority of the transthoracic esophageal dissection is preformed through the hiatus. Much of the mediastinal component of the dissection is done manually without the ability to visualize the dissection or to do a directed lymph node dissection. The advantage of this approach is that it does not involve a separate thoracic incision. The left cervical incision allows mobilization of the cervical esophagus and transection of the esophagus at the thoracic inlet. Completion of the esophagectomy is achieved via the laparotomy and the gastric conduit is carefully drawn up through the mediastinum and externalized in the cervical incision where the esophagogastric anastomosis is performed (Fig. 16.1). The NCCN treatment guideline mentions that transhiatal approach is applicable for lesions at any thoracic location, but might not be feasible for dissection of bulky, mid esophageal cancers adjacent to the trachea. Other studies have suggested that transhiatal esophagectomy is best suited for tumors centered at the esophagogastric junction, as survival of true esophageal cancers is improved with transthoracic operations [16].

Ivor Lewis Esophagogastrectomy

This is the most common utilized approach worldwide. It involves a laparotomy followed by a right thoracotomy with the anastomosis typically done in the upper thorax at or above the level of the azygos vein. Gastric mobilization is performed as described for the transhiatal approach. This approach involves two standard incisions and all the dissection is done under direct vision including a directed lymph node dissection (Fig. 16.2). This approach is appropriate for most lower and lower middle level tumors and has the additional advantage that this approach can be performed with minimal cardiac manipulation, which is of hypothetical benefit in patients with cardiac comorbidities.

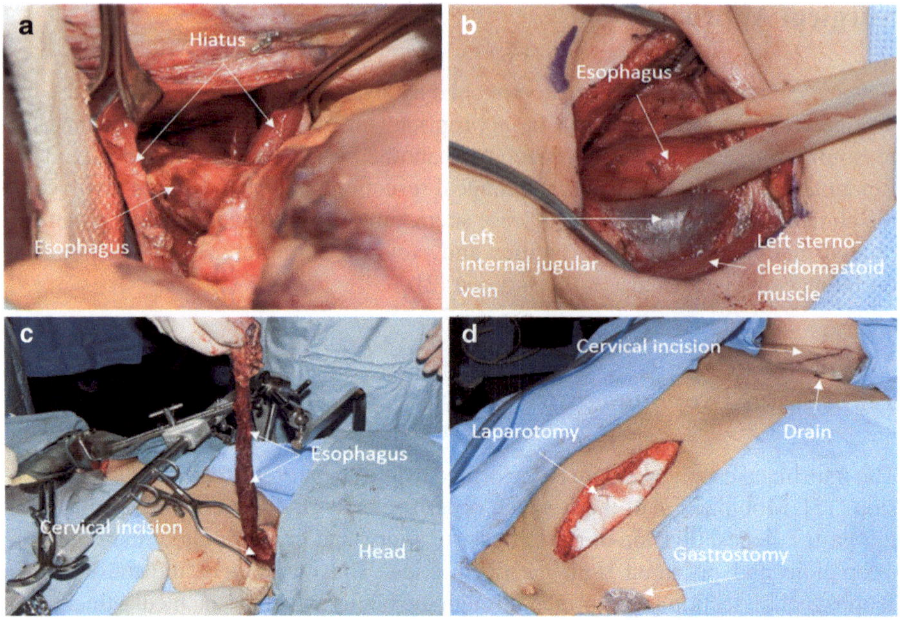

Fig. 16.1 Transhiatal esophagectomy. (**a**) Mediastinal esophageal dissection through the hiatus via midline laparotomy. (**b**) Preparation of cervical esophagus through left cervical incision. (**c**) Dissected esophagus completely excavated through cervical incision. (**d**) Upper midline laparotomy and closed left cervical incision after cervical anastomosis, placement of cervical wound drain, and gastrostomy tube

McKeown (Three-Stage) Esophagogastrectomy

This approach begins with a right-sided thoracotomy for complete mobilization of the esophagus and dissection of the thoracic lymph nodes under direct vision, followed by abdominal and left cervical incisions after repositioning the patient from the left lateral decubitus to the supine position. Gastric mobilization and cervical anastomosis are performed as described for the transhiatal approach. With this approach large mid and upper thoracic tumors can be mobilized under direct vision and resectability can be assured prior to gastric mobilization (Fig. 16.3).

Left Thoracoabdominal Esophagogastrectomy

The left thoracoabdominal esophagectomy utilizes a contiguous incision from the upper abdomen to the left thorax typically through the eighth intercostal space (Fig. 16.4). Mobilization of the stomach is similar to the description in previous procedures. Esophagectomy is accomplished through the left chest and the anastomosis can be performed in either the intrathoracic or cervical location. The anastomosis can be performed just inferior to the aortic arch, or following dissection under

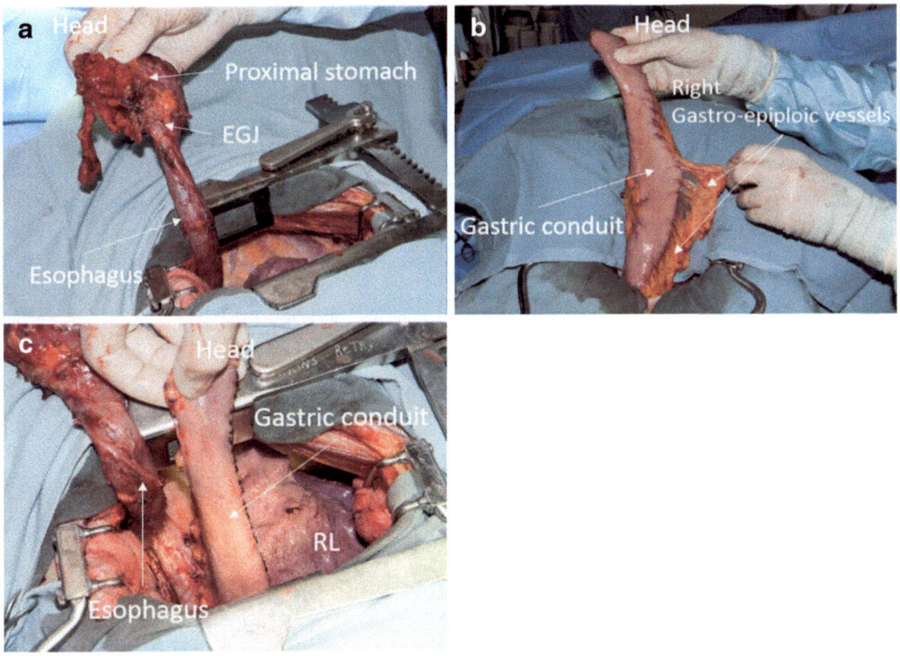

Fig. 16.2 Ivor Lewis esophagectomy. (**a**) Dissected esophagus and esophagogastric junction (*EGJ*) excavated through the right thoracotomy. (**b**) Upper midline laparotomy; prepared gastric conduit after resecting cardia and portion of lesser curvature to provide a 5–10 cm resection margin around the esophagogastric junction (*EGJ*); preserved right epiploic vessels. (**c**) Gastric conduit pulled through hiatus and dissected esophagus, both excavated through thoracotomy. Right lung (*RL*) deflated

the aorta can be accomplished above the arch. The intrathoracic dissection can be continued into the neck through a window made in the pleura above the aortic arch and lateral to the subclavian artery. The dissection separates the vagus nerves from the esophagus making the mobilization in the neck more straightforward and decreasing the incidence of recurrent nerve injuries. This approach provides superior exposure to the distal esophagus and allows a complete abdominal and thoracic lymph node dissection. It also provides the significant advantage of providing exposure to the chest and abdomen at the same time which facilitates modifying the operation according to intraoperative findings. Specifically not only can the level of the anastomosis be changed but also the colon or small bowel can be used if the stomach is found to be unavailable or inappropriate.

Transhiatal Esophagectomy Versus Transthoracic Esophagectomy

Several studies have compared the outcomes between transthoracic and transhiatal approaches. The only randomized trial showed significantly higher pulmonary morbidity and wound infections in patients who underwent a transthoracic resection

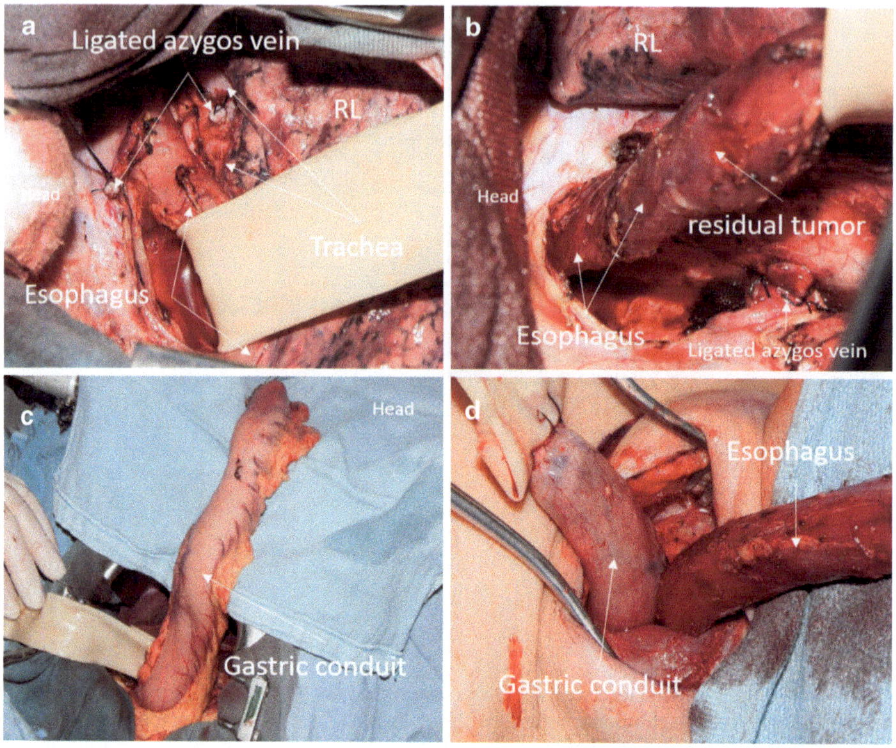

Fig. 16.3 McKeown esophagectomy after neoadjuvant chemoradiotherapy for a previously bulky squamous cell esophageal cancer with extensive contact plane to posterior trachea. (**a**) Right thoracotomy, esophagus partly dissected and secured with loop, ligated azygos vein, deflated right lung (*RL*), extensive adherence to trachea. (**b**) Complete dissection of the esophagus into the apex of the thorax, proximal location of residual tumor at the level of the azygos vein. (**c**) Prepared gastric conduit excavated through upper midline laparotomy. (**d**) Gastric conduit and dissected esophagus seen through the cervical incision before performing cervical anastomosis

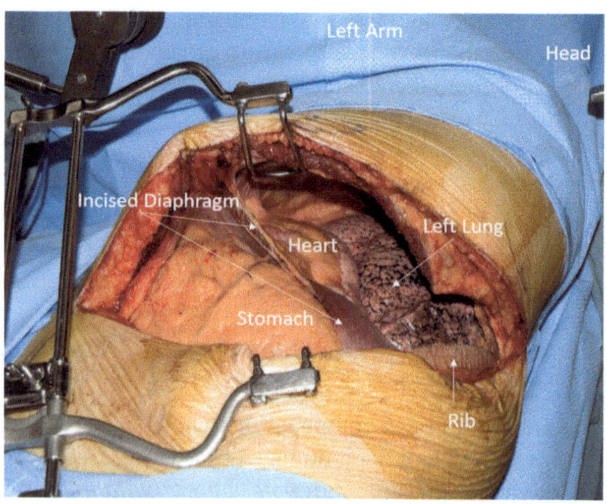

Fig. 16.4 Left thoracoabdominal esophagectomy: Patient in right semi-lateral decubitus position. View through contiguous incision from the upper abdomen to the left thorax in abdominal and thoracic cavity. The diaphragm has been incised

[17]. Additionally perioperative mortality rates were nonsignificantly higher when compared to transhiatal esophageal resections. However, transhiatal resections were associated with higher incidences of recurrent laryngeal nerve palsy as well as anastomotic leak and stricture rates. Despite a higher average lymph node harvest in the transthoracic approach, no difference was demonstrated in overall survival between the transhiatal and the transthoracic patients. These results may reflect a selection bias as patients who underwent transhiatal resections had significantly lower tumor stages and tumors were more commonly located in the distal esophagus. This was given added credibility following a subsequent subanalysis which revealed a survival advantage of 14 % for the subgroup of patients undergoing transthoracic resection for esophageal cancers not including those cancers at the esophagogastric junction [16].

Minimally Invasive Esophagectomy

In the last decade the utilization of minimally invasive and hybrid techniques for esophageal resections has increased. National and international audits suggest that currently 15–30 % of all esophageal resections are performed with at least a component of the operation utilizing minimally invasive approaches [18]. Decreased blood loss, lower incidence of respiratory complications, as well as shorter hospital stay have been described in the literature as potential advantages of the minimally invasive approach over the transhiatal or transthoracic operations [19]. Initial concerns as to whether minimally invasive resections would negatively impact the integrity of the oncologic resection have not been proven as there has been no differences identified between open and minimally invasive studies comparing in-hospital mortality, complete resection rates, and total number of lymph nodes harvested. Additionally studies have shown no difference in overall survival between minimally invasive and open procedures [19–21]. Patients with more advanced diseases or those who have undergone extensive prior abdominal and/or thoracic surgery are currently felt to be less suitable for minimally invasive surgery.

Salvage Esophagectomy

The best initial management for early and locoregional esophageal squamous cell carcinoma continues to evolve. Studies have shown no overall survival benefit between surgery and definitive chemoradiation in patients with squamous cell cancer [22, 23]. These reports have resulted in many patients undergoing definitive chemoradiation and reserving salvage esophagectomy for patients with persistent or recurrent disease [24, 25]. This treatment course is currently not well established and at the present time no definitive methodology for identifying patients with complete response after definitive chemoradiotherapy is available. In addition the majority of publications suggest that secondary to the late effects of radiotherapy salvage esophagectomy is associated with significant higher levels of perioperative morbidity and mortality [26, 27].

Summary

The most appropriate approach will continue to vary between centers and surgeons. Specialized centers capable of providing a diversified surgical approach, depending on physiologic factors and tumor characteristics, while applying standardized recovery pathways and enhanced recovery programs will be in the best position to provide superior outcomes.

Technical Aspects of Esophageal Resection

Lymphadenectomy

Discussion continues as to whether the extent of lymph node dissection has a therapeutic and survival benefit rather than being of only prognostic significance as a marker for systemic disease. Several studies support both a therapeutic and prognostic benefit as they document a link between the number of lymph nodes removed at the time of surgery and survivorship [28–31]. One study using the SEER database identified the total nodal count as an independent predictor of overall survival regardless of the extent of lymphatic metastasis and independently of tumor histology [28]. Subsequently, there have been several studies targeting the appropriate extent of nodal dissection and although opinions continue to vary one paper indicates that removal of 23 or more nodes provides the optimal threshold for survival [30]. Another report based recommendations for the optimal number of resected lymph nodes on the T-stage, ranging from 10 to 12 nodes for pT1 tumors to 30–50 nodes for pT3/4 tumors [31].

These targets raised the question as to which of the approaches to esophageal resection provides the most appropriate opportunity for adequate nodal dissection. Multiple papers have advocated the single-field (transhiatal) versus two-field (Ivor Lewis) versus three-field (McKeown) lymphadenectomy and failed to demonstrate a clear superiority for any one approach. One randomized trial comparing single-field versus two-field dissection showed a nonsignificant trend for the transthoracic two-field en bloc approach [17]. Analysis of the subset of adenocarcinomas of the distal tubular esophagus showed a significant improvement in survival for the more extensive transthoracic procedure [32]. Three-field lymphadenectomy has been advocated mainly in Asia in studies dominated by squamous cell cancer. A Japanese randomized trial comparing two- and three-field dissections showed a nonsignificant improvement in 2- and 5-year survival following three-field dissection [33]. However, incidences of tracheostomies and phrenic and laryngeal nerve palsies were increased following three-field dissection.

The current NCCN treatment guideline recommends a two-field lymphadenectomy with the goal of resecting at least 15 nodes. The optimum number of nodes that should be removed after neoadjuvant therapy is currently unknown, although similar lymph node resection is recommended.

Resection Margins

Although there is a lack of data addressing the adequacy of resection margins, evidence from large retrospective case series demonstrates that R1 (microscopic tumor at margin) and R2 (macroscopic tumor at margin) resection margins are associated with a poor prognosis [34–36]. There is general agreement that achieving negative proximal and distal margins is considered a prerequisite for a curative esophagectomy. Squamous cell carcinoma is associated with intramural cancer spread and satellite lesions in up to 30 % of patients [37] and in adenocarcinoma a similar incidence in submucosal lymphatic spread has been found [35]. In a prospective study including only SCC patients, an intraoperatively measured proximal margin of 5 cm was associated with a 20 % recurrence probability at the anastomosis. Recurrence rate decreased with extended resection margins with recurrence probabilities of 8 % for 5–10 cm margins and 0 % for >10 cm margins [38]. The resection margins in adenocarcinoma were assessed in a retrospective study including 500 patients. In this series all tumors were located at the esophagogastric junction and an intraoperatively measured resection margin of 7 cm or more was independently associated with survival in patients who had R0 resections and at least 15 lymph nodes resected [35]. The current NCCN treatment guideline recommends, where feasible, resection margins of at least 10 cm proximally and 5 cm distally regardless of tumor histology [36].

The assessment of the circumferential resection margins (CRM) in esophageal cancer remains unclear and currently two different definitions for CRM from the College of American Pathologists (CAP) and the Royal College of Pathology (RCP) are utilized. CRM is generally defined as the distance of the outer tumor edge to the lateral surface of the surgical specimen in millimeters. While the CAP defines a positive CRM as tumor presence at the circumferential transection margin, the RCP defines positive CRM as tumor cells within a 1 mm radius of the surface. Irrespective of which pathologic criteria are used, it has been shown that positive CRM is associated with increased local recurrence rates and decreased survival [39–42]. It remains unclear to what extent surgery can affect CRM and the impact of positive CRM after neoadjuvant treatment needs to be further evaluated (Fig. 16.5). Current guidelines recommend the pathologic assessment of CRM in all cases.

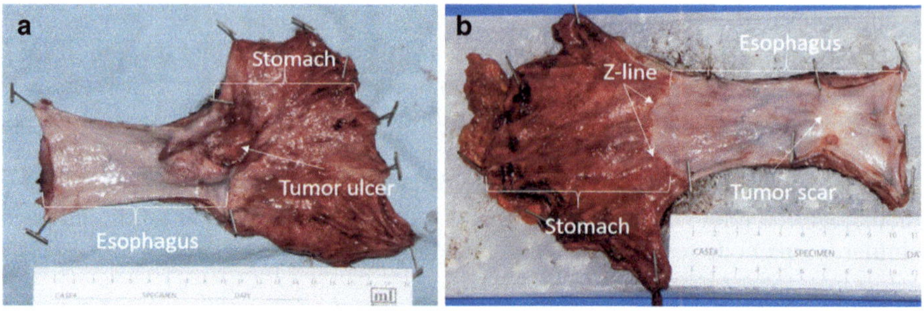

Fig. 16.5 Surgical specimen after esophagectomy. (**a**) Esophagogastric junction with ulcerated tumor, no previous neoadjuvant therapy. (**b**) Distal esophageal scaring in the region of primary tumor after neoadjuvant chemoradiotherapy

Choice of Conduit

Surgery in esophageal cancer patients aims to remove all primary and residual cancer and to provide a functional reconstruction of upper gastrointestinal continuity. Most commonly the stomach is utilized for reconstruction; however, no randomized trials currently exist. Clear advantages for the utilization of the stomach are the requirement for only one anastomosis, shorter operative time, and quicker return to oral alimentation. The most appropriate width of the gastric conduit has been debated and remains unclear with most surgeons preferring a wide tube of at least 5 cm. Potential disadvantages of the use of a gastric conduit are loss of gastric reservoir function with the risks of early satiety, dumping syndrome, and most commonly gastroesophageal reflux. Reflux symptoms can be reduced by performing a cervical anastomosis or a high intrathoracic anastomosis above the level of the azygos vein. After reconstruction with a gastric conduit, postoperative delayed gastric emptying is common and has been shown to increase pulmonary complications. A meta-analysis comparing outcomes in patients with and without a pyloric drainage procedure showed a nonsignificant benefit for those who underwent a drainage procedure with regard to gastric emptying, ability to eat, and postoperative nutrition [43]. Additionally no increase in complications associated with that procedure was reported. However, pyloric drainage did not affect late complications such as dumping or bile reflux. More recently the utilization of a botulinum toxin injection into the pylorus and endoscopic pyloric balloon dilation for the treatment of delayed gastric emptying has been reported, but none of these procedures has yet been compared to surgical division of the pylorus [44–46].

If the stomach is not available or inappropriate as a conduit, other alternatives include pedicled or free jejunal conduits or the left and the right colon. Utilizing a bowel interposition will always result in multiple anastomoses and add to the complexity of the procedure. As colonic blood supply is generally robust, ischemic complications are reduced. Colonic grafts can be associated with the development of redundancy over time which can impact oral nutrition and quality of life.

The application of pedicled jejunal grafts is largely limited due to the extent to which the jejunal segment can be mobilized into the mediastinum [47]. Although depending on the mesenteric blood supply and the fatty content of the small bowl mesentery, pedicled jejunal grafts can typically extend up to the inferior pulmonary vein. The Merendino procedure, first described in 1955, interposes a pedicled jejunal segment as a reconstruction following a limited distal esophageal resection. Primarily introduced for the treatment of benign strictures of the distal esophagus, very few case reports describe the utilization of the Merendino procedure in the setting of early limited disease in patients with esophageal cancer [48–51]. Possible advantages that have yet to be proven are to achieve free margins and removal of underlying Barrett's esophagus with a limited resection as well as a near total preservation of functional and anatomic upper GI continuity. The authors of one case report describe an evolutionary laparoscopic vagal-sparing procedure and propose that the Merendino procedure may play a greater role in early adenocarcinoma of the distal esophagus and the esophagogastric junction [51]. Additionally it may fill the gap of a limited resection when endoscopic mucosal resection is not feasible and limited esophageal resection is appropriate. Free jejunal grafts have been utilized for reconstruction of the cervical esophagus to interpose short segments. However, no randomized trials comparing the outcomes of different conduits are available. The decision regarding the most suitable conduit will most often be based on type and location of tumor and the availability of conduit options. High volume centers should be familiar with all of the reconstructive options to be able to apply appropriate approaches when the stomach is not available.

Anastomosis

Previous studies have compared cervical and intrathoracic anastomoses (Figs. 16.6 and 16.7) regarding leak and stricture rates. A recent meta-analysis including 267 patients showed a significantly higher risk of anastomotic leakage and recurrent nerve injuries in cervical anastomoses [52]. Pulmonary complications, perioperative mortality, and anastomotic stricture rates were comparable with intrathoracic anastomoses. However, the choice of the location of the anastomoses is dictated by the surgical approach utilized, which varies according to a variety of factors but mainly on tumor location. It must be highlighted that a low intrathoracic anastomosis should be avoided whenever possible as impaired gastric emptying as well as severe gastroesophageal reflux and the development of peptic strictures are common sequels.

A meta-analysis of five randomized trials found that in contrast to circular stapled anastomoses, hand-sewn anastomoses were associated with higher risks of anastomotic leakage and anastomotic strictures [53]. Another meta-analysis including 1,407 patients compared hand-sewn versus circular stapled anastomoses showed no difference in anastomotic leak rates or mortality rates [54]. Contrary to the previous review, this study showed that circular stapled anastomoses were associated with a higher stricture rate. Two studies reviewed the outcomes of a hybrid approach, with a longitudinal

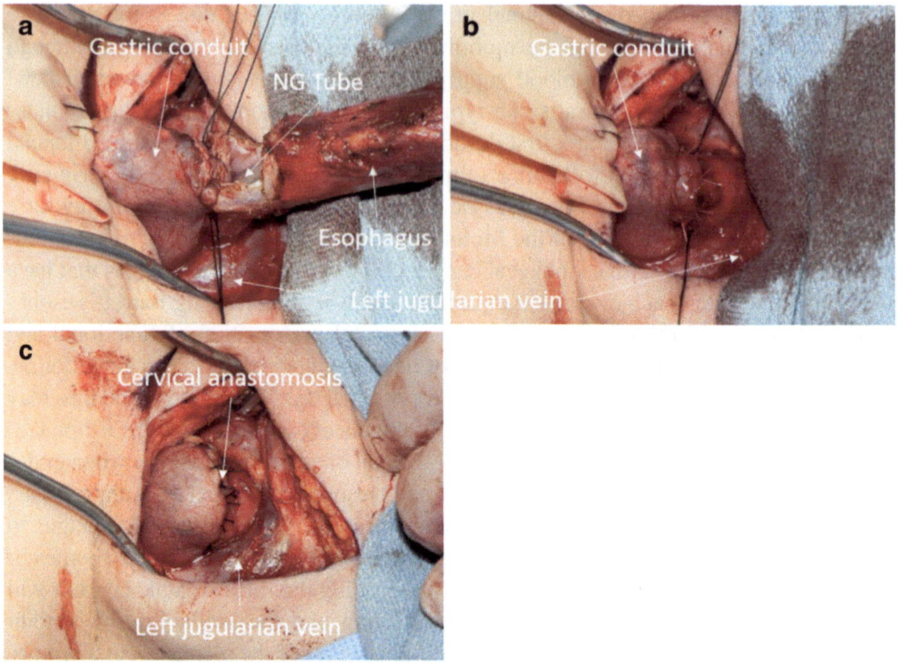

Fig. 16.6 (**a**) Begin of cervical anastomosis though a 5–6 cm incision anterior to the left sterno-cleidomastoid muscle. (**b**) Completed first layer of anastomosis with interrupted sutures. (**c**) Completed cervical esophagogastric anastomosis, hand sewn in two layers. The anastomosis is placed back into the prevertebral space following completion of the anastomosis

stapled back wall and a hand-sewn front wall (Fig. 16.7), with a low incidence of anastomotic complications [55, 56]. This technique has found a wide adaption among esophageal surgeons and a recent randomized trial comparing stricture rates at 3 months after hand-sewn, circular stapled, or hybrid anastomoses showed no strictures in the hybrid anastomoses whereas the circular stapled anastomoses had the highest stricture rate of 19 % [57]. Results of both hand-sewn and stapled anastomoses are acceptable. Although randomized trials are not consistent, postoperative stricture rates seem more common in hand-sewn anastomoses. Circular stapled anastomoses may be associated with a higher complication rate than linear stapled anastomoses.

Complications and Outcome

Common Major Complications Associated with Esophageal Resection

Esophagectomy is historically associated with high morbidity rates and remains one of the most demanding surgical procedures in thoracic surgery. Although mortality rates are decreasing in the United States, morbidity rates remain high at

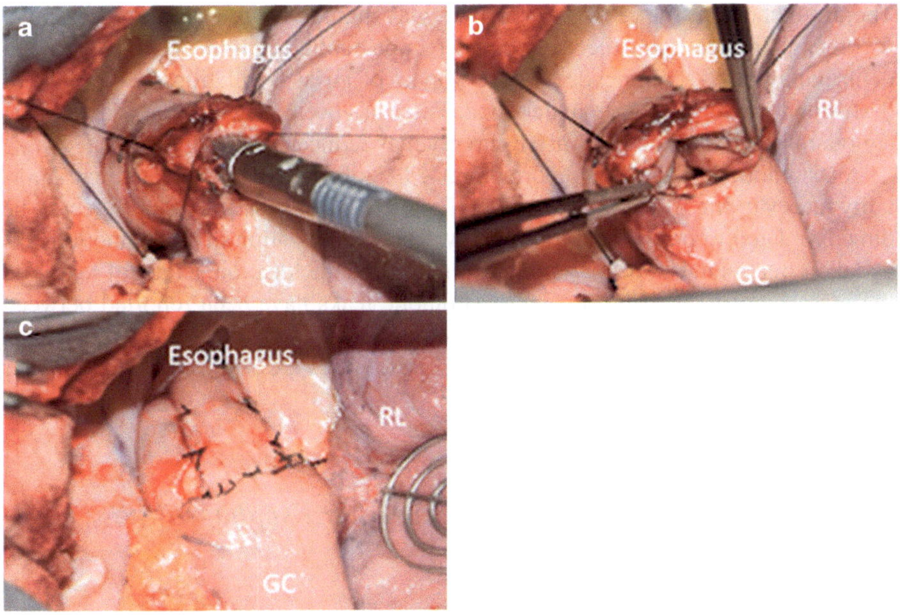

Fig. 16.7 Intrathoracic hybrid chest anastomosis during Ivor Lewis esophagectomy, deflated right lung (*RL*). (**a**) Linear stapler with upper arm in the esophageal lumen and lower arm in the gastric conduit (*GC*) lumen. (**b**) Completed stapled common wall of esophagogastric anastomosis. (**c**) Hand sewn front wall of the completed esophagogastric anastomosis

approximately 50 % [58]. The most common complications associated with esophagectomy are pneumonia, atrial arrhythmia, and anastomotic leakage [59]. Pulmonary complications are the most common complications and are thought to be responsible for 50–65 % of mortalities associated with esophagectomy [60]. Patients who develop pneumonia have a sixfold increased risk of perioperative mortality [61]. The incidence of pneumonia is directly linked to technical complications associated with the surgical procedure and is lower in transhiatal procedures and, more recently, in minimally invasive approaches [62]. Other factors associated with increased respiratory complications are recurrent nerve injuries and poor gastric emptying [43]. Perioperative factors that have been highlighted to decrease pulmonary complications include advanced regional anesthetic techniques, especially thoracic epidurals, minimizing blood loss and transfusion requirements and restricting perioperative fluid administration as well as avoidance or early recognition of vocal cord dysfunction [63–66]. Currently there is no evidence that neoadjuvant chemoradiotherapy increases the incidence of short-term pulmonary complications or overall morbidity [67].

Atrial arrhythmia occurs in up to 17 % of cases during the perioperative period and appears to occur more commonly in elderly patients and in those who are undergoing neoadjuvant therapy [68, 69]. Reports demonstrated an association between the occurrence of atrial fibrillation and perioperative complications, specifically anastomotic leakage and pneumonia as well as an increased mortality [70, 71].

Therefore, the appearance of atrial arrhythmias should lead to a careful assessment of other complications. Electrolytes correction, antiarrhythmic medication, and defibrillation are recommended as the impact of atrial fibrillation on the conduit perfusion is currently poorly understood. There has been evidence that prophylactic amiodarone and minimally invasive surgery may reduce atrial arrhythmias [72, 73].

Anastomotic leakages are reported in 3–21 % of cases and associated with mortality rates varying from 0 to 35 % [74]. The incidence of leaks does not seem to be directly related to prior induction therapy. The manifestation of anastomotic leaks and their treatment can be extremely diverse due to the location, extent of leak, and the presence of a systemic sepsis. Anastomotic leaks have been reported between postoperative day 1 and 30, but are most commonly seen between day 4 and 8. There is increasing evidence that cervical anastomoses are associated with a higher leak rate.

Effects of Complications on Outcome After Esophageal Resection

Evolving evidence has shown a direct impact of complications on perioperative outcomes such as mortality, length of stay, and postoperative quality of life [61, 68, 75, 76]. Many studies assessing the impact of complications on survival have shown an effect on timing and incidence of cancer recurrence as well as long-term survival [77]. However, disease-free survival seems less affected by complications [61].

The evolution of staging modalities leading to an improved patient selection as well as the performance of the operation in high volume centers or by high volume surgeons has been linked to decreased complications and improved outcomes [9]. The Leapfrog Group (http://www.leapfroggroup.org) currently defines high volume surgeons or units as those performing 13 or more cases per year. However, this definition remains elusive as other international groups set the definition of "high volume" at 20–50 cases per year [6, 78].

Standardized Clinical Pathway and Enhanced Recovery

Although surgery remains an important component to the management of early and locoregional esophageal cancer, standardized clinical pathways and enhanced recovery programs are now recognized as an important framework for optimizing the treatment process and improving recovery [5, 79]. These pathways should ideally include all participating disciplines in the treatment of esophageal cancer such as surgery, anesthesiology, gastroenterology, medical oncology, radiology and oncologic radiology, pathology, nurses, dietary services, and physical therapy. The pathway should include standardized approaches to all key factors associated with improved recovery, starting from the perioperative management with the utilization of thoracic epidurals, restrictive fluid management, as well as approaches to shorten operation time and minimize blood loss to the postoperative management including early nutritional support, early mobilization, and effective pain control. It has been shown that standardized pathways specifically developed for esophagectomy led to a significant improvement in length of stay, mortality rates, and complications [80].

Quality of Life Following Esophagectomy

Overall the 5-year survival rate of esophageal cancers remains poor; however, an increasing number of patients are presenting with early disease making evaluation of quality of life measures following esophagectomy more important. Historically there was the general impression that quality of life remains poor after surgical resection, due to the extent and invasiveness of the procedure. Multiple studies have shown that after initial postoperative deterioration of quality of life, an improvement at 3 months and return to a comparable baseline at 6 months after surgery can be expected [81]. However, it has also been shown that the occurrence of perioperative complications had significant deleterious effects on quality of life [76]. These data suggests that comparable levels of quality of life following esophageal resection can be achieved most likely in high volume and experienced centers, where complication rates tend to be lower.

References

1. Siegel R, Naishadham D, Jemal A. Cancer statistics, 2012. CA Cancer J Clin. 2012;62(1):10–29.
2. D'Amico TA. Outcomes after surgery for esophageal cancer. Gastrointest Cancer Res. 2007;1(5):188–96.
3. Varghese Jr TK, Wood DE, Farjah F, Oelschlager BK, Symons RG, MacLeod KE, et al. Variation in esophagectomy outcomes in hospitals meeting Leapfrog volume outcome standards. Ann Thorac Surg. 2011;91(4):1003–9.
4. Ajani JA, Barthel JS, Bekaii-Saab T, Bentrem DJ, D'Amico TA, Fuchs CS, et al. Esophageal cancer. J Natl Compr Canc Netw. 2008;6(9):818–49.
5. Low DE. Evolution in surgical management of esophageal cancer. Dig Dis. 2013;31(1):21–9.
6. Kohn GP, Galanko JA, Meyers MO, Feins RH, Farrell TM. National trends in esophageal surgery – are outcomes as good as we believe? J Gastrointest Surg. 2009;13(11):1900–10.
7. Birkmeyer JD, Dimick JB. Potential benefits of the new Leapfrog standards: effect of process and outcomes measures. Surgery. 2004;135(6):569–75.
8. Birkmeyer JD, Siewers AE, Finlayson EV, Stukel TA, Lucas FL, Batista I, et al. Hospital volume and surgical mortality in the United States. N Engl J Med. 2002;346(15):1128–37.
9. Markar SR, Karthikesalingam A, Thrumurthy S, Low DE. Volume-outcome relationship in surgery for esophageal malignancy: systematic review and meta-analysis 2000–2011. J Gastrointest Surg. 2012;16(5):1055–63.
10. Derogar M, Orsini N, Sadr-Azodi O, Lagergren P. Influence of major postoperative complications on health-related quality of life among long-term survivors of esophageal cancer surgery. J Clin Oncol. 2012;30(14):1615–9.

11. Moraca RJ, Low DE. Outcomes and health-related quality of life after esophagectomy for high-grade dysplasia and intramucosal cancer. Arch Surg. 2006;141(6):545–9.
12. Parameswaran R, McNair A, Avery KN, Berrisford RG, Wajed SA, Sprangers MA, et al. The role of health-related quality of life outcomes in clinical decision making in surgery for esophageal cancer: a systematic review. Ann Surg Oncol. 2008;15(9):2372–9.
13. Pech O, Manner H, Ell C. Endoscopic resection. Gastrointest Endosc Clin N Am. 2011;21(1):81–94.
14. Rice TW, Mason DP, Murthy SC, Zuccaro Jr G, Adelstein DJ, Rybicki LA, et al. T2N0M0 esophageal cancer. J Thorac Cardiovasc Surg. 2007;133(2):317–24.
15. Orringer MB, Marshall B, Chang AC, Lee J, Pickens A, Lau CL. Two thousand transhiatal esophagectomies: changing trends, lessons learned. Ann Surg. 2007;246(3):363–72.
16. Hulscher JB, van Lanschot JJ. Individualised surgical treatment of patients with an adenocarcinoma of the distal oesophagus or gastro-oesophageal junction. Dig Surg. 2005;22(3):130–4.
17. Hulscher JB, van Sandick JW, de Boer AG, Wijnhoven BP, Tijssen JG, Fockens P, et al. Extended transthoracic resection compared with limited transhiatal resection for adenocarcinoma of the esophagus. N Engl J Med. 2002;347(21):1662–9.
18. Boone J, Livestro DP, Elias SG, Borel Rinkes IH, van Hillegersberg R. International survey on esophageal cancer: part I surgical techniques. Dis Esophagus. 2009;22(3):195–202.
19. Hoppo T, Jobe BA, Hunter JG. Minimally invasive esophagectomy: the evolution and technique of minimally invasive surgery for esophageal cancer. World J Surg. 2011;35(7):1454–63.
20. Luketich JD, Schauer PR, Christie NA, Weigel TL, Raja S, Fernando HC, et al. Minimally invasive esophagectomy. Ann Thorac Surg. 2000;70(3):906–11.
21. Singh RK, Pham TH, Diggs BS, Perkins S, Hunter JG. Minimally invasive esophagectomy provides equivalent oncologic outcomes to open esophagectomy for locally advanced (stage II or III) esophageal carcinoma. Arch Surg. 2011;146(6):711–4.
22. Murakami M, Kuroda Y, Okamoto Y, Kono K, Yoden E, Kusumi F, et al. Neoadjuvant concurrent chemoradiotherapy followed by definitive high-dose radiotherapy or surgery for operable thoracic esophageal carcinoma. Int J Radiat Oncol Biol Phys. 1998;40(5):1049–59.
23. Chiu PW, Chan AC, Leung SF, Leong HT, Kwong KH, Li MK, et al. Multicenter prospective randomized trial comparing standard esophagectomy with chemoradiotherapy for treatment of squamous esophageal cancer: early results from the Chinese University Research Group for Esophageal Cancer (CURE). J Gastrointest Surg. 2005;9(6):794–802.
24. Smithers BM, Cullinan M, Thomas JM, Martin I, Barbour AP, Burmeister BH, et al. Outcomes from salvage esophagectomy post definitive chemoradiotherapy compared with resection following preoperative neoadjuvant chemoradiotherapy. Dis Esophagus. 2007;20(6):471–7.
25. Swisher SG, Wynn P, Putnam JB, Mosheim MB, Correa AM, Komaki RR, et al. Salvage esophagectomy for recurrent tumors after definitive chemotherapy and radiotherapy. J Thorac Cardiovasc Surg. 2002;123(1):175–83.
26. Marks J, Rice DC, Swisher SG. Salvage esophagectomy in the management of recurrent or persistent esophageal carcinoma. Thorac Surg Clin. 2013;23(4):559–67.
27. Markar SR, Karthikesalingam A, Penna M, Low DE. Assessment of short-term clinical outcomes following salvage esophagectomy for the treatment of esophageal malignancy: systematic review and pooled analysis. Ann Surg Oncol. 2014:21(3):922–31.
28. Schwarz RE, Smith DD. Clinical impact of lymphadenectomy extent in resectable esophageal cancer. J Gastrointest Surg. 2007;11(11):1384–93.
29. Groth SS, Virnig BA, Whitson BA, DeFor TE, Li ZZ, Tuttle TM, et al. Determination of the minimum number of lymph nodes to examine to maximize survival in patients with esophageal carcinoma: data from the Surveillance Epidemiology and End Results database. J Thorac Cardiovasc Surg. 2010;139(3):612–20.
30. Peyre CG, Hagen JA, Demeester SR, Altorki NK, Ancona E, Griffin SM, et al. The number of lymph nodes removed predicts survival in esophageal cancer: an international study on the impact of extent of surgical resection. Ann Surg. 2008;248(4):549–56.
31. Rizk NP, Ishwaran H, Rice TW, Chen LQ, Schipper PH, Kesler KA, et al. Optimum lymphadenectomy for esophageal cancer. Ann Surg. 2010;251(1):46–50.

32. Omloo JM, Lagarde SM, Hulscher JB, Reitsma JB, Fockens P, van Dekken H, et al. Extended transthoracic resection compared with limited transhiatal resection for adenocarcinoma of the mid/distal esophagus: five-year survival of a randomized clinical trial. Ann Surg. 2007;246(6):992–1000.
33. Nishihira T, Hirayama K, Mori S. A prospective randomized trial of extended cervical and superior mediastinal lymphadenectomy for carcinoma of the thoracic esophagus. Am J Surg. 1998;175(1):47–51.
34. Law S, Wong J. What is appropriate treatment for carcinoma of the thoracic esophagus? World J Surg. 2001;25(2):189–95.
35. Barbour AP, Rizk NP, Gonen M, Tang L, Bains MS, Rusch VW, et al. Adenocarcinoma of the gastroesophageal junction: influence of esophageal resection margin and operative approach on outcome. Ann Surg. 2007;246(1):1–8.
36. Casson AG, Darnton SJ, Subramanian S, Hiller L. What is the optimal distal resection margin for esophageal carcinoma? Ann Thorac Surg. 2000;69(1):205–9.
37. Tsutsui S, Kuwano H, Watanabe M, Kitamura M, Sugimachi K. Resection margin for squamous cell carcinoma of the esophagus. Ann Surg. 1995;222(2):193–202.
38. Tam PC, Siu KF, Cheung HC, Ma L, Wong J. Local recurrences after subtotal esophagectomy for squamous cell carcinoma. Ann Surg. 1987;205(2):189–94.
39. Khan OA, Cruttenden-Wood D, Toh SK. Is an involved circumferential resection margin following oesphagectomy for cancer an important prognostic indicator? Interact Cardiovasc Thorac Surg. 2010;11(5):645–8.
40. Pultrum BB, Honing J, Smit JK, van Dullemen HM, Van Dam GM, Groen H, et al. A critical appraisal of circumferential resection margins in esophageal carcinoma. Ann Surg Oncol. 2010;17(3):812–20.
41. Dexter SP, Sue-Ling H, McMahon MJ, Quirke P, Mapstone N, Martin IG. Circumferential resection margin involvement: an independent predictor of survival following surgery for oesophageal cancer. Gut. 2001;48(5):667–70.
42. Deeter M, Dorer R, Kuppusamy MK, Koehler RP, Low DE. Assessment of criteria and clinical significance of circumferential resection margins in esophageal cancer. Arch Surg. 2009;144(7):618–24.
43. Urschel JD, Blewett CJ, Young JE, Miller JD, Bennett WF. Pyloric drainage (pyloroplasty) or no drainage in gastric reconstruction after esophagectomy: a meta-analysis of randomized controlled trials. Dig Surg. 2002;19(3):160–4.
44. Kent MS, Pennathur A, Fabian T, McKelvey A, Schuchert MJ, Luketich JD, et al. A pilot study of botulinum toxin injection for the treatment of delayed gastric emptying following esophagectomy. Surg Endosc. 2007;21(5):754–7.
45. Martin JT, Federico JA, McKelvey AA, Kent MS, Fabian T. Prevention of delayed gastric emptying after esophagectomy: a single center's experience with botulinum toxin. Ann Thorac Surg. 2009;87(6):1708–13.
46. Sebastian JJ, Pena E, Blas JM, Cena G, Diez M. Management of gastric outlet obstruction after esophagectomy using forced pyloric dilation. Rev Esp Enferm Dig. 2008;100(9):594–5.
47. Blackmon SH, Correa AM, Skoracki R, Chevray PM, Kim MP, Mehran RJ, et al. Supercharged pedicled jejunal interposition for esophageal replacement: a 10-year experience. Ann Thorac Surg. 2012;94(4):1104–11.
48. Gutschow CA, Schroder W, Wolfgarten E, Holscher AH. Merendino procedure with preservation of the vagus for early carcinoma of the gastroesophageal junction. Zentralbl Chir. 2004;129(4):276–81.
49. Staiger WI, Ronellenfitsch U, Kaehler G, Schildhaus HU, Dimitrakopoulou-Strauss A, Schwarzbach MH, et al. The Merendino procedure following preoperative imatinib mesylate for locally advanced gastrointestinal stromal tumor of the esophagogastric junction. World J Surg Oncol. 2008;6:37.
50. Holscher AH, Vallbohmer D, Gutschow C, Bollschweiler E. Reflux esophagitis, high-grade neoplasia, and early Barrett's carcinoma-what is the place of the Merendino procedure? Langenbecks Arch Surg. 2009;394(3):417–24.

51. Pring C, Dexter S. A laparoscopic vagus-preserving Merendino procedure for early esophageal adenocarcinoma. Surg Endosc. 2010;24(5):1195–9.
52. Biere SS, Maas KW, Cuesta MA, van der Peet DL. Cervical or thoracic anastomosis after esophagectomy for cancer: a systematic review and meta-analysis. Dig Surg. 2011;28(1):29–35.
53. Hsu HH, Chen JS, Huang PM, Lee JM, Lee YC. Comparison of manual and mechanical cervical esophagogastric anastomosis after esophageal resection for squamous cell carcinoma: a prospective randomized controlled trial. Eur J Cardiothorac Surg. 2004;25(6):1097–101.
54. Honda M, Kuriyama A, Noma H, Nunobe S, Furukawa TA. Hand-sewn versus mechanical esophagogastric anastomosis after esophagectomy: a systematic review and meta-analysis. Ann Surg. 2013;257(2):238–48.
55. Orringer MB, Marshall B, Iannettoni MD. Eliminating the cervical esophagogastric anastomotic leak with a side-to-side stapled anastomosis. J Thorac Cardiovasc Surg. 2000;119(2):277–88.
56. Collard JM, Romagnoli R, Goncette L, Otte JB, Kestens PJ. Terminalized semimechanical side-to-side suture technique for cervical esophagogastrostomy. Ann Thorac Surg. 1998;65(3):814–7.
57. Wang WP, Gao Q, Wang KN, Shi H, Chen LQ. A prospective randomized controlled trial of semi-mechanical versus hand-sewn or circular stapled esophagogastrostomy for prevention of anastomotic stricture. World J Surg. 2013;37(5):1043–50.
58. Bailey SH, Bull DA, Harpole DH, Rentz JJ, Neumayer LA, Pappas TN, et al. Outcomes after esophagectomy: a ten-year prospective cohort. Ann Thorac Surg. 2003;75(1):217–22.
59. Low DE, Bodnar A. Update on clinical impact, documentation, and management of complications associated with esophagectomy. Thorac Surg Clin. 2013;23(4):535–50.
60. Bakhos CT, Fabian T, Oyasiji TO, Gautam S, Gangadharan SP, Kent MS, et al. Impact of the surgical technique on pulmonary morbidity after esophagectomy. Ann Thorac Surg. 2012;93(1):221–6.
61. Hii MW, Smithers BM, Gotley DC, Thomas JM, Thomson I, Martin I, et al. Impact of postoperative morbidity on long-term survival after oesophagectomy. Br J Surg. 2013;100(1):95–104.
62. Ferri LE, Law S, Wong KH, Kwok KF, Wong J. The influence of technical complications on postoperative outcome and survival after esophagectomy. Ann Surg Oncol. 2006;13(4):557–64.
63. Law S, Wong KH, Kwok KF, Chu KM, Wong J. Predictive factors for postoperative pulmonary complications and mortality after esophagectomy for cancer. Ann Surg. 2004;240(5):791–800.
64. Tsui SL, Law S, Fok M, Lo JR, Ho E, Yang J, et al. Postoperative analgesia reduces mortality and morbidity after esophagectomy. Am J Surg. 1997;173(6):472–8.
65. Dumont P, Wihlm JM, Hentz JG, Roeslin N, Lion R, Morand G. Respiratory complications after surgical treatment of esophageal cancer. A study of 309 patients according to the type of resection. Eur J Cardiothorac Surg. 1995;9(10):539–43.
66. Kita T, Mammoto T, Kishi Y. Fluid management and postoperative respiratory disturbances in patients with transthoracic esophagectomy for carcinoma. J Clin Anesth. 2002;14(4):252–6.
67. Atkins BZ, Shah AS, Hutcheson KA, Mangum JH, Pappas TN, Harpole Jr DH, et al. Reducing hospital morbidity and mortality following esophagectomy. Ann Thorac Surg. 2004;78(4):1170–6.
68. Carrott PW, Markar SR, Kuppusamy MK, Traverso LW, Low DE. Accordion severity grading system: assessment of relationship between costs, length of hospital stay, and survival in patients with complications after esophagectomy for cancer. J Am Coll Surg. 2012;215(3):331–6.
69. Rao VP, Addae-Boateng E, Barua A, Martin-Ucar AE, Duffy JP. Age and neo-adjuvant chemotherapy increase the risk of atrial fibrillation following oesophagectomy. Eur J Cardiothorac Surg. 2012;42(3):438–43.
70. Stawicki SP, Prosciak MP, Gerlach AT, Bloomston M, Davido HT, Lindsey DE, et al. Atrial fibrillation after esophagectomy: an indicator of postoperative morbidity. Gen Thorac Cardiovasc Surg. 2011;59(6):399–405.

71. Murthy SC, Law S, Whooley BP, Alexandrou A, Chu KM, Wong J. Atrial fibrillation after esophagectomy is a marker for postoperative morbidity and mortality. J Thorac Cardiovasc Surg. 2003;126(4):1162–7.
72. Tisdale JE, Wroblewski HA, Wall DS, Rieger KM, Hammoud ZT, Young JV, et al. A randomized, controlled study of amiodarone for prevention of atrial fibrillation after transthoracic esophagectomy. J Thorac Cardiovasc Surg. 2010;140(1):45–51.
73. Turaga KK, Shah KU, Neill EO, Mittal SK. Does laparoscopic surgery decrease the risk of atrial fibrillation after foregut surgery? Surg Endosc. 2009;23(1):204–8.
74. Sarela AI, Tolan DJ, Harris K, Dexter SP, Sue-Ling HM. Anastomotic leakage after esophagectomy for cancer: a mortality-free experience. J Am Coll Surg. 2008;206(3):516–23.
75. Rizk NP, Bach PB, Schrag D, Bains MS, Turnbull AD, Karpeh M, et al. The impact of complications on outcomes after resection for esophageal and gastroesophageal junction carcinoma. J Am Coll Surg. 2004;198(1):42–50.
76. Viklund P, Lindblad M, Lagergren J. Influence of surgery-related factors on quality of life after esophageal or cardia cancer resection. World J Surg. 2005;29(7):841–8.
77. Lerut T, Moons J, Coosemans W, Van RD, De LP, Decaluwe H, et al. Postoperative complications after transthoracic esophagectomy for cancer of the esophagus and gastroesophageal junction are correlated with early cancer recurrence: role of systematic grading of complications using the modified Clavien classification. Ann Surg. 2009;250(5):798–807.
78. van Lanschot JJ, Hulscher JB, Buskens CJ, Tilanus HW, ten Kate FJ, Obertop H. Hospital volume and hospital mortality for esophagectomy. Cancer. 2001;91(8):1574–8.
79. Zehr KJ, Dawson PB, Yang SC, Heitmiller RF. Standardized clinical care pathways for major thoracic cases reduce hospital costs. Ann Thorac Surg. 1998;66(3):914–9.
80. Low DE, Kunz S, Schembre D, Otero H, Malpass T, Hsi A, et al. Esophagectomy – it's not just about mortality anymore: standardized perioperative clinical pathways improve outcomes in patients with esophageal cancer. J Gastrointest Surg. 2007;11(11):1395–402.
81. Parameswaran R, Blazeby JM, Hughes R, Mitchell K, Berrisford RG, Wajed SA. Health-related quality of life after minimally invasive oesophagectomy. Br J Surg. 2010;97(4):525–31.

Chapter 17
Esophageal Cancer: Neoadjuvant and Adjuvant Therapy

Shuang Qin Zhang and Victoria M. Villaflor

Abstract The incidence of esophageal cancer has increased more than 15 % in the past 20 years. It ranks fifth in mortality rate among cancers. Squamous cell carcinoma (SCC) and adenocarcinoma (AC) account for the majority of all esophageal cancers. In developed countries, the incidence of AC of the esophagus has increased dramatically over the past couple of decades, whereas the incidence of SCC has decreased. Distinction on how the different histology should dictate treatment approach is not clear. For now, there is little evidence to support different treatment regimens for these two carcinomas. Based on calculations from a pool of cancer registries, the survival rate for patients with esophageal cancer is 33 % at 1 year and 10 % at 5 years. Survival rate of patients with local resectable disease after curative resection at 3 years was 20 %.

Keywords Esophageal cancer • Chemotherapy • Radiotherapy • Neoadjuvant therapy • Adjuvant therapy

S.Q. Zhang, MD
Division of Medical Oncology, Department of Medicine, Center for Esophageal Diseases, University of Chicago Pritzker School of Medicine, Chicago, IL, USA

V.M. Villaflor, MD (✉)
Division of Medical Oncology, Department of Medicine, Center for Esophageal Diseases, University of Chicago Pritzker School of Medicine, Chicago, IL, USA

Department of Internal Medicine, Section of Hematology/Oncology, University of Chicago Medicine, 5841 S. Maryland Avenue, MC 2115, Chicago, IL 60637, USA
e-mail: vvillfl@medicine.bsd.uchicago.edu

P.M. Fisichella et al. (eds.), *Esophageal Diseases*,
DOI 10.1007/978-3-319-04337-1_17,

Introduction

The incidence of esophageal cancer has increased more than 15 % in the past 20 years. It ranks fifth in mortality rate among cancers. Squamous cell carcinoma (SCC) and adenocarcinoma (AC) accounts for the majority of all esophageal cancers. In developed countries, the incidence of AC of the esophagus has increased dramatically over the past couple of decades, whereas the incidence of SCC has decreased. Distinction on how the different histology should dictate treatment approach is not clear. For now, there is little evidence to support different treatment regimens for these two carcinomas. Based on calculations from a pool of cancer registries, the survival rate for patients with esophageal cancer is 33 % at 1 year and 10 % at 5 years. Survival rate of patients with local resectable disease after curative resection at 3 years was 20 %. Advances in surgical techniques have improved survival with the caveat that these complex oncologic operations should be performed in specialized, high-volume hospitals, since there is a direct correlation between outcome and hospital volume. Despite advances in surgical technique, it is now well accepted that patients benefit most from a multimodality treatment approach.

In this chapter, we will provide an evidence-based review with the intent to examine the role of radiation therapy, chemotherapy—both as neoadjuvant (preoperative) and adjuvant (postoperative) therapies, in the management of locally advanced esophageal cancer.

What Is the Big Picture?

Based on guidelines set forth by the Union for International Cancer Control, primary local resection is indicated for cT1-2 N0 disease. In contrast, the accepted standard of care for patients with locally advanced esophageal cancer (cT3-4 and or N positive) is preoperative therapy followed by surgical resection. Having stated this, you will quickly realize that there is a wealth of conflicting data regarding the optimal treatment sequence in managing locally advanced esophageal cancer. While resection is the cornerstone of therapy, the aggressiveness of this malignancy requires the addition of systemic therapy. A number of authors have attempted to define a standard approach in how to administer systemic therapy, yet their data have yielded conflicting results. These discrepancies may be attributed to the heterogeneous patient populations, tumor histology in addition to the different chemotherapy regimen, dosing schedules, and radiation schedules used in the plethora of studies. Despite the discrepancies, it is well accepted that improved survival is directly correlated with R0 resections and pathologic complete response.

Table 17.1 Adenocarcinoma: clinical trials of neoadjuvant chemotherapy versus surgery alone

Study	Histology	*N*	Chemoradiation regimen	Median survival (m)	3 year OS	*p*-value
Tepper et al. [37]	75 % AC	30	Cis/5-FU + 50 Gy (5.5 wks) + surgery	54	39 % (5 y)	0.002
		26	Surgery	21	16 % (5 y)	
Walsh et al. [41]	100 % AC	58	Cis/5-FU + 40 Gy (3 wks) + surgery	16	32 %	<0.05
		55	Surgery	11	6 %	
Urba et al. [38]	75 % AC	47	Cis/5-FU/Vinb + 45 Gy (1.5 Gy BID) + surgery	17	30 %	NS
		50	Surgery	18	16 %	
Burmeister et al. [7]	62 % AC	128	Cis/5-FU + 35 Gy (3 wks) + surgery	22	17 % (5 y)	NS
		128	Surgery	19	13 % (5 y)	
Van Hagen et al. [40]	75 % AC	175	Carbo/Tax + 41 Gy (4.5 wks) + surgery	49	59 %	0.011
		188	Surgery	24	44 %	

AC adenocarcinoma, *Cis* cisplatin, *5-FU* 5-fluorouracil, *Tax* taxol, *Vinb* vinblastine, *BID* twice daily, *OS* overall survival, *NS* not significant, *wks* weeks, *m* months, *y* year

Is There a Role for Neoadjuvant Chemoradiotherapy?

Several randomized trials have been conducted to determine the benefit of preoperative chemoradiotherapy as opposed to surgery alone. Table 17.1 outlines 5 clinical trials, which are mostly AC. Table 17.2 outlines 7 clinical trials, which are mostly SCC in histology. Of the 12 clinical trials, 4 contemporary studies, 3 including adenocarcinoma esophageal cancer patients showed a survival benefit.

The CALGB 9781 study by Tepper et al. in 2008 randomized only 56 patients to neoadjuvant chemoradiotherapy (cisplatin plus 5-FU infusion plus radiation) versus surgery alone. The study is criticized for its poor accrual and subsequent low power. Despite its lack of accrual, the results were impressive. It showed a 5-year overall survival of 39 % for patients who received preoperative multimodality treatment and 16 % for patients who received surgery alone ($p=0.002$).

In the 1996 Irish trial by Walsh et al., 113 patients were randomized to receive neoadjuvant chemoradiotherapy (cisplatin plus 5-FU infusion plus radiation) versus surgery alone. This study is criticized for the very low survival in the surgery arm as compared to other trials. Other criticisms include inadequate staging, radiation dose (40 Gy), 5-FU dose, and premature closure. Similarly, despite these criticisms, the study yielded impressive results. It showed a significant survival benefit with a

Table 17.2 Squamous cell carcinoma: clinical trials of neoadjuvant chemotherapy versus surgery alone

Study	Histology	*N*	Chemoradiation regimen	Median survival (m)	3 year OS	*p*-value
Nygaard et al. [28]	100 % SCC	47	Bleo/Cis + 35 Gy + surgery	8	11.5 %	NS
		41	Surgery	7	9.5 %	
Bosset et al. [6]	100 % SCC	143	Cis + 37 Gy + surgery	19		NS
		139	Surgery	19	9 % (5 y)	
Le Prise et al. [21]	100 % SCC	41	Cis/5-FU + 20 Gy (split) + surgery	10	19 %	NS
		45	Surgery	10	14 %	
Apinop et al. [3]	100 % SCC	35	Cis/5-FU + 20 Gy + surgery	10	24 % (5 y)	NS
		34	Surgery	7	10 % (5 y)	
Lee et al. [22]	100 % SCC	51	Cis/5-FU + 45 Gy (1.2 Gy BID) + surgery	28	49 %	NS
		50	Surgery	27	51 %	
Mariette et al. [26]	71 % SCC	97	Cis/5-FU + 45 Gy (5 wks) + surgery	32	48 %	NS ($p = 0.68$)
		98	Surgery	45	55 %	
Lv et al. [24]	100 % SCC	80	Cis/Tax + 40 Gy (4 wks) + surgery	53	44 % (5 y)	0.04
		80	Surgery	36	34 % (5 y)	
		78	Surgery + Cis/Tax + 40 Gy (4 wks)	48	42 % (5 y)	

wks weeks, *m* months, *y* year

3-year survival of 32 % for the chemoradiotherapy group versus 6 % for the surgery-only group ($p = 0.01$).

In 2012, a phase III Dutch study randomized 363 patients to receive either neoadjuvant chemoradiotherapy (carboplatin plus paclitaxel plus radiation) or surgery alone. This study demonstrated that patients who received preoperative therapy benefited from higher rate of R0 resection; R0 resection was achieved in 92 % patients in the preoperative chemoradiotherapy arm versus 69 % in the surgery arm ($p < 0.001$). Notably, patients who received neoadjuvant chemoradiotherapy had a significant benefit in 3-year survival (59 vs. 48 %, $p = 0.011$).

Neoadjuvant chemoradiotherapy is currently the standard of care in the USA for locally advanced esophageal cancer due to the benefit of reducing micrometastatic disease and facilitating surgical resection by downstaging primary tumor. The first randomized controlled trials (RTCs) of preoperative chemoradiotherapy appeared in 1992 followed by many other studies. Using data from these RCTs, there have been several meta-analyses that have suggested a significant survival benefit for neoadjuvant chemoradiotherapy over surgery alone. Prior to these publications, esophagectomy alone was the standard treatment for patients with resectable esophageal cancer, though most patients recurred due to incomplete resections from proximity of esophagus to vital organs, and more commonly, at the time of primary

Table 17.3 Meta-analyses of neoadjuvant chemoradiotherapy versus surgery alone

Study	No. of studies	No. of patients	HR (95 % CI)	*p*-value
Urschel and Vasan [39]	9	1,116	0.66 (0.47–0.92) (3 yr)	0.016
Fiorica et al. [14]	6	764	0.53 (0.31–0.93) (3 yr)	0.03
Gebski et al. [16]	10	1,209	0.81 (0.70–0.93) (2 yr)	0.002
Sjoquist et al. [33]	12	1,864	0.78 (0.70–0.88)	<0.0001

HR hazard ratio, *CI* confidence interval, *yr* year, *No* number

diagnosis, micrometastatic systemic disease was often present which would show up as either peritoneal implants or appear shortly following surgical resection. Despite the limitations of surgery, there was still concern that preoperative chemoradiotherapy may cause not only delay in possible definitive treatment with surgery but also unacceptable increase in perioperative mortality and even death independent of surgery. The following are the four largest meta-analyses, which have provided a foundation for today's clinical practice (Table 17.3).

In 2002, Urschel and Vasan identified RTCs, yielding data on 1,116 patients, which compared neoadjuvant chemoradiotherapy (study arm) and surgery with surgery alone (control arm) for esophageal cancer. The data showed a 3-year survival benefit for patients who received neoadjuvant chemoradiotherapy treatment compared with surgery alone. Data was generated from trials, which administered chemotherapy and radiotherapy concurrently, rather than sequentially, which theoretically allowed for maximal antineoplastic synergy. In addition, patients who received neoadjuvant chemoradiotherapy had reduced local-regional cancer recurrence and were more likely to have a complete (R0) resection, further suggesting that preoperative chemoradiotherapy downstages tumors and facilitates complete resection.

In 2004, Fiorica et al. published a second meta-analysis. The authors reviewed six RCTs, totaling 764 patients, and also showed a survival benefit at 3 years in the study arm compared to the control arm. Of concern, they found a significant increase in postoperative mortality in patients who received neoadjuvant chemoradiotherapy.

A third meta-analysis published in 2007 by Gebski and colleagues pooled 1,209 patients from 10 RCTs that compared neoadjuvant chemoradiotherapy (study arm) versus surgery alone (control arm) in locally resectable esophageal carcinoma. The hazard ratio for all-cause mortality in the study arm versus control arm was 0.81 (95 % CI 0.70–0.93; $p=0.002$) with 13 % absolute difference in survival at 2 years.

The most recent meta-analysis by Sjoquist et al. in 2011, an update of the meta-analysis by Gebski, pooled 1,854 patients from 12 RCTs and came to similar conclusions. The hazard ratio for all-cause mortality in the study arm versus control arm was 0.78 (95 % CI 0.70–0.88; $p<0.0001$), corresponding to absolute survival benefit at 2 years of 8.7 % and a number needed to treat of 11. Of note, the survival benefits for the treatment arm were similar in both tumor subtypes—SCC and AC. In contrast to the study by Fiorica et al., this study concluded that there were little association between risk of postoperative mortality (in-hospital or 30-day postoperative death) and the neoadjuvant treatment.

Because the RCTs evaluated in the meta-analyses used different drugs, doses, and schedules of chemotherapy and radiotherapy (Table 17.1), the optimum neoadjuvant treatment regimen has not been established. Despite this, it is well noted that most regimens used cisplatin, typically with 5-fluorouracil since 1988 [16]. In short, there appears to be an advantage of preoperative chemoradiotherapy over surgery alone in patients with resectable esophageal cancer.

Is There a Role for Perioperative Chemotherapy?

There are convincing data to show that perioperative chemotherapy increases the likelihood of an R0 resection and significantly improves progression-free and overall survival in resectable esophageal cancer. In 2006, Cunningham and colleagues published in New England Journal of Medicine a landmark study called the Medical Research Council Adjuvant Gastric Infusional Chemotherapy (MAGIC) trial, where they assigned patients with resectable adenocarcinoma of the stomach, EGJ, or lower esophagus to either perioperative chemotherapy (study arm) or surgery alone (control arm). Of the 250 patients in the study arm, 25 % had distal esophageal and GEJ AC. The patients in the study arm received three preoperative and three postoperative cycles of intravenous epirubicin, cisplatin, and continuous intravenous infusion of 5-FU (ECF). Only half of the patients were able to complete postoperative ECF. Patients randomized to ECF had higher R0 resections, higher overall survival at 5 years (36 % vs. 23 %, HR 0.75; CI 0.60–0.93; $p=0.009$) and higher progression-free survival (HR 0.66; CI 0.53–0.81; $p<0.001$). Despite the impressive data, it should be noted that criticisms of this study include non-standardized surgery, inaccurate preoperative staging due to absence of laparoscopy, different population of patients, and relatively poor outcome in the surgery alone arm.

In a similar trial published in 2011, Ychou et al. assigned patients with resectable adenocarcinoma of the lower esophagus, stomach, and gastroesophageal junction (GEJ) to either perioperative chemotherapy (study arm) or surgery alone (control arm). Of the 113 patients in the study arm, 75 % had AC of the distal esophagus and GEJ. The patients in the study arm received cisplatin and 5-FU (CF): 2–3 cycles preoperatively and 3–4 cycles postoperatively. Again, only half of the patients completed postoperative therapy. Patients who received CF had higher overall survival at 5 years (38 % vs. 24 %; HR 0.69, CI 0.5–0.95; $p=0.02$) and a higher progression-free survival at 5 years (34 % vs. 19 %; HR 0.65 CI 0.48–0.89; $p=0.003$). Despite perioperative toxicity from chemotherapy (primarily neutropenia), postoperative morbidity was similar in the two groups.

Several meta-analyses have also been performed to determine the survival benefit of perioperative chemotherapy for resectable esophageal cancer [16, 33] (Table 17.4). In 2007, Gebski et al. pooled eight RCTs, totaling 1,724 patients, and found a small but significant reduction in mortality for perioperative chemotherapy (HR 0.90; 95 % CI, 0.81–1.00; $p=0.05$). Interestingly, the benefit was limited to adenocarcinomas only—(HR 0.78; 95 % CI, 0.64–0.95; $p=0.014$) and not

Table 17.4 Meta-analyses of neoadjuvant chemotherapy versus surgery alone

Study	No. of studies	No. of patients	HR (95 % CI)	*p*-value
Gebski et al. [16]	8	1,724	0.90 (0.81–1.00)	0.05
Sjoquist et al. [33]	9	1,981	0.87 (0.79–0.96)	0.005

HR hazard ratio, *CI* confidence interval, *yr* year, *No* number

squamous cell carcinomas (HR 0.88; 95 % CI, 0.75–1.03; $p=0.12$). In 2011, Sjoquist et al. pooled 9 RCTs, totaling 1,981 patients, and showed a significant reduction in mortality with perioperative chemotherapy (HR 0.87; 95 % CI, 0.79–0.96; $p=0.005$), which corresponded to an absolute 2-year survival benefit of 5.1 %. Similarly, the benefit was limited to AC (HR 0.83; 95 % CI, 0.71–0.95; $p=0.01$) and not SCC (HR 0.9295 % CI, 0.81–1.04; $p=0.18$). The data clearly show that perioperative cisplatin and 5-FU-based chemotherapy improve overall and disease-free survival compared with surgical resection alone in patients with resectable esophageal cancer.

Is There a Difference in Survival in Patients Receiving Preoperative Chemoradiotherapy or Perioperative Chemotherapy?

There have been primarily two RTCs which have compared neoadjuvant chemoradiotherapy with perioperative chemotherapy: a German study by Stahl et al. (POET) and an Australian study by Burmeister et al. published in *Eur J Cancer* 2011. The POET trial included 126 patients, all of which had AC of the EGJ, who received chemotherapy alone (cisplatin/5-FU/leucovorin) for 15 or 12 weeks of the same regimen followed by low-dose radiotherapy concurrent with cisplatin and etoposide. The Australian trial included only 75 patients with AC of the esophagus. The authors used a similar design but used two cycles of cisplatin/fluorouracil and radiotherapy of 35 Gy in 15 fractions starting on day 22. Both trials, unfortunately, were closed prematurely due to poor accrual, and neither showed a statistical advantage for neoadjuvant chemoradiotherapy over perioperative chemotherapy due to lack of power, but there was a trend toward improvement with chemoradiotherapy.

Despite paucity of sufficient data generated by individual RTCs, meta-analysis by Gebski et al. and Sjoquist et al. have shed some light on how these two modalities compare. In 2007, Gebski and colleagues found that a significant survival benefit was evident for preoperative chemoradiotherapy and, to a less extent, for chemotherapy in patients with adenocarcinoma of the esophagus. Specifically, there was a 13 % absolute difference in survival at 2 years in favor of chemoradiotherapy versus perioperative chemotherapy with a 7 % absolute difference versus surgery alone. The updated meta-analysis by Sjoquist in 2011 confirmed these findings, with an absolute benefit of 8.7 % chemoradiotherapy and 5.1 % perioperative chemotherapy at 2 years. This analysis pooled results of 2,220 patients receiving either neoadjuvant chemoradiotherapy or perioperative chemotherapy. The HR from the randomized comparisons was 0.77 (CI 0.53–1.12; $p=0.17$) in favor of neoadjuvant chemoradiotherapy as opposed to perioperative chemotherapy alone.

Is There a Role for Adjuvant Chemoradiotherapy?

Based on a landmark publication by MacDonald in 2001, it became standard of care for postoperative chemoradiotherapy to be considered for high-risk patients with AC of the GEJ who had not received preoperative therapy. High-risk patients were defined by lymph node involvement, T3 or 4 tumors, or positive margins. In this study, 556 patients with resected GEJ (comprised 20 % of the patients) or gastric AC were randomly assigned to surgery alone or surgery plus postoperative chemoradiotherapy (45 Gy with 5-FU). The median overall survival in the surgery-only group was 27 months, as compared with 36 months in the chemoradiotherapy group. More than a decade later in 2012, Smalley and colleagues provide an updated analysis of the MacDonald study and reported that patients who had received postoperative chemoradiotherapy continued to benefit from significant reduction in both overall relapse and locoregional relapse. Notably, patients in this group did suffer a higher incidence of secondary malignancies (21 patients who had received postoperative chemotherapy arm compared to 8 patients who received surgery alone), but the authors interpreted it to be acceptable given the significant overall survival benefit.

Is There a Difference in Survival Between Preoperative and Postoperative Chemoradiotherapy?

A Chinese study published in 2010 by Lv and colleagues showed a benefit of perioperative chemoradiotherapy in treatment of locally advanced SCC of esophagus (Table 17.2). In this study, patients were randomized into three groups: surgery alone, preoperative chemoradiotherapy, and postoperative chemoradiotherapy. In the treatment groups (preoperative CRT and postoperative CRT), patients received 40 Gy concurrent with cisplatin and taxol. The local recurrence rates for preoperative CRT, postoperative CRT, and S group were 11.3, 14.1, and 35 %, respectively. Though there were no significant differences in overall survival (OS) or progression-free survival (PFS) between the treatment groups, there was a significant overall survival benefit between the treatment groups and control (surgery only). Based on these data, it is reasonable to offer adjuvant chemoradiotherapy to patients with locally advanced esophageal cancer who did not already receive preoperative therapy, though esophageal cancer patients seem to tolerate preoperative chemoradiotherapy better than postoperative chemoradiotherapy.

Is Neoadjuvant or Adjuvant Radiotherapy Appropriate?

There has been a lack of convincing data to justify treating patients with resectable esophageal cancer with either preoperative or postoperative radiotherapy. Multiple RTCs have been published, each using different radiation doses and techniques, none of which have shown significant survival benefit. In a meta-analysis by Arnott and colleagues, the authors pooled 5 RCTs, totaling 1,147 patients to determine whether preoperative radiotherapy improves overall survival. They concluded that there was no clear evidence of survival advantage: at 9-year follow-up, HR 8.9, CI 0.78–1.01, but p value was 0.062, indicating lack of statistical significance. Randomized controlled trials and meta-analyses of trials have not shown a significant survival advantage for any combinations of surgery and radiotherapy alone.

Is There a Role for Radiation Alone in the Treatment of Unresectable Esophageal Cancer?

Radiation therapy alone for localized disease has resulted in poor local control and poor survival. Earlam and Cuhna-Melo in a well-cited 1980 publication reviewed 122 articles that documented surgical outcomes of 83,783 patients with SCC of esophagus. They calculated only a 4 % survival rate at 5 years. In a separate study reviewing the role of RT, they calculated a similar 6% survival rate at 5 years.

The Radiation Therapy Oncology Group (RTOG) launched RTOG 85-01, a prospective, randomized stratified phase III trial that assessed whether primary treatment with chemoradiotherapy was superior to radiation alone in patients with localized esophageal carcinoma. In the combined therapy arm, RT was given in 25 fractions over 5 weeks to total 50 Gy in addition to cisplatin and 5-FU chemotherapy. In the control arm, RT was given in 32 fractions over 6.4 weeks to total 64 Gy. One hundred and twenty-nine patients were enrolled. Patients who received combined therapy had a significant survival advantage over patients who received radiation alone. Survival rates at 12 and 24 months were 33 and 10 % for radiation and 50 and 38 % for chemoradiotherapy, respectively. It is suggested that chemotherapy may not only enhance local effects of radiation but may also reduce micrometastases. In short, combined therapy increases survival of patients with SCC or AC of esophagus as opposed to radiation alone. Hence, radiation alone should only be considered for palliative intent.

Is There a Role for Targeted Therapy in Chemoradiotherapy?

Molecular-targeted therapy for management of unresectable esophageal cancer has attracted promising research. Targeted therapy against EGFR, VEGF, and HER2 has already been approved for other malignancies (Table 17.5).

Table 17.5 Targets for cancer therapy

Target	Drug	Mechanism	Approved use
EGFR	Cetuximab	Anti-EGFR monoclonal antibody	CRC, HNC
	Panitumumab	Anti-EGFR monoclonal antibody	CRC
	Gefitinib	Small molecule EGFR TKI	NSCLC
	Erlotinib	Small molecule EGFR TKI	NSCLC, pancreatic cancer
VEGF	Bevacizumab	Anti-VEGF monoclonal antibody	CRC, breast, GB, RCC, NSCLC
	Sunitinib	VEGF receptor TKI	pNET, GIST, RCC
	Sorafenib	VEGF receptor TKI	Thyroid, HCC, RCC
HER2	Trastuzumab	Anti-HER2 monoclonal antibody	*AC of gastric or GEJ, breast*
	Lapatinib	Dual EGFR/HER2 TKI	Breast

EGFR epidermal growth factor receptor, *HER2* human epidermal growth factor receptor 2, *VEGF* vascular endothelial growth factor, *TKI* tyrosine kinase inhibitor, *CRC* colorectal cancer, *NSCLC* nonsmall cell lung carcinoma, *HNC* head and neck cancer, *GB* glioblastoma, *RCC* renal cell carcinoma, *pNET* pancreatic neuroendocrine tumor, *GIST* gastrointestinal stromal tumor, *HCC* hepatocellular carcinoma, *AC* adenocarcinoma, *GEJ* gastroesophageal junction

The epidermal growth factor receptor (EGFR) is a member of the ErbB tyrosine kinase family that has been identified as a target for cancer therapy. Ligand-induced EGFR tyrosine kinase activation leads to upregulation of downstream signals via the RAS, ERK1/2, PI3K/Akt, and STAT pathways, inducing cell proliferation and angiogenesis. Cetuximab is a monoclonal IgG1 antibody, which binds to the extracellular domain of EGFR and competes for receptor binding, thereby inducing EGFR internalization, downregulation, and degradation. High levels of EGFR expression have been detected in 50–70 % of esophageal cancer and have been correlated with poor prognosis. Initial studies in esophageal cancer appeared promising. For example, in a phase II study, 62 patients with histologically confirmed, EGFR-expressing, unresectable, advanced esophageal SCC were randomized to receive cisplatin/5-FU (control) with or without cetuximab. The median overall survival (OS) for control and study arm was 9.5 and 5.5 months, respectively, indicating that cetuximab may increase efficacy of standard cisplatin/5-FU chemotherapy. Unfortunately, the recent phase III RTOG 0436 trial-evaluating patients with unresectable esophageal advanced esophageal cancer did not confirm these findings. Patients were randomized to cisplatin, paclitaxel, and radiation with or without cetuximab with OS as primary endpoint. The study was to enroll 420 patients to detect an increase in 2-year overall survival from 41 to 53 %. The study stopped accruing adenocarcinoma patients in 2012 as it became clear that was not meeting efficacy goals. The 2-year overall survival for AC and SCC patients receiving cisplatin/paclitaxel/radiation is 42 and 43 % (without cetuximab) and 44 and 46 % (with cetuximab), respectively.

The human epidermal growth factor receptor 2 (HER2) is another member of the tyrosine kinase receptor family, associated with tumor cell proliferation, adhesion, migration, and differentiation. Overexpression in AC of the GEJ has been detected between 0 and 43 % associated with aggressive disease. Trastuzumab, a monoclonal antibody, targets HER2 and inhibits HER2-mediated signaling. In a phase III study,

594 patients with HER2-positive advanced gastric or GEJ cancers were randomized to receive standard chemotherapy (control) or chemotherapy plus intravenous trastuzumab (study). Median overall survival for control and study arm was 11.1 and 13.8 months, respectively (HR 0.74; 95 % CI 0.6–0.01; $p = 0.0046$). It has since been FDA approved for treatment of metastatic HER2-positive metastatic gastric or GEJ cancers. Studies are now ongoing evaluating the efficacy of Her-2 inhibition with chemoradiotherapy.

Another molecular target that is overexpressed in esophageal cancer is vascular endothelial growth factor (VEGF). VEGF is a signaling protein which mediates both physiologic and pathologic angiogenesis. Bevacizumab is a monoclonal antibody that binds to VEGF and prevents interaction with VEGF-receptors on endothelial cells. A phase III study to compare the capecitabine/cisplatin combination ± bevacizumab in 774 patients with unresectable, locally advanced or metastatic stomach/GEJ AC yielded negative results; no survival difference was appreciated between the two study arms. Studies adding this molecule to radiation have shown increased toxicity and fistula formation hence have been abandoned.

What Pressing Questions Are Still Left Unanswered?

Treatment of resectable esophageal cancer has significantly evolved in the past few decades. Despite the multiple clinical trials comparing chemotherapy, chemoradiotherapy, radiation, and surgery, there remains a paucity of phase III trials with multiple arms directly comparing the different treatment modalities. Aside from that, the clinical trials from which we are basing clinical practice are generated from heterogeneous groups of patients with GEJ/AC and SCC, different organs, different radiation dosing and schedules, and different chemotherapy usually without uniform staging studies.

There needs to be further discussion regarding the clinical difference between GEJ/AC and SCC of esophagus, specifically the influence of on response to therapy.

Conclusions

Based on findings from clinical trials and meta-analyses, it is a standard of care to offer patients with locally advance esophageal cancer preoperative chemoradiotherapy or at minimum perioperative chemotherapy. Preoperative combination chemoradiotherapy appears to yield a higher survival benefit and increased pathologic complete response at resection when compared to perioperative chemotherapy. The role of adjuvant therapy is not as well defined. Patients with adenocarcinoma who undergo surgery alone and have positive margins, high T stage or lymph node involvement should be offered postoperative chemoradiotherapy. There is a paucity of data to support postoperative chemotherapy, though it may be reasonable to offer to patients with positive lymph nodes after preoperative chemoradiotherapy. There is no curative role for radiation therapy alone in the management of esophageal cancer. Ongoing research on integrating targeted therapy based on tumor profiles with neoadjuvant treatment may improve outcomes of this disease.

Summary

- Neoadjuvant chemoradiotherapy or perioperative chemotherapy provides a significant overall survival benefit over surgery alone in esophageal adenocarcinoma.
- The data suggest that neoadjuvant chemoradiotherapy is more effective than perioperative chemotherapy in achieving optimal survival benefit.
- In contrast, data on adjuvant therapy have shown limited benefits. Patients with high-risk resected disease (pathologically positive margins and lymph nodes) who did not receive neoadjuvant therapy may benefit from adjuvant chemoradiotherapy.
- There are limited data to support adjuvant chemotherapy aside from a role in treatment for patients with residual node positive disease after preoperative chemoradiotherapy.
- Radiation alone should be reserved for the palliative setting.
- Treatment decisions should be individualized based on each patient's performance status, comorbidities, and goals of care.

Selected Reading

1. al-Kasspooles M, Moore JH, Orringer MB, Beer DG. Amplification and over-expression of the EGFR and erbB-2 genes in human esophageal adenocarcinomas. Int J Cancer. 1993;54:213–9.
2. Almhanna K, Shridhar R, Meredith KL. Neoadjuvant or adjuvant therapy for resectable esophageal cancer: is there a standard of care? Cancer Control. 2013;20:89–96.
3. Apinop C, Puttisak P, Preecha N. A prospective study of combined therapy in esophageal cancer. Hepatogastroenterology. 1994;41:391–3.
4. Arnott SJ, Duncan W, Gignoux M, et al. Preoperative radiotherapy for esophageal carcinoma. Cochrane Database Syst Rev. 2005:CD001799.
5. Bang YJ, Van Cutsem E, Feyereislova A, et al. Trastuzumab in combination with chemotherapy versus chemotherapy alone for treatment of HER2-positive advanced gastric or gastro-oesophageal junction cancer (ToGA): a phase 3, open-label, randomised controlled trial. Lancet. 2010;376:687–97.
6. Bosset JF, Gignoux M, Triboulet JP, et al. Chemoradiotherapy followed by surgery compared with surgery alone in squamous-cell cancer of the esophagus. N Engl J Med. 1997;337:161–7.
7. Burmeister BH, Thomas JM, Burmeister EA, et al. Is concurrent radiation therapy required in patients receiving preoperative chemotherapy for adenocarcinoma of the oesophagus? A randomised phase II trial. Eur J Cancer. 2011;47:354–60.

8. Cooper JS, Guo MD, Herskovic A, et al. Chemoradiotherapy of locally advanced esophageal cancer: long-term follow-up of a prospective randomized trial (RTOG 85–01). Radiation Therapy Oncology Group. JAMA. 1999;281:1623–7.
9. Cunningham D, Allum WH, Stenning SP, et al. Perioperative chemotherapy versus surgery alone for resectable gastroesophageal cancer. N Engl J Med. 2006;355:11–20.
10. Earlam R, Cunha-Melo JR. Oesophageal squamous cell carcinoma: I. A critical review of surgery. Br J Surg. 1980;67:381–90.
11. Earlam R, Cunha-Melo JR. Oesophogeal squamous cell carcinomas: II. A critical view of radiotherapy. Br J Surg. 1980;67:457–61.
12. Earle CC, Maroun JA. Adjuvant chemotherapy after curative resection for gastric cancer in non-Asian patients: revisiting a meta-analysis of randomised trials. Eur J Cancer. 1999;35:1059–64.
13. Feo CV, Villaflor VM, Patti MG. Should esophageal resections for cancer be performed in high-volume centers only? Updates Surg. 2011;63:147–50.
14. Fiorica F, Di Bona D, Schepis F, et al. Preoperative chemoradiotherapy for oesophageal cancer: a systematic review and meta-analysis. Gut. 2004;53:925–30.
15. Fujita H, Sueyoshi S, Yamana H, et al. Optimum treatment strategy for superficial esophageal cancer: endoscopic mucosal resection versus radical esophagectomy. World J Surg. 2001;25:424–31.
16. Gebski V, Burmeister B, Smithers BM, et al. Survival benefits from neoadjuvant chemoradiotherapy or chemotherapy in oesophageal carcinoma: a meta-analysis. Lancet Oncol. 2007;8:226–34.
17. Gibault L, Metges JP, Conan-Charlet V, et al. Diffuse EGFR staining is associated with reduced overall survival in locally advanced oesophageal squamous cell cancer. Br J Cancer. 2005;93:107–15.
18. Hermans J, Bonenkamp JJ, Boon MC, et al. Adjuvant therapy after curative resection for gastric cancer: meta-analysis of randomized trials. J Clin Oncol. 1993;11:1441–7.
19. Herskovic A, Martz K, al-Sarraf M, et al. Combined chemotherapy and radiotherapy compared with radiotherapy alone in patients with cancer of the esophagus. N Engl J Med. 1992;326:1593–8.
20. Inoue K, Ozeki Y, Suganuma T, Sugiura Y, Tanaka S. Vascular endothelial growth factor expression in primary esophageal squamous cell carcinoma. Association with angiogenesis and tumor progression. Cancer. 1997;79:206–13.
21. Le Prise E, Etienne PL, Meunier B, et al. A randomized study of chemotherapy, radiation therapy, and surgery versus surgery for localized squamous cell carcinoma of the esophagus. Cancer. 1994;73:1779–84.
22. Lee JL, Park SI, Kim SB, et al. A single institutional phase III trial of preoperative chemotherapy with hyperfractionation radiotherapy plus surgery versus surgery alone for resectable esophageal squamous cell carcinoma. Ann Oncol. 2004;15:947–54.
23. Lorenzen S, Schuster T, Porschen R, et al. Cetuximab plus cisplatin-5-fluorouracil versus cisplatin-5-fluorouracil alone in first-line metastatic squamous cell carcinoma of the esophagus: a randomized phase II study of the Arbeitsgemeinschaft Internistische Onkologie. Ann Oncol. 2009;20:1667–73.
24. Lv J, Cao XF, Zhu B, Ji L, Tao L, Wang DD. Long-term efficacy of perioperative chemoradiotherapy on esophageal squamous cell carcinoma. World J Gastroenterol. 2010;16:1649–54.
25. Macdonald JS, Smalley SR, Benedetti J, et al. Chemoradiotherapy after surgery compared with surgery alone for adenocarcinoma of the stomach or gastroesophageal junction. N Engl J Med. 2001;345:725–30.
26. Mariette C, Seitz J, Maillard E, Mornex F, Thomas PA, Raoul J, Boige V, Pezet D, Genet C, Bedenne L. Surgery alone versus chemoradiotherapy followed by surgery for localized esophageal cancer: analysis of a randomized controlled phase III trial FFCD 9901. Proc ASCO. J Clin Oncol. 2010;28:15s (suppl; abstr 4005).
27. Minsky BD, Pajak TF, Ginsberg RJ, et al. INT 0123 (Radiation Therapy Oncology Group 94-05) phase III trial of combined-modality therapy for esophageal cancer: high-dose versus standard-dose radiation therapy. J Clin Oncol. 2002;20:1167–74.

28. Nygaard K, Hagen S, Hansen HS, et al. Pre-operative radiotherapy prolongs survival in operable esophageal carcinoma: a randomized, multicenter study of pre-operative radiotherapy and chemotherapy. The second Scandinavian trial in esophageal cancer. World J Surg. 1992;16:1104–9; discussion 10.
29. Ohtsu A, Shah MA, Van Cutsem E, et al. Bevacizumab in combination with chemotherapy as first-line therapy in advanced gastric cancer: a randomized, double-blind, placebo-controlled phase III study. J Clin Oncol. 2011;29:3968–76.
30. Shimada H, Nabeya Y, Matsubara H, et al. Prediction of lymph node status in patients with superficial esophageal carcinoma: analysis of 160 surgically resected cancers. Am J Surg. 2006;191:250–4.
31. Shridhar R, Imani-Shikhabadi R, Davis B, Streeter OA, Thomas Jr CR. Curative treatment of esophageal cancer; an evidenced based review. J Gastrointest Cancer. 2013;44:375–84.
32. Siegel R, Naishadham D, Jemal A. Cancer statistics, 2013. CA Cancer J Clin. 2013;63:11–30.
33. Sjoquist KM, Burmeister BH, Smithers BM, et al. Survival after neoadjuvant chemotherapy or chemoradiotherapy for resectable oesophageal carcinoma: an updated meta-analysis. Lancet Oncol. 2011;12:681–92.
34. Smalley SR, Benedetti JK, Haller DG, et al. Updated analysis of SWOG-directed intergroup study 0116: a phase III trial of adjuvant radiochemotherapy versus observation after curative gastric cancer resection. J Clin Oncol. 2012;30:2327–33.
35. Stahl M, Walz MK, Stuschke M, et al. Phase III comparison of preoperative chemotherapy compared with chemoradiotherapy in patients with locally advanced adenocarcinoma of the esophagogastric junction. J Clin Oncol. 2009;27:851–6.
36. Suntharalingam M. The initial report of RTOG 0436: a phase III trial evaluating the addition of cetuximab to paclitaxel, cisplatin, and radiation for patients with esophageal cancer treated without surgery. 2014 Gastrointestinal Cancers Symposium. San Francisco; 2014.
37. Tepper J, Krasna MJ, Niedzwiecki D, et al. Phase III trial of trimodality therapy with cisplatin, fluorouracil, radiotherapy, and surgery compared with surgery alone for esophageal cancer: CALGB 9781. J Clin Oncol. 2008;26:1086–92.
38. Urba SG, Orringer MB, Turrisi A, Iannettoni M, Forastiere A, Strawderman M. Randomized trial of preoperative chemoradiation versus surgery alone in patients with locoregional esophageal carcinoma. J Clin Oncol. 2001;19:305–13.
39. Urschel JD, Vasan H, Blewett CJ. A meta-analysis of randomized controlled trials that compared neoadjuvant chemotherapy and surgery to surgery alone for resectable esophageal cancer. Am J Surg. 2002;183:274–9.
40. van Hagen P, Hulshof MC, van Lanschot JJ, et al. Preoperative chemoradiotherapy for esophageal or junctional cancer. N Engl J Med. 2012;366:2074–84.
41. Walsh TN, Noonan N, Hollywood D, Kelly A, Keeling N, Hennessy TP. A comparison of multimodal therapy and surgery for esophageal adenocarcinoma. N Engl J Med. 1996;335:462–7.
42. Westerterp M, Koppert LB, Buskens CJ, et al. Outcome of surgical treatment for early adenocarcinoma of the esophagus or gastro-esophageal junction. Virchows Arch. 2005;446: 497–504.
43. Wiedmann MW, Mossner J. New and emerging combination therapies for esophageal cancer. Cancer Manag Res. 2013;5:133–46.
44. Ychou M, Boige V, Pignon JP, et al. Perioperative chemotherapy compared with surgery alone for resectable gastroesophageal adenocarcinoma: an FNCLCC and FFCD multicenter phase III trial. J Clin Oncol. 2011;29:1715–21.

Index

A
Abdominal esophagus
EGJ, 42
and LES, 43
lymphatic drainage, 4
Ablative therapies
APC, 182
cryotherapy, 183–184
endoscopic eradication, 171
PDT, 182–183
RFA, 181–182
AC. *See* Adenocarcinoma (AC)
Achalasia
Allgrove syndrome, 134
Auerbach myenteric plexus, 134
barium esophagogram, 111, 112
classic "bird's beak" appearance, esophagogastric junction, 137
DES, 18
description, 133
diagnostic findings, manometry, 138
diffuse esophageal spasm (DES), 18, 24
dilated and sigmoid-shaped esophagus, 18, 21–22
Dor fundoplication, 147
endoscopic botulinum toxin injection, 144
end-stage, barium swallow, 135, 136
epiphrenic diverticulum, 19
esophageal, 18, 20
functional lumen imaging probe (FLIP), 140
heartburn and chest pain, 136
HLA-DR and-DQalleles, 135
impaired LES relaxation, 144
inflammatory response, 134–135
LHM (*see* Laparoscopic Heller myotomy (LHM))
malnutrition and recurrent aspiration pneumonia, 137
minimally invasive surgery, 145
motility disorder, 17, 19
non-propulsive contractions, 10
normal LES muscle strips, 134
pneumatic dilatation, 144–145
POEM (*see* Peroral endoscopic esophageal myotomy (POEM))
postoperative dysphagia, 92
primary, 55, 104, 134
respiratory symptoms, 136–137
solids and liquids, dysphagia, 135–136
stages, 135, 136
swallowing and esophageal peristalsis, 17
tertiary waves, 8
treatment modalities, 144
type I, II and III, 138–140
Adenocarcinoma (AC)
Barrett's esophagus, 169
distal esophagus, 21
and HGD, 166, 178
mucosal, 184
stage grouping, 196
Adjuvant chemoradiotherapy, 234
Allgrove syndrome, 134, 135
Ambulatory pH monitoring
abnormal, 60, 61
clinical diagnosis, GERD, 62
diagnosis, GERD, 99
esophageal motility profile, 62
gastroesophageal reflux, 12
heartburn and regurgitation, 113
normal, 60, 61
postoperative GERD, 147
reflux theory, 98
wireless, 63

P.M. Fisichella et al. (eds.), *Esophageal Diseases*,
DOI 10.1007/978-3-319-04337-1, © Springer International Publishing Switzerland 2014

Anastomosis
cervical *vs.* intrathoracic, 216
gastric mobilization, 210
hand-sewn and stapled, 217
intrathoracic hybrid chest, 29, 217
left sternocleidomastoid muscle, 217, 218
meta-analysis, 217
tumor location, 217
upper thorax, 209
Antireflux surgery
angle of His, 44–45
clinical response, PPIs, 55
delayed gastric emptying, 64, 65
diaphragm, 44
esophageal peristalsis, 167
and hiatal hernia, 49
indications, 71
LES and abdominal esophagus, 43
manometry, 57
metaplasia, 169
MSA, 70
natural antireflux mechanisms, 42
pH monitoring, 62
phrenoesophageal membrane, 45, 46
primary esophageal motility disorders, 55
psychiatric disorder, 106
APC. *See* Argon plasma coagulation (APC)
Argon plasma coagulation (APC), 12, 182

B

Barium swallow. *See also* Esophagram, barium
achalasia (*see* Achalasia)
benign esophageal masses, 161
classic "bird's beak" appearance, 137
and endoscopy, 141
end-stage achalasia, 135, 136
esophageal duplication cyst, 155, 156
esophagogastric junction, 137
GERD (*see* Gastroesophageal reflux disease (GERD))
hemangioma, 158
hiatal hernias (*see* Hiatal hernias)
LES relaxation and esophageal emptying, 149
paraesophageal hernias (*see* Paraesophageal Hernias)
Schatzki's ring, 18
ZD, 131
Barrett's esophagus (BE)
acid suppression therapy, 178
aspirin and nonsteroidal anti-inflammatory drug, 178
description, 178
and EAC, 177
endoscopic treatment, 179
and esophageal adenocarcinoma, 169
and HGD, 170–172
and LGD, 170
metaplasia, 169–170
surveillance, 179–181
upper endoscopy, 56, 65, 99
BE. *See* Barrett's esophagus (BE)
Belafsky clinical scoring system, laryngopharyngeal reflux, 100–102
Benign esophageal tumors
classification, 154
cysts and fibrovascular polyps, 154
diagnostic testing, 154–155
epidemiology, 154
indications, surgery, 155–161
leiomyomas, 20, 30–31, 153
polyps, 20, 29–30
Bernstein test
acid dripping, esophagus, 101
chloridric acid instillation, distal esophagus, 98
esophageal sensitivity, 98
Botulinum toxin injection
and balloon dilatation, UES, 122
endoscopic, 144
vs. pneumatic dilatation, 145

C

Cardiac and noncardiac chest pain, 104
Cervical esophagus
free jejunal grafts, 217
inferior thyroid veins, 4
left cervical incision, 209
lipomas, 159
myotomy, 122
Chemotherapy
neoadjuvant, 203
perioperative, 232–234
and radiotherapy, 231, 232
stent-related complications, 194
vs. surgery, 229
Chloridric acid instillation, 98
CO_2 laser diverticulotomy, 128
Cough
ambulatory pH monitoring, 65
defined, 102
distal GERD, 98

CP. *See* Cricopharyngeal (CP) myotomy
Cricopharyngeal (CP) myotomy
  bougie dilator, 122–123
  endoscopic repair, 125–126
  proximal cervical esophagus, 122
  risks, 123
Cryotherapy, 172, 183–184

D
Diaphragm
  diverticulum, 19
  hiatal hernia, 44
  high-resolution manometry images, 44
  LES resting pressure, 9
  and posterior vagus nerve, 73
  synergistic action, 168
Distal esophageal tumor
  Barrett's segment, 197
  endoscopic aspect, 198
  mediastinum, 199
  metastatic diseases, 201
  primary staging, 199
Diverticulectomy
  CP myotomy, 122
  dissection, left transcervical incision, 123
  and diverticular inversion, 130
  excised nasogastric tube, 123, 124
Diverticulopexy
  description, 124
  and diverticular inversion, 122, 131
Dor fundoplication, 146–148
Duplication cysts, 156, 160–161
Dysphagia
  endoscopy, 138
  LPF *vs.* LTF, 78
  patients, achalasia, 135–136
  stages, 135, 136
Dysplasia
  biomarkers, 180
  HGD (*see* High-grade dysplasia (HGD))
  LGD (*see* Low-grade dysplasia (LGD))

E
EMR. *See* Endoscopic mucosal resection (EMR)
Endoscopic approach
  and barium swallow, 141
  CO_2 laser diverticulotomy, 128
  CP myotomy, 125–126
  cricopharyngeal bar, 127
  dilatation, 77, 145, 148
  dysphagia, 138
  equipment, 126, 127
  flexible endoscopic diverticulotomy, 129
  harmonic scalpel diverticulotomy, 129
  mediastinitis and death, 125
  operating room setup, 126
  residual food and debris, 127
  stapler diverticulotomy, 128
  vs.open endoscopic approaches, 122, 129–130
  zero-degree telescope, 126
Endoscopic mucosal resection (EMR)
  cap-assisted technique, 184
  and EUS, 171
  and IMC, 185
  neoplastic epithelium, 184
  staging tool, 179
Epiphrenic diverticula
  barium swallow, 19, 27–28
  characteristics, 110
  contralateral cardiomyotomy, 113, 115
  diagnostic workup, 111
  epidemiology, 110–111
  esophageal musculature defect, 113, 114
  laparoscopic approach, 116
  longitudinal staple line, esophageal submucosa, 113, 114
  management, postoperative, 117
  manometry, 112–113
  motility disorder, 110
  mucosal, submucosal and muscular layers, 110
  myotomy, 116
  odynophagia and weight loss, 111
  partial anterior 180° fundoplication, 113, 115
  postoperative complications and recurrences, 109
  pulsion/false diverticula, 110
  surgical management, patient, 113, 114
  symptoms, 111
  transthoracic approach, right thoracotomy incision, 115–116
  upper endoscopy, 112
  vagal nerve injury/transection, 116
Epithelial protection, 46–47
EPT. *See* Esophageal pressure topography (EPT)
Erosive esophagitis, 99
Esophageal cancer
  achalasia, 17–24
  age, 192–193
  benign tumors, 20, 29–31

Esophageal cancer (*cont.*)
 cardiopulmonary status, 193–194
 chest/abdominal CT scan, 21, 36–37
 diverticula, 19, 25–28
 endoscopy and endoscopic ultrasound, 21, 35
 epidemiology, 190–191
 etiology and pathophysiology, 190–191
 GERD, 12–17
 malignant tumors, 21, 32–38
 medical history, 192
 mid-thoracic esophageal squamous cell cancer, 21, 32–33
 morbidity and mortality rates, 208
 nutrition, 194
 PET scan, 21, 37–38
 RTOG, 235
 staging (*see* Staging)
 surgical approach (*see* Esophagogastrectomy)
 symptoms, 192
Esophageal clearance
 DeMeester score, 167
 motility, 46
 mucosal injury, 45
 pathophysiology, 166–167
 peristalsis and saliva production, 167
 psychotropic medication, 106
 saliva production, 46
Esophageal diverticula
 epidemiology, 110–111
 epiphrenic diverticulum, 19, 27–28
 pathophysiology, 110
 ZD, 19, 25–26
Esophageal function tests
 ambulatory pH monitoring, 99
 LES and UES, 99
 SAP, 100
 SI, 99–100
 SSI, 100
Esophageal pressure topography (EPT), 138
Esophagectomy. *See also* Esophagogastrectomy
 esophageal cancer (*see* Esophageal cancer)
 HGD and intramucosal carcinoma, 186
 indications, 171
 LHM failure, 147
 nodal involvement, 187
 T1b cancer patients, 171
 treatment, HGD, 170
Esophagogastrectomy. *See also* Esophagectomy
 anastomosis, 217–218
 complications, 218–220
 conduit choice, 216–217
 esophagogastrectomy (*see* Esophagogastrectomy)
 ivor lewis, 209, 211
 left thoracoabdominal, 210–212
 lymphadenectomy, 214–215
 McKeown/three-stage, 210, 212
 perioperative outcomes, 220
 quality of life, 221
 resection margins, 215, 216
 salvage, 213–214
 standardized clinical pathway and recovery, 220–221
 transhiatal, 209, 210
 transthoracic *vs.* transhiatal, 211, 213
Esophagogastric junction (EGJ)
 diagnostic algorithm, 138
 FLIP, 140
 gastric cancer staging system, 191
 Gubaroff valves, 45
 valve mechanism, 42
Esophagram, barium. *See also* Barium swallow
 epiphrenic diverticulumm esophageal motility disorder, 111, 112
 esophageal emptying, 138
 gastric content reflux, 55
 hiatal hernias, 112
 radiological abnormalities, 56
 surgical planning, 111
 test sensitivity, 100
Esophagus
 architecture, 2–3
 blood supply, 3–4
 innervation, 4–5
 laparoscopic view, 7, 8
 left thoracoscopy, 5–7
 lymphatic drainage, 4
 physiology, 8–9
 right thoracoscopic view, 5
Eustachian tube dysfunction, 98

F

Fibrovascular polyps, 159–160
Flexible endoscopic diverticulotomy, 129
FLIP. *See* Functional lumen imaging probe (FLIP)
Functional lumen imaging probe (FLIP)
 clinical practice, 140
 description, 140
Fundoplication
 acid exposure, 185–186
 gastroesophageal barrier, 168

laparoscopic partial (*see* Partial fundoplication)
peristalsis, 167
refractory reflux symptom, 185
RFA, 170
total fundoplication (*see* Laparoscopic total fundoplication)
treatment, GERD, 63

G

Gastroesophageal reflux disease (GERD)
age, 48
ambulatory 24-h pH monitoring, 60–63
anterior (180° and 90°) LPF *vs.* LTF, 78
antireflux mechanisms, 42–45
barium esophagram, 55–56, 100
Barrett's esophagus, 166
causative factors, 50
chest x-ray, 15, 16
definition, 96
diagnosis, 12
drugs, diet and hormones, 48
epiphrenic diverticula, management, 113
esophageal function tests, 99–100
extraesophageal, symptom pathophysiology, 96, 97
gastric hydrochloric acid, 42
gastric volvulus, 15, 16
heartburn and regurgitation, 54, 113
Helicobacter pylori, 48
hiatal hernias, 13–16, 49
indirect involvement, 98
laryngoscopy, 100, 101
LTF, 70
manometry, 56–60
medical therapy, 70–71
MII-pH, 63–64
"mixed" hiatal hernia, 15, 16
MSA, 79
myotomy incision, 114–115
oropharyngeal pH testing, 100
paraesophageal hernia, 13, 14
partial fundoplication, 75–76
pathophysiology, 166–172
physiological, 41
posterior LPF *vs.* LTF, 78
postoperative complications, 77
protective mechanisms, 45–47
radiolabeled gastric emptying study, 64–65
radiologic abnormalities, 12–13
reflex theory, 98
reflux theory, 98
rolling hernia, 13, 14
Schatzki's rings, 17–19
sensitivity, 98
sliding hiatal hernia, 13, 14
symptomatic evaluation, 55
target organs (*see* Target organs, GERD)
thoracoabdominal gradient, 47
total fundoplication, 71–75
transient dysphagia, 77
type III paraesophageal hernia, 15
type IV hiatal hernia, 15, 17
upper endoscopy, 56, 99
GERD. *See* Gastroesophageal reflux disease (GERD)
Granular cell tumor, 154, 157–158

H

Harmonic scalpel diverticulotomy, 129
Heartburn
cancer (*see* Gastroesophageal reflux disease (GERD))
and chest pain, 136
and regurgitation, 55, 84
sexual intercourse, 105
Hemangioma, 154, 158
HGD. *See* High-grade dysplasia (HGD)
Hiatal hernias
Barrett's esophagus, 168
chest X-ray, 88, 90
classification, 84–86
epiphrenic diverticula, 112
GERD symptoms, 48
Helicobacter pylori, 49
high-resolution manometry, 44
pathophysiology, 86–87
types, 13–17
upper digestive endoscopy, 99
High-grade dysplasia (HGD)
ablative therapies, 171
and adenocarcinoma, 178
cryotherapy, 172
EMR and EUS, 171
eradication therapy, 180
esophagectomy, 170
intramucosal carcinoma, 186
and neoplasia, 178
neoplastic lesion, 171
High-resolution manometry (HRM)
and EPT, 138
esophageal achalasia, classification, 139
FLIP, 140

Hoarseness
Belafsky clinical scoring system, laryngopharyngeal reflux, 101, 102
chronic inflammation, 99
HRM. *See* High-resolution manometry (HRM)
Hybrid therapy, BE, 185

I
Idiopathic pulmonary fibrosis (IPF), 102
IPF. *See* Idiopathic pulmonary fibrosis (IPF)

L
Laparoscopic Heller myotomy (LHM)
crus, right and left pillars, 146
dysphagia, 146–147
gastric fundus and traction, 146
vs. pneumatic dilatation, 147–148
postoperative gastroesophageal reflux, 147
surgical approaches, 148
symptoms, 147
trocars placement, 145, 146
Laparoscopic total fundoplication
Babcock clamp, 74
crura closure, 74
gastric fundus wrapping, 74–75
gastroesophageal reflux, 92
gastrohepatic ligament division, 73
instrumentation, 72
manometry, 93
patient positioning, 71–72
peritoneum and phreno-esophageal membrane, 73
short gastric vessels, 73–74
trocars placement, 71–73
Laryngoscopy
Belafsky reflux score system, 100, 101
ENT surgeons, 100
Leiomyoma, esophagus, 31, 155, 157
LES. *See* Lower esophageal sphincter (LES)
LGD. *See* Low-grade dysplasia (LGD)
LHM. *See* Laparoscopic Heller myotomy (LHM)
Lipoma, 159, 160
Lower esophageal sphincter (LES)
and abdominal esophagus, 43
achalasia, 133
cyclic phasic contractile activity, 9
EGJ, 42
gastric content reflux prevention, 9
hiatal hernias, 87
inhibitory ganglionic neurons, 134
intra-abdominal portion, 43
laparoscopic fundoplication, 54
manometry, 99
muscle strips, 134
myenteric plexus, 4
myotomy incision, 115
pan-esophageal motor disorder, 62
pathologic reflux, 9
periodic relaxations, 9, 43
psychotropic medication, 106
reflux control, 43
relaxation, 9, 144
resting pressure, 43
and TLESR, 168
transient relaxations, 9
Low-grade dysplasia (LGD)
annual surveillance endoscopy, 180
biopsies, 180
regression, 185
Lung manifestations
asthma, 102
chronic cough, 102
extraesophageal GERD complaints, 102
idiopathic pulmonary fibrosis (IPF), 102
medical therapy, acid-reducing medications, 103
Lymphadenectomy, 214–215

M
Magnetic sphincter augmentation (MSA)
gastric anatomy, 79
laparoscopic implantation, 79
LINX Reflux Management System, 70
Manometry, esophagus
achalasia, 57, 59–60, 138
advantages, HRM, 59–60
ambulatory pH monitoring, 113
definition, 12
diagnostic testing, 111
dysmotility, 113
esophageal motility, 56
function tests (*see* Esophageal function tests)
gastroesophageal junction, 87, 89
HRM and EPT, 138
ineffective motility, 57–59
motility disorders, 112–113
normal peristalsis, 57, 58
Metaplasia
and dysplasia, 187
eradication rates, 185
goblet cells, 166
intestinal, 178
neoplasia, 178

RFA, 170
surgical approach, 169
MII. *See* Multichannel intraluminal impedance (MII)
MSA. *See* Magnetic sphincter augmentation (MSA)
Multichannel intraluminal impedance (MII)
acid-suppressive therapy, 64
liquids and gas flow, 63
medical therapy, 64
pathologic gastroesophageal reflux, 71

N
NCCN treatment guidelines
limited locoregional disease, 202
locoregional disease, 202–203
metastatic disease, 203
Neoadjuvant therapy
adenocarcinoma, 229
esophageal cancer, 231
5-fluorouracil, 232
meta-analysis, 231
RTCs, 230
SCC, 230
vs. surgery, 229
New surgical approaches, LHM. *See* Laparoscopic Heller myotomy (LHM)

O
Open transcervical resection
CP (*see* Cricopharyngeal (CP) myotomy)
diverticular inversion, 125
diverticulectomy, 123–124
diverticulopexy, 124
myotomy, 122
SCM and carotid sheath, 122
ZD and CP, comparison, 125
Oral manifestations, GERD
dental erosions, 103
halitosis, 103–104
Otorhinolaryngology manifestations
Belafsky clinical scoring system, laryngopharyngeal reflux, 101, 102
chronic sinusitis and otitis media, 101

P
Paraesophageal hernias
classification, 84–86
clinical presentation, 87
diagnostic testing, 87–90
"mixed" hiatal hernia, 15
pathophysiology, 86–87
peritoneum, 83
postoperative management, 93
surgical approaches, 91–92
worrisome symptoms, 91
Partial fundoplication
anterior, 75–76, 147
esophageal motility disorder, 93
gastroesophageal junction, 116
laparoscopic Heller myotomy, 143
posterior, 75
proton pump inhibitors, 147
Partial posterior fundoplication, 147
PDT. *See* Photodynamic therapy (PDT)
Perioperative chemotherapy
ECF, 232
GEJ, 232
meta-analysis, 232, 233
Peristalsis, esophagus
antireflux mechanism, 167
conventional manometry, 57
fundoplication, 167
peristaltic wave, 9
pharyngeal contraction, 12
primary, 8
and saliva production, 167
secondary, 8
sensory receptors stimulation, 10
Peroral endoscopic esophageal myotomy (POEM)
advantages, 149
description, 148
and LHM, 150
pneumoperitoneum, 149
postoperative manometry and barium swallows, 149
procedure, 150
Photodynamic therapy (PDT), 182–183
Pneumatic dilatation
vs. botulinum toxin injection, 145
vs. LHM, 147–148
recurrent dysphagia after Heller myotomy, 145
Rigiflex balloons, 144–145
POEM. *See* Peroral endoscopic esophageal myotomy (POEM)

R
Radiation Therapy Oncology Group (RTOG), 235
Radiofrequency ablation (RFA), 170, 181–182

Radiolabeled gastric emptying study, 54, 64–65
Reflex theory, GERD, 98
Reflux theory, GERD, 98
RFA. *See* Radiofrequency ablation (RFA)
Roux-en-Y gastric bypass, 92

S
SAP. *See* Symptom-AssociationProbability (SAP)
SCC. *See* Squamous cell carcinoma (SCC)
Schatzki's rings, 13, 17–19, 55
Sexual manifestations, GERD, 105
Sleep manifestations, GERD, 104–105
Smith and Knight classification, dental erosion (tooth wear), 103
Squamous cell carcinoma (SCC)
  and AC, 228
  systemic therapy, 228
SSI. *See* Symptom Sensitivity Index (SSI)
Staging
  adenocarcinoma, 195, 196
  AJCC system, 190
  cancer, 21
  M category, 200–201
  N category, 198–200
  squamous cell carcinoma, 195, 196
  T category, 196–198
  TNMG descriptors, 194, 195
Symptom-association probability (SAP), 100
Symptom sensitivity index (SSI), 100

T
Target organs, GERD
  cardiac and noncardiac chest pain, 104
  lung manifestations, 102–103
  oral manifestations (*see* Oral manifestations, GERD)
  otorhinolaryngology manifestations, 101–102
  psychologic/psychiatric manifestation, 105–106
  sexual manifestations, 105
  sleep manifestations, 104–105
Thoracic esophagus
  lipomas, 159
  mediastinal pleura, 5
  pericardium and left atrium, 2
  tracheal bifurcation, 2
Thoracoabdominal pressure, 47, 168–169
Thoracoscopic repair
  and laparoscopic, 116
  postoperative complaints, 117
Torax Medical, 70, 77

U
UES. *See* Upper esophageal sphincter (UES)
Upper digestive endoscopy, 99
Upper esophageal sphincter (UES)
  esophageal manometry, 56
  functional obstruction, 19
  hypotonic, 99
  motor innervation, 8
  resting pressures, 122

Z
Zenker's diverticulum (ZD)
  barium swallow demonstration, 120, 121
  carotid artery, 120
  cervical esophageal lipoma, 160
  CP myotomy, 122
  description, 119
  dysphagia, 120
  endoscopic approach (*see* Endoscopic approach)
  esophageal, 19, 25–26
  Killian's triangle, 120
  muscular wall weakness, 120
  presentation, evaluation and treatment, 120, 121
  symptomatic, 121–122
  UES dysfunction, 120

MIX
Papier aus verantwortungsvollen Quellen
Paper from responsible sources
FSC® C105338

If you have any concerns about our products,
you can contact us on
ProductSafety@springernature.com

In case Publisher is established outside the EU,
the EU authorized representative is:
Springer Nature Customer Service Center GmbH
Europaplatz 3, 69115 Heidelberg, Germany

Printed by Libri Plureos GmbH
in Hamburg, Germany